Industrial Psychology

Ankur Negi

Design Engineer
Larsen and Toubro
Vadodara (Gujarat) India

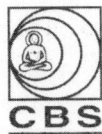

CBS

CBS PUBLISHERS & DISTRIBUTORS PVT. LTD.
New Delhi • Bengaluru • Chennai • Kochi • Mumbai • Pune

Industrial Psychology

ISBN: 978-81-239-2290-4

CBS First Edition: 2013

Reprint: 2015

Published by Satish Kumar Jain and produced by Varun Jain for

CBS Publishers & Distributors Pvt Ltd

4819/XI Prahlad Street, 24 Ansari Road, Daryaganj, New Delhi 110 002, India.

Ph: 23289259, 23266861, 23266867   Website: www.cbspd.com

Fax: 011-23243014   e-mail: delhi@cbspd.com; cbspubs@airtelmail.in.

Corporate Office: 204 FIE, Industrial Area, Patparganj, Delhi 110 092

Ph: 4934 4934   .   Fax: 4934 4935   e-mail: publishing@cbspd.com; publicity@cbspd.com

Branches

- **Bengaluru:** Seema House 2975, 17th Cross, K.R. Road,
  Banasankari 2nd Stage, Bengaluru 560 070, Karnataka
  Ph: +91-80-26771678/79   Fax: +91-80-26771680   e-mail: bangalore@cbspd.com
- **Chennai:** 7, Subbaraya Street, Shenoy Nagar, Chennai 600 030, Tamil Nadu
  Ph: +91-44-26260666, 26208620   Fax: +91-44-42032115   e-mail: chennai@cbspd.com
- **Kochi:** Anshan House, No. 39/1904, AM Thomas Road, Valanjambalam, Eranakulam 682 018,
  Kochi Kerala
  Ph: +91-484-4059061-65   Fax: +91-484-4059065   e-mail: kochi@cbspd.com
- **Mumbai:** 83-C, Dr E Moses Road, Worli, Mumbai-400018, Maharashtra
  Ph: +91-22-24902340/41   Fax: +91-22-24902342   e-mail: mumbai@cbspd.com
- **Pune:** Bhuruk Prestige, Sr. No. 52/12/2+1+3/2 Narhe, Haveli
  (Near Katraj-Dehu Road Bypass), Pune 411 041, Maharashtra
  Ph: +91-20-64704058/59, 32392277   Fax: +91-20-24300160   e-mail: pune@cbspd.com

Representatives

- **Hyderabad** 0-9885175004   • **Kolkata** 0-9831437309, 0-9051152362
- **Nagpur** 0-9021734563   • **Patna** 0-9334159340
- **Vijayawada** 0-9000660880

Printed at: India Binding House, Noida, UP

Dedicated

To

MY PARENTS

Whose Love Is The Foundation Of My Life

Special Thanks

I would like to thank SANDEEP BALIYAN aka "BALLI", Mechanical Engineer from *H.B.T.I Kanpur*, who is a friend, a colleague and batch mate in my course of engineering, without whose help it would have been very difficult to complete the book. He contributed by sharing his industrial experiences in context of various topics discussed in this book. He was my companion in brainstorming sessions in an effort to make this book interesting without compromising on technical aspects. To sum up, I must say that he has whole heartedly backed and supported my efforts.

Preface

Industrial Psychology has always been an area of interest among the researchers and managers as it influences various parameters in actual productivity of the organization. Lot of research has been done on this topic and many books have been written. This book is conceived in an effort to make the concepts easy to understand in the lucid flow of language.

The objective that has been tried to achieve is to make the book as much interesting as possible so as to repulse the boredom in students and avoid the feeling of "Just another theoretical course book". For realization of above, few new approaches towards effective learning have been introduced.

Learning Objectives: Each chapter starts with the purpose of learning.

The Insight: The Insight is a short introduction mostly by means of real examples, given in the beginning of each chapter. The purpose is to "preheat the system before the actual combustion starts".

Wisdom Tooth: "Golden words are said but once, but should reverberate for generations to come". This section shares the words of wisdom told by great people who were either directly related to the topics being discussed or their words are relevant in context of the topic being discussed.

You Should Know: This section is more of a general awareness session. It includes facts and figures relating to the topic being discussed, that may not be directly asked in examination but are good for better understanding of the subject.

Test Your Grey Matter: It is aimed at testing knowledge base formed by the end of a topic, group of topics or the chapter itself. The distribution of these sections is done so as to segregate the chapter into subdivisions, so that important topics are given due weightage and are highlighted separately.

Thinking Time: This section is incorporated to increase involvement of the reader. It includes the activities and tasks which require creative and conscious effort.

Besides this, effective use of pictures, flowcharts and flow diagrams has been made for better understanding and easy learning. These will be very useful at the time of revision and will save a lot of time while going through a particular topic.

Point-wise structure is followed throughout the book to give a concise and direct approach to the whole learning process.

Every effort has been made to make this book a students' delight, on which they can rely for accuracy, quality and time saving approach. It is hoped that faculty members will also find it in line with contemporary teaching methodologies and of value for students.

The comments and suggestions of readers are always welcome for further improvement of the book.

The author can be contacted at ankur.negi.author@gmail.com

Author

Acknowledgement

Firstly I would like to thank the person who motivated me as well as supported me with the idea of writing this book, Mr. Sushant Gomber, Director, Word-Press. He has shown interest and believed in my knowledge and conceptual capabilities. Without his help and support it would have been virtually impossible to complete this task.

I acknowledge the efforts of Miss Preeti Vats, whose valuable suggestions regarding the prevalent teaching methodologies as well as improvisation of the same has been quite instrumental in making this book coherent with the expectation of students.

Best wishes of my parents Mr. Surendra Singh Negi & Mrs. Suman Negi and the blessings of my Grandma Mrs. Maheshwari fueled me physically as well as mentally to complete this work with perfection. They have inculcated in me the sense of independent thinking which has helped me in all spheres of life. My brother, Akansh Negi constantly motivated me to deliver my best.

I am also thankful to my friends Shobhit Srivastava, Puneet Mittal, Hemu Gupta, Gaurav Bansal and Parmesh Singh for their continuous support. Each one of them helped me in their own ways.

Contents

"My philosophy, in essence, is the concept of man as a heroic being,
With his own happiness as the moral purpose of his life,
With productive achievements as his noblest activity,
And reason as his only absolute."

Ayn Rand

1 | Introduction to Industrial Psychology

By the end of this chapter, you would be able to :

- Understand Industrial Psychology and its emergence as an independent field of science.
- Know the historical developments which resulted in the present form of Industrial Psychology.
- Appreciate the importance of Industrial Psychology and learn about its scope.
- Acquaint yourself with the careers in Industrial Psychology to pursue it as a career in future.
- Learn about the concepts applied and the problems faced in Industrial Psychology.

The chapter contains :

- Psychology
- Industry
- Industrial Psychology
- History of Industrial Psychology
- Scope/Application of Industrial Psychology
- Concepts of Industrial Psychology
- Careers in Industrial Psychology
- Major problems of Industrial Psychology

A. THE INSIGHT

- "I love my job very much and I wish to give the best in me for my organisation."
- "My office is one of the best places on earth and I cannot wait to go to office and start working."
- "My organisation is the best organisation in the world."
- "My aim in life is to take my organisation to its zenith."

Wouldn't the bosses be happy if their employees gave such pleasing statements?

Actually, this was the reason why Industrial Psychology came into existence, i.e. to develop techniques that provided a way towards the goal of a joyous and productive workforce.

B. CONCEPTS

Industrial Psychology, the subject of our study can be clearly broken down into two words, Industry and Psychology.

Psychology

- Psychology is a branch of science that helps us to understand ourselves and others.
- It answers our basic questions in life, as to why people become sad, happy, angry, motivated etc. and most importantly, why do people get attracted and fall in love!!!
- By understanding the psychology of the teacher, you can even get good marks by presenting the answers in the way he/she wants it.

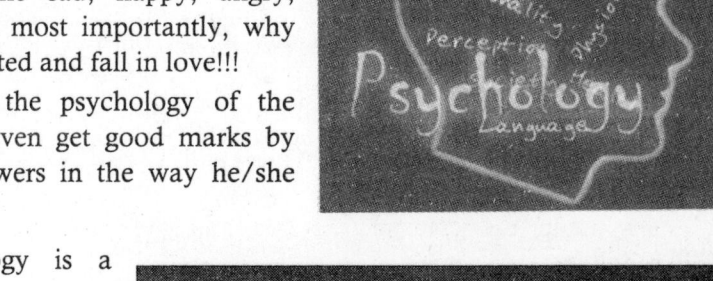

Definition: Psychology is a scientific study of mental processes, experiences and behaviour.

Fields of Psychology

There are various fields in which psychology is applied, such as:

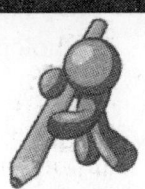

Wisdom Tooth

"Know thyself, for once we know ourselves, we may know how to care for ourselves, otherwise we never shall"

- Socrates

- Cognitive Psychology
- Comparative Psychology
- Abnormal Psychology
- Clinical & Counselling Psychology
- Cross-Cultural & Cultural Psychology
- Educational & School Psychology
- Environmental Psychology
- Health Psychology
- Life Span Development Psychology
- Social Psychology
- Aviation Psychology

- Military Psychology, Rural Psychology, Engineering Psychology, Sports Psychology, Peace Psychology (yes, it exists) etc., and
- Industrial/Organisational Psychology (I.O)

Industry

Definition: "Industry means any systematic activity carried on by co-operation between an employer and his workmen for the production, supply or distribution of goods or services with a view to satisfy human wants or wishes."

Thus, industry is a type of Economic Activity producing Goods or Services.

Industrial Psychology

We can now combine both the words Industry and Psychology to understand Industrial Psychology.

Definition: "Industrial Psychology is a branch of psychology that applies principles of psychology to the workplace, to explain and enhance the effectiveness of human behaviour and cognition in the workplace."

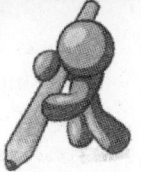

Wisdom Tooth

"Everything that irritates us about others can lead us to an understanding about ourselves".

Carl Gustav

Principles of Psychology

- It refers to the methods which psychologists use in gaining knowledge. These methods or means are thus applied to the workplace in Industrial Psychology to achieve some results.
- Methods used by psychologists -
  - It begins with a description of the goals of a psychological inquiry.
  - Then, the nature and characteristics of scientific research are given.
  - This is followed by details of some of the main types of investigations carried out by psychologist i.e. observational, experimental, non-experimental, cross-sectional and longitudinal, case study and survey.
  - Psychological tools such as tests, interviews and questionnaires used in investigations are also described.
  - Finally, the ethical issues in conducting psychological investigations are described.

Cognition

Definition: Cognition is the mental process of knowing, which includes aspects such as awareness, perception, reasoning and judgement.

C. HISTORY OF INDUSTRIAL PSYCHOLOGY

Psychology was formally established as a science in 1879 (when Wilhelm Wundt established the first psychology laboratory). So, obviously, Industrial and Organisational Psychology was established sometime after that. Yet, many of the issues important to I/O psychology had been discussed long before then. Below are just a few examples.

- **Aristotle**, in *Politics*, developed foundations for many modern management concepts, including specialisation of labour, delegation of authority, departmentalisation, decentralisation, and leadership selection.

- **Machiavelli** (in *The Prince*, 1527) offered practical advice for developing authoritarian structures within organisations.

- **Thomas Hobbes** (1651) advocated strong centralised leadership as a means for "bringing order to the chaos created by man". He provided a justification for autocratic rule that helped establish the pattern for organisations through the nineteenth century.

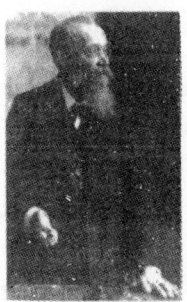

Wilhelm Wundt

- **John Locke** (1690) outlined the philosophical justification later manifested in the U.S. Declaration of Independence, which in effect, advocates participatory management, in his argument that leadership is granted by the governed.

- **Jean Jacques Rousseau**, in *The Social Contract* (1762), in effect supported Locke's position.

- **Adam Smith** (1776), in *The Wealth of Nations* revolutionised economic and organisational thought by suggesting the use of centralisation of labour and equipment in factories, division of specialised labour, and management of specialisation in factories.

The Early Years (Pre-WW1)

- **1881:** The first school of professional management was started at the University of Pennsylvania when Joseph Wharton donated $100,000 for it.

- **1883: Frederick W. Taylor** began experiments at the Midvale and Bethlehem Steel plant, which later led to the development of his "Scientific Management" philosophy

- **1903: W.L. Bryan**, prior to the formation of I/O psychology, gave a presidential address to APA in which he encouraged psychologists to study "concrete activities and functions as they appear in everyday life". Although he didn't cite industry directly, he did encourage such "real life" applications of the science of psychology.

- **Walter Dill Scott** gave a talk to Chicago business leaders on the application of psychology to advertising, which led to books on the topic being published in 1903 & 1908.

By 1911 he had published two more books (*Influencing Men in Business* and *Increasing Human Efficiency in Business*), and became the first to apply the principles of psychology to motivation and productivity in the workplace.

He also became instrumental in the application of personnel procedures within the army during World War I.

You should know

"The term 'Industrial Psychology first appeared in a 1904 article of Bryan s APA address. Ironically, it appeared in print only as a typographical error. Bryan was quoting a sentence he had written five years earlier in which he spoke of the need for more research in individual psychology. Instead, Bryan wrote industrial psychology and did not catch his mistake."
(source: Muchinsky, 1997, p10)

- **Hugo Munsterberg**, considered by many as **"The Father of Industrial Psychology"**, pioneered the application of psychological findings from laboratory experiments to practical matters
  - ❑ In 1911, he cautioned managers to be concerned with "all the questions of the mind...like fatigue, monotony, interest, learning, work satisfaction, and rewards."
  - ❑ He was also the first to encourage government-funded research in the area of industrial psychology.
  - ❑ In 1913, his book *Psychology and Industrial Efficiency* addressed such things as personnel selection and equipment design.

Munsterberg's early I/O psychology became influential well into the 1950s. It assumed that people need to fit into the organisation, thus, applied behavioural sciences largely consisted of helping organisations shape people to serve as replacement parts for organisational machines

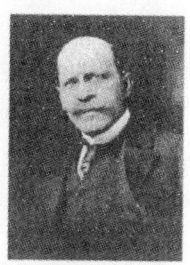

Hugo Munsterberg (1863 - 1916)

About the same time as Munsterberg, Frederick W. Taylor began publishing similar philosophies on management which had a tremendous impact on organisational management

- **Frederick W. Taylor**
  - ❑ Taylor realised the value of redesigning the work situation (through use of time and motion studies) to achieve both higher output for the company and higher wages for the worker
  - ❑ His writings were one of the first reasonably comprehensive philosophies of management
  - ❑ 1909 Taylor's book on Shop Management explained the management's role in motivating workers to avoid "natural soldiering", i.e., the natural tendency of people to "take it easy"
  - ❑ 1911 Taylor published the book *The Principles of Scientific Management.*
  - ❑ We will read about F.W Taylor in Chapter 2.

World War I (1917-1918)

- **Robert Yerkes** was the most influential psychologist in getting psychology into the war. He proposed ways of screening recruits for mental deficiency and assigning selected recruits to army jobs
- Committees of psychologists also investigated soldier motivation, morale, psychological problems of physical incapacity ("shell shock") and discipline.
- The Army was sceptical and approved only a modest number of proposals, primarily in the assessment of recruits — which Yerkes and others developed as a general intelligence test
- Meanwhile **Walter Dill Scott** was doing research on the best placement of soldiers in the Army. He classified and placed enlistees, conducted performance evaluations of officers, and developed and prepared job duties and qualifications for over 500 jobs.
- However, the final authorisation for the testing program came in August 1918, only three months before the Armistice was signed — thus the intelligence tests were not utilised as much as Yerkes had hoped
- 1917: *Journal of Applied Psychology* began publication. Today, it is still perhaps the most respected, representative journal in I/O field

Between the Wars (1919-1940)

- Psychological Corporation was started by **James Cattell** in 1921.The main purpose was to advance psychology and promote its usefulness to industry.
- 1920s: Doctoral degrees specialising in industrial psychology begin to be offered at U.S. universities. Among the first: Ohio State, Carnegie Institute of Technology, Univ. of Minnesota, and Stanford University.
- **The Hawthorne Studies**
  We will read about Hawthorne Experiments and Elton Mayo in Chapter 4.

Between the Wars: During and Shortly After the Hawthorne Studies

- Major advances in measurement of attitudes during 1920s and 1930s
- Likert and Thurstone among those particularly prominent.
- One of the earliest with clinical roots to enter I/O psychology was Morris Viteles
  - **Viteles** was a student of **Lightner Witmer** (who many consider the father of clinical psychology)
  - Among Viteles' books were:
    - *Industrial Psychology* (1932) (perhaps the first book to use that term in its title)
    - *The Science of Work* (1934)
    - *Motivation and Morale in Industry* (1953)
- In 1939, **Kurt Lewin** led the first publication of an empirical study of the effects of leadership styles; this work initiated arguments for the use of participative management techniques.

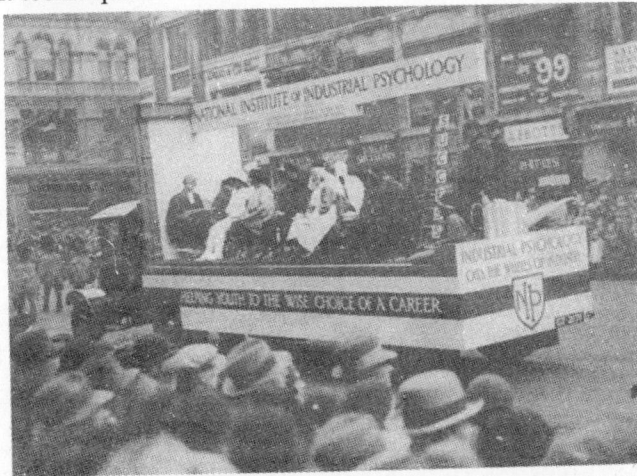

1931 Lord Mayor's Parade explained that industrial psychology was to 'Oil the Wheels of Industry' by 'helping youth to the wise choice of a career.'

World War II (1941-1945)

- By this time industrial psychologists had improved many of their techniques for employee selection and placement, and were sought after by the army for their help with these functions.
- Successful I/O contributions included development of:
  - Army General Classification Test
  - Used to classify an estimated 12 million soldiers into military jobs.

- ❑ Tests of performance under situational stress for U.S. Office of Strategic Services. The tests were highly successful in identifying the best candidates to be OSS agents.
- 1945: **Kurt Lewin** formed the Research Centre for Group Dynamics at MIT to perform experiments in group behaviour. In 1948, the research centre moved to the University of Michigan and became a branch of the Institute for Social Research.

1950s and 1960s

- Late 40s & early 50s: Clinical psychologists **Carl Rogers'** and **Abraham Maslow's** theories of motivation supported the human relations movement.
- **Skinner** initiated discussions of behaviourism's applications to organisational settings.
- 1954: **Peter F. Drucker** outlined his Management by Objectives (MBO) approach and **John C. Flanigan** outlined his Critical Incidents Technique.
- **Rise of Motivation Theories in late 1950s through 1960s**
  - ❑ Late 1950s: **Douglas McGregor** proposed his Theory X and Theory Y assumptions of the relations between employees and organisations.
  - ❑ Early 1960s: Contingency models of leadership proposed a need for different styles under different circumstances — a view that rose with the work of **Fred Fiedler** in mid 1960s.
  - ❑ 1964: **Vroom's** VIE theory (valence, instrumentality, expectancy) of motivation proposed. It was influential in the development of later expectancy theories
  - ❑ Mid 1960s: **David McClelland** proposed the need for achievement theory which argues that there are two groups of people, the majority who are not concerned about achieving and the minority who are challenged by achieving.
  - ❑ Late 1960s: **Frederick Herzberg** proposed his two-factor theory of motivation (satisfiers/motivators & hygiene factors).
  - ❑ **Edwin Locke** outlined his goal-setting approach to motivation.
- 1964: Civil Rights Act is passed. Title VII, section 703a states: "it is unlawful to discriminate in any employment practice on the basis of race, colour, religion, sex, or national origin."
- 1966: **Katz & Kahn** published classic text outlining theory and research of organisational behaviour as embedded in open, socio-technical systems.
- Mid 1960s to early 1970s: Advances in job analysis techniques, including:
  - ❑ 'Task inventory' approach developed from research with U.S. Air Force.

❑ *Dictionary of Occupational Titles* published in 1965 (third edition).

❑ 1960s research at Purdue Occupational Research Centre led to publication of the *Position Analysis Questionnaire* in 1972.

❑ **Edwin Fleishman** developed 'ability requirements' approach.

1970s

- 1971: **B.F. Skinner**, in *Beyond Freedom and Dignity*, advocated behaviour modification strategies to motivate people in organisations.

- Organisational behaviour modification's successes increasingly demonstrated e.g., in **Luthans & Kreitner's** (1975) and **Frederiksen's** (1982) books

- Rise of cognitive approaches to studying topics in psychology (which grew in 1960s) continued in 1970s, including their influence on a wide range of I/O research.

- Early 1970s: **Porter & Lawler** proposed revised expectancy model of motivation.

- Early/mid 1970s: Civil rights laws and related Supreme Court decisions led to increasing research on bias in organisations.

1980s & 1990s

- In the1980s, the rigidity of classical theories of management produced harsh consequences for American businesses (e.g. in the automobile industry).During these times of rapid change in the technological and business environments the Japanese were prospering with the methods first proposed by Americans.

- 1984 article in the *Academy of Management Review* outlined explanations for the success of Japanese management techniques as:
  i)   Superior manufacturing processes
  ii) Increased quality and quantity coupled with reduced cost
  iii) Participatory management techniques
  iv) Use of statistical quality control techniques
  v)   Consensus decision making
  vi) Lifetime job security (although in the 1990s some Japanese companies moved away from this guarantee)
  vi) Long-term planning

- Mid 1980s: increasing attention to use of *quality circles* and other participatory management techniques.

- Late 1980s: renewed interest in organisational climate and groups .

- Late 1980s: rise of participatory management techniques known by such terms as Total Quality Management (TQM), Continuous Quality Improvement (CQI), and Continuous Process Improvement (CPI)

- 1990s: rise of *meta-analysis* as a statistical technique (spurred by Hunter & Schmidt's 1990 book — an extension of their 1977 Schmidt & Hunter journal article).
- Late 1980s & into the 1990s: work stress received increasing attention in I/O research, theory and practice.
- Balancing work and family lives received increasing attention in I/O research in late 1980s, and again in mid/late 1990s.
- Workplace aggression/workplace violence emerged as topic of study in mid/late 1990s

TEST YOUR GREY MATTER

Q1) Define Psychology. Name some of its major fields.

Q2) Define Industrial Psychology. What is the difference between psychology and industrial psychology?

Q3) What are the principles of Psychology which are used in Industrial Psychology?

Q4) Briefly describe the history of development of industrial psychology, mentioning only those events and persons who drastically changed the course of thinking.

Q5) Write an explanatory note on the evolution and growth of industrial psychology.

D. SCOPE/APPLICATION OF INDUSTRIAL PSYCHOLOGY

Industrial Psychology provides two approaches to solve the problem of increasing productivity.

i) Industrial Approach

It focuses on determining competencies needed to perform a job, staffing the organisation with employees who have those competencies and increasing these competencies through training.

ii) Organisational Approach

This involves creating an organisational structure and culture that will motivate employees to perform weil, provide them with necessary information to do their jobs and provide working conditions that are safe and results in an enjoyable and satisfying work environment.

Thus, the Scope of Industrial Psychology can be further divided into 3 major groups and their sub-groups as follows:

1. Personnel Psychology

It involves study and practice in the areas as

- **Job analysis**

Job Analysis is the process of collecting information about various components of a job. It includes both, duties and conditions of work and individual qualifications of the worker. This information is used to prepare the job description and job specification.

It is dealt with in detail in Chapter 14.

- **Recruitment**

Recruitment refers to the process of attracting, screening and selecting qualified people for a job at an organisation or company.

It is dealt with in detail in Chapter 15.

- **Selection**

Selection is basically, picking applicants from a pool of job applicants, who have the appropriate qualifications and competency to do the job in the organisation.

It is dealt with in detail in Chapter 15.

- **Employee performance appraisal and determination of salaries**

It is the process of obtaining, analysing and recording information about the relative worth of an employee.

It is dealt with in detail in Chapter 17.

- **Training and development of employees**

Training and development is an attempt to improve a current or future employees' performance by increasing the employee's ability to perform through learning, usually by changing the employee's attitude or increasing his/ her skills and knowledge.

It is dealt with in detail in Chapter 18.

2. Organisational Psychology

It is concerned with the basic issues of:

- **Leadership**

Leadership is a process of social influence in which one person can enlist the aid and support of others in the accomplishment of a common task.

It is dealt with in detail in Chapter 9.

- **Job Satisfaction**

  Job satisfaction is the amount of contentment (or lack of it) arising from the interplay of the employee's positive and negative feelings towards his or her job.

  It is dealt with in detail in Chapter 6.

- **Employee Motivation**

  Motivation is a term referring to a family of concepts used to explain initiation, direction, maintenance & termination of activities taken up by living organisms.

  It is dealt with in detail in Chapter 5.

- **Organisational Communication**

  Organisational communication is defined as the process of exchange of information and understanding among the people of the organisation.

- **Conflict Management**

  Conflict is the psychological and behavioural reaction to a perception that another person is either keeping you away from reaching the goal, taking away your right to behave in a particular way or violating the expectancies of a relationship.

  Conflict management is the practice of identifying and handling conflict in a sensible, fair, and efficient manner. Conflict management requires such skills as effective communication, problem solving, and negotiating with a focus on interests.

- **Organisational Culture**

  Organisational culture is defined as the specific collection of values and norms that are shared by people and groups in an organisation and that control the way they interact with each other and with stakeholders outside the organisation.

  It is dealt with in detail in Chapter 8.

- **Group Dynamics**

  Group Dynamics is a social process by which people interact face-to-face in small groups.

  It is dealt with in detail in Chapter 10.

3. Human Factor/Ergonomics

It mainly focuses on:

- **Fatigue and Boredom**

  Fatigue is a condition characterised by the decrease in output of an activity due to previous activity and is directly proportional to poorness of the output.

  Boredom refers to the dull, uninterested and unfavourable state of mind or attitude of a worker towards his work.

  It is dealt with in detail in Chapter 12.

- **Stress**

  Stress is a person's adaptive response to a stimulus that places excessive psychological and physical demands on him or her.

  It is dealt with in detail in Chapter 7.

- **Accident and Safety**

  An occurrence in an industrial establishment causing bodily injury to a person, which makes him unfit to resume his duties in the next 48 hours.

  It is dealt with in detail in Chapter 13.

- **Work Environment**

  Work Environment comprises of the surroundings in which a worker does his work. It includes Physical Environment, Psychological/Mental Environment and Social Environment.

  It is dealt with in detail in Chapter 11.

- **Ergonomics**

  It is defined as the scientific study of the relationship between man and his working environment.

  It is dealt with in detail in Chapter 11.

E. CONCEPTS OF INDUSTRIAL PSYCHOLOGY

Two basic concepts used in Industrial Psychology are:

i. Individual Difference

- Industrial Psychology assumes that every individual is different.
- Each individual has his own characteristics such as intelligence, attitude, physical strength, skills etc.

- These differences make the work of industrial psychology difficult as different behaviour results in different on-the-job behaviour, and thus different methods to control it to direct it towards productivity.
- It also calls for identifying these factors of individual differences so that proper selection, placement and training techniques could be developed.

ii. Causation of Behaviour

- Industrial Psychology assumes that behind every human behaviour there is a cause or a reason.
- Thus, it strives at finding the cause for a particular behaviour and then changing the cause to change the behaviour of the employee in favour of the organisation.
- This concept is very useful in motivating employees.

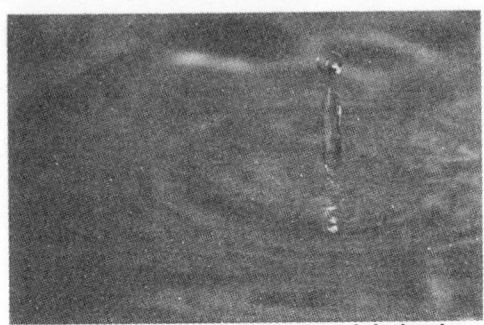

There is a cause behind each behaviour

F. CAREERS IN INDUSTRIAL PSYCHOLOGY

- An Industrial Psychologist is a person who studies and predicts human behaviour with the help of scientific methods.
- An Industrial Psychologist can be employed in the following major areas:
  - i) Consultant
  - ii) Employee of a company or government called **"Staff Psychologist"**
  - iii) University teacher
  - iv) Combination of two of the three of the above mentioned roles
- Following are the locations where an industrial psychologist is placed:

i. Academic Institutions & Consulting Firms

- According to a 1997 membership survey of the Society for Industrial-Organisational Psychology, nearly two-thirds of U.S. Industrial Psychologists are employed by academic institutions and consulting firms.
- Employment at consulting firms has been the growth in the profession, while the percentage of Industrial Psychologists employed by academic and private organisations has declined somewhat.

ii. Private Companies

- About 15 percent work for private companies, and the rest work for government agencies or other organisations.

- Large organisations are the primary users of industrial psychological methods, either directly by employing an Industrial/ Organisational Psychologist's services or indirectly by using information from the field (e.g., published articles, books, seminars).
- Numerous large American corporations such as AT&T, IBM, Unisys Corp., General Motors Corp., Ford Motor Co., PepsiCo Inc., to name just a few, maintain a staff of Industrial Psychologists.
- Many other companies regularly use Industrial Psychologists as consultants on an as-needed basis.

iii. Government

Industrial Psychologists are also employed by the government. The Federal Office of Personnel Management in U.S.A has an active test development program for civil service test construction.

iv.Military

All branches of the military employ Industrial Psychologists to conduct research and design applications in leadership, personnel placement testing, human factors, and for improving motivation and morale. The U.S. Army Research Institute is an example of one such military agency.

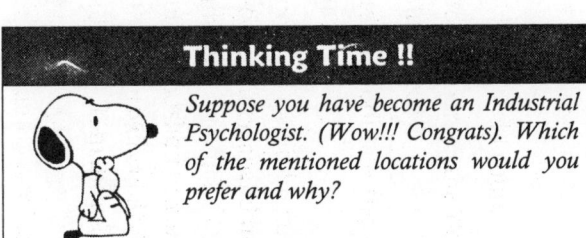

Thinking Time !!

Suppose you have become an Industrial Psychologist. (Wow!!! Congrats). Which of the mentioned locations would you prefer and why?

v. State and Municipal Governments

They also employ psychologists, especially for personnel selection purposes in the context of local civil service requirements.

G. MAJOR PROBLEMS OF INDUSTRIAL PSYCHOLOGY

i. Resistance to Change

- Human beings have a tendency to resist change and this problem causes a major hurdle for industrial psychologists.
- Resistance may not come from the employee only but also from all levels of management and the employer
- Resistances may take the form of hostility and aggression against the change itself or against the administration.

50 Reasons Not To Change

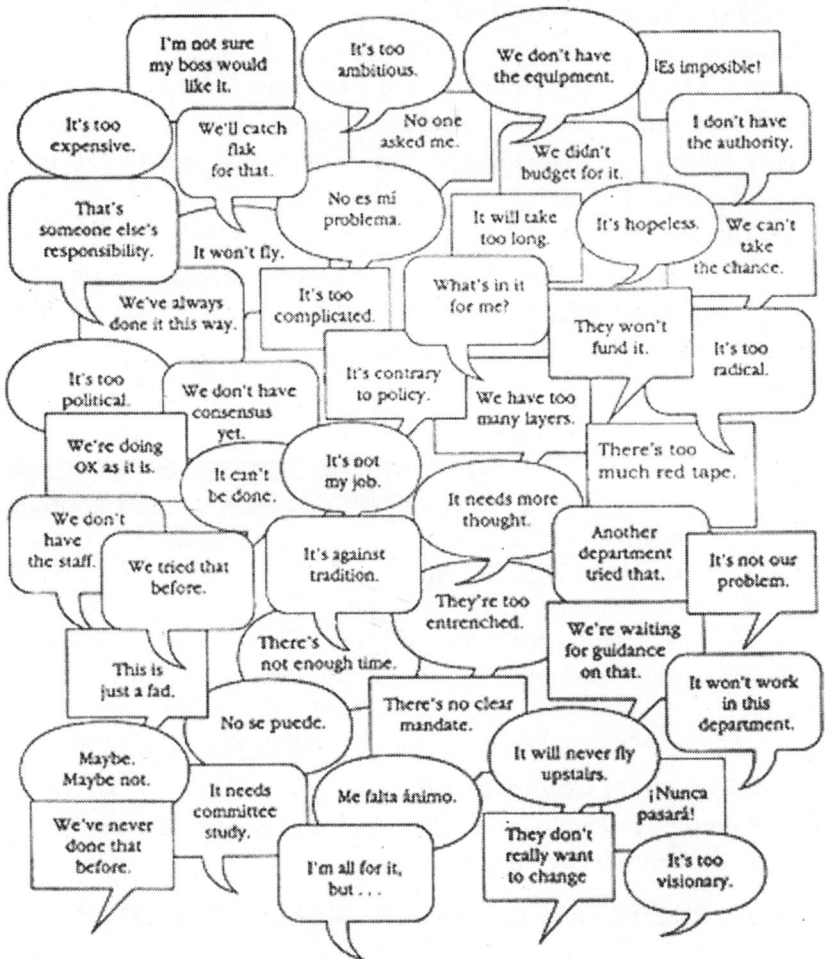

So, before introducing a change, the following should be done:

- The reason for change should be explained.
- Those involved in the change should have an opportunity to participate in the implementation of the change.
- The change should not force all to agree to a one-sided decision; rather it should be a two-way affair.
- The administrator of the change should recognise that the change is a real, imagined or potential threat and must do everything to eliminate or reduce the possible threat.

ii. Communication

- The language and techniques used by an industrial psychologist are sometimes too hard for others to understand. Thus, other people who are also related to the problem are left out.
- Hence, language that is clearly understood by everyone should be used so that everyone can participate in problem solving.

TEST YOUR GREY MATTER

Q1) Describe the scope of Industrial Psychology. Discuss the activities and functions which are to be performed by Industrial Psychology.

Q2) What are the basic concepts of Industrial Psychology

Q3) What are the career prospects of an Industrial Psychologist? Where is he mostly placed?

Q4) Mention the hurdles faced by an industrial psychologist while applying the discoveries, theories or principles in real life?

2 | Scientific Management

By the end of this chapter, you would be able to :

- Understand why Scientific Management came into existence.
- Know about F.W Taylor and his contributions.
- Learn about Scientific Management as a theory and also about its principles and elements.
- Appreciate the benefits that Workers, Management and Society derive from the application of the principles of Scientific Management.
- Critically examine and evaluate the Scientific Management Theory from different viewpoints.

The chapter contains :

- F.W Taylor-His Life and Work
- Definition of Scientific Management
- Principles of Scientific Management
- Elements of Scientific Management
- Mental Revolution
- Benefits of Scientific Management
- Experiments conducted to prove the importance of Scientific Management
- Critical Evaluation of Scientific Management

A. THE INSIGHT

President Roosevelt, in his address to the Governors at the White House, prophetically remarked that "The conservation of our national resources is only preliminary to the larger question of national efficiency."

This was the statement which gave one man the reason to point out the problems faced by the industries at that time and propose solutions.

This man was **Fredrick Winslow Taylor** and he is called the Father & Founder of Scientific Management.

We will see the life and work of F.W Taylor to find out how he actually gave one of the most important theory in the history of Industrial Psychology.

B. F.W. TAYLOR

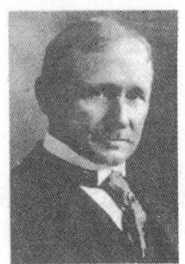

- He began his career in 1871 as an apprentice machinist and turner at the cramp shipyard at Philadelphia, U.S.A. After 3 years he joined Midvale Steel Works as a machine shop worker. Because of his hard work, he progressed rapidly to become machinist gang boss, foreman and finally Chief Engineer in 1884. He served company till 1889.

- To satisfy his hunger for technical know-how Taylor joined Stevens Institute and obtained Masters Degree in Engineering.

- Then he joined Bethlehem Steel Company, where he served from 1898-1901.

- During his career as a machinist and foreman, Taylor saw -

  i. Much disorder and wastage of human and other resources at the work place.

  ii. The workers did not produce more than one third of a day's work.

  iii. Workmen did not want the management to know about how much work they could do because they feared that their wages would be cut.

  iv. Moreover, the management did not have any idea of the capacity of the workers.

  v. And also, the management did not want to pay more to the workers.

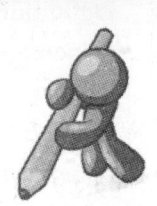

> ### Wisdom Tooth
>
> *Hardly a competent workman can be found who does not devote a considerably amount of time to studying just how slowly he can work and convince his employer that he is going at a good price.*
>
> **Frederick Winslow Taylor**

- Therefore, to solve these problems, Taylor came up with some solutions and made the following contributions –

  i. He developed the **'Principle of Breaking of task'** into elements for timing it.

  ii. He explored the causes of inefficiency and labour difficulties in the Industry. He developed **'Time Studies'** to recognise losses of efficiency.

  iii. He evolved certain principles of

    a) Investigating work on scientific basis.

    b) Selecting the best worker for a task and training him to further acquire the desired skill.

   c) Developing co-operative spirit between management and workers.

   d) Almost equal division of work between workers and management etc.

iv. He also developed a concept of **'A Fair Day's Task'**.

He experimented on the fatigue incurred by workers and the time necessary to complete a task. Taylor suggested that for increasing the production rate, work of each person should be planned at least one day in advance and he should be allotted a definite work to complete within a given time using a pre-explained method.

v. Taylor developed Functional Organisation in which one foreman was made in charge of each function to be performed.

vi. He established 'Work Standards' by 'Time studies'.

vii. He introduced various costing systems.

viii. Taylor also proposed 'Wage Incentive Scheme' known as 'Taylor's Differential Piece Rate Plan'.

> ### Thinking Time !!
>
>
>
> *Great men are not born but they become great by the work and effort they put in. We just now saw how F.W Taylor started from the lowest job and ended up being one of the most influential thinkers of our time.*
>
> *Do we ever consciously see the world around us? Problems which exists? Problems still unidentified? Solutions still undiscovered? Knowledge still waiting to be found? World shouting, wanted to be explored?*

TEST YOUR GREY MATTER

Q1) Give a brief description of the life and work of F.W Taylor?

Q2) What were the problems faced by industries at the time of F.W Taylor?

Q3) Explain briefly the solutions proposed by F.W Taylor to the problems he identified in industries?

C. SCIENTIFIC MANAGEMENT

Definition:

"Scientific Management is the substitution of exact scientific investigations and knowledge for the old individual judgments or opinions in all matters relating to the work done in shop". – F.W. Taylor

> ### You should know
>
> - In 1910 Louis Brandeis coined the word Scientific Management.
> - F.W. Taylor wrote a book 'The Principles of Scientific Management in year 1911.

Thus, Taylor introduced scientific methods in decision making and replaced **'Rule of Thumb'** or **'Trial and Error'** or **'Common Believes'**. This was the major theme of his theory. He wanted science to be the guiding force behind all the actions and decisions taken in an organisation.

Therefore, he not only propounded the theory but also laid down the Principles to be followed to practice Scientific Management.

C.1. Principles of Scientific Management

In Chapter 2 of his book *'The Principles of Scientific Management* , Taylor enlists his 4 principles of Scientific Management –

i.   Replace 'Rule of Thumb' work methods with methods based on scientific study of the task. This is 'Standardisation of Work'.
ii. Scientifically select and train workers.
iii. Co-operate with workers to ensure that scientifically developed methods are being followed.
iv. Divide work and responsibility nearly equally between managers and workers, so that managers apply scientific management principles for planning the work and workers for performing the work.

We will now discuss the techniques which are to be applied to follow the 4 principles and also understand their meaning and application –

C.2. Techniques to follow the Principles

1. Standardisation of Work

While doing any work, Taylor says that a scientific method must be found for doing that work which should be more efficient and effective and this should replace the old rule of thumb or the traditional way of doing it.

It has two advantages
a.   Improved methodology of production is developed.
b.   It also sets the standards which determine work performance of workers.

Various techniques used for standardisation of work are –

Work Study

Work study investigates the work done in an organisation and it aims at finding the best and most efficient way of using the available resources i.e. man, material, money and machinery.

Various aspects of work study are –

i. Method Study

It is defined as the systematic investigation of the existing method of doing a job in order to develop an easy, efficient, effective and less fatiguing procedure for doing the same job at lower cost. This is generally achieved by eliminating unnecessary motions involved in a certain procedure or by changing the sequence of operation or the process itself.

ii. Motion Study

It is the study of the movement of a machine operator and his machine on job. The purpose of motion analysis is to design an improved method which eliminates unnecessary motions and uses human effort more productively.

iii. Time Study

It is the study to find out minimum time required to do a job, once the best way of doing a job is determined. It is used to determine the standard time to do a job. It helps to determine a fair day's work of worker.

iv. Fatigue Study

It is the study to find out a method of doing work which causes minimum fatigue to workers so that they can maintain their operational efficiency. It determines both, mental & physical fatigue caused by working conditions and monotonous job (due to specialisation). Fatigue study is in precise sense a part of Motion Study.

2. Scientific Selection and Training

In the past, worker chose his own work and trained himself, as best as he could. But Taylor introduced the principle of scientific selection and then training, teaching and developing the workman.

All the men who refused to, or were unable to adopt the best methods were eliminated. He explained the two processes as follows:

i. Scientific Selection

When persons are recruited for a particular job, it should be based on work i.e. one must have similar education and experience that is required for the work and workers must have same tastes and preferences with which work is concerned.

ii. Scientific Training

Training is introduced to develop skills in artificial conditions which eliminated possibility of time, money and raw material wastage. By this process, the standardisation of work and scientific selection were brought together.

3. Co-operation with Workers

This principle was introduced so that the first two principles could be followed i.e. management should co-operate with the workers to ensure that all the work is being done in accordance with the principles of science which have been developed.

i. Task Idea

Taylor said that - The work of each worker should be fully planned out by the management at least one day in advance, and each worker should receive in most cases, complete written instructions, describing in detail the task which he is to accomplish, as well as the means to be used in doing the work. And work planned in this way constitutes a task which is to be solved, not by the worker alone, but almost in all cases, by the joint effort of the worker and the management. This task specifies not only what is to be done, but how it is to be done and the exact time allowed for doing it. And whenever the worker succeeds in doing his task right and within the time specified, he receives additional money.

ii. Differential Piece–Rate System

Taylor introduced this system to motivate workers to increase production. In this method of wage payment, two different rates were fixed for efficient and inefficient workers. Those who failed in attaining the standard, were to be paid at a lower rate and those exceeding the standard or just attaining the standard were to get a higher rate.

E.g. The standard is fixed at 50 units per day and piece rate are Rs. 5 and Rs. 6 per unit. If a worker produces say 50 units he gets

50 x 6 = 300 Rs. per day

and if he produces less than 50 say 49, he gets –

49 x 5 = 245 Rs. per day

4. Division of Responsibility

In the fourth principle, Taylor says that there must be almost equal division of work and responsibility between management and worker. He says that all the planning work must be done by the management in accordance with the laws of science and the execution work is to be done by the worker.

i. Principle of Exception

If anything exceptional occurs in the organisational functioning i.e. which is not routine activity or which is innovative or creative, it should be undertaken by management.

ii. Functional Foremanship

Taylor developed this concept in order to apply specialisation at supervisor level. Under this, system planning and execution are separated from each other and the job of planning is entrusted to a specialised planning department. As a single supervisor cannot be expected to be an expert in all the aspects of work, therefore, Taylor suggested different experts in different phases of the job. He advocated appointment of 8 foremen, 4 of them being responsible for planning the work and 4 concerned with the execution of work in the shop.

Four Foremen at Management Level

i.   Route Clerk

He gives the instructions about the way in which the work is to be done i.e. he fixes the route of production, the route through which the raw materials have to pass and the sequence of operations.

ii.   Instruction Card Clerk

He lays down the instructions to the worker describing the manner of doing the work.

iii.   Time and Cost Clerk

He determines the standard time for completion of work and sets the time table for doing various jobs and maintains record of the work. He also specifies material and labour cost in each operation.

iv.   Shop Disciplinarian

He enforces rules and regulations and maintains proper discipline among workers. He deals with the cases of conflicts and offers solutions.

Four Foremen at Execution or Shop Level

i.   Gang Boss

He has to keep the stage ready for work performance i.e. ensure that all materials and things are available for the workers, machine is set, tools are in place etc.

ii.   Repair Boss

He is responsible for the maintenance, renewal and repair of the machine, such as cleaning the machine, oiling it, repairing it etc.

iii.   Speed Boss

He looks after the time management, that is, whether worker would attain his targets or not. He guides the worker as to how best they can do their job and determines the speed at which work is to be done for its completion in time.

iv.   Inspector

He checks the quality of work turned out by workers and certifies the standards of workmanship of each job. Thus, workers become quality conscious.

After understanding all the principles and techniques, we can see that it does not involve any new invention or discovery. Taylor says it just involved a certain combination of elements which have not existed in the past.

TEST YOUR GREY MATTER

Q1) What is Scientific Management and briefly state its principles?

Q2) What is Standardisation of Work and what are the various techniques used to follow this principle?

Q3) How does Taylor propose to achieve co-operation of workers?

Q4) Describe different types of Foremen and explain why Taylor separates Foreman for Management level and Shop level?

Q5) What is the principle of exception?

C.3. Elements of Scientific Management

1. Science not thumb rule

Old conversations and beliefs to be replaced by scientific investigations and analysis.

2. Harmony not Discord

According to Taylor, there must be harmony between workers and management and prosperity of the organisation should be their only objective. Workers must contribute to their best level and management should share the gains of the company with the worker.

Thus, he calls for a 'mental revolution' i.e. a complete change in outlook and attitude for each other, as earlier, management considered workers to be good for nothing and workers felt that they were exploited, underpaid and overburdened. We will read about mental revolution later in this chapter.

3. Co-operation, No Individualism

In this context Taylor says "The time is fast going for the great personal or individual achievement of any one man standing alone and without the help of those around him. And the time is coming when all great things will be done by the type of cooperation in which each man performs the function for which

> ### Wisdom Tooth
>
> "In the past the man has been first; in the future the system must be first... The first object of any good system must be that of developing first class men."
>
> *-F.W Taylor*

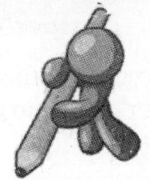

he is best suited, each man preserves hiś own individuality and is supreme in his particular function, and each man at the same time loses none of his originality and proper personal initiative, and yet is controlled by and must work harmoniously with many other men."

4. Maximum Output in place of Restricted Output

Taylor says that both management and workers should aim at maximum output. He says that as each worker has been systemically trained to the highest state of efficiency, and management and workers co-operate, there will be higher output, which will lead to increased profits and lower production costs as a result of increased labour productivity. For the worker, it also means higher wages.

5. The development of each man to his greatest efficiency and prosperity

This result from the selection and training principle laid down by Taylor. After proper selection of worker for a job, he is sent for training from time to time to update his knowledge. This will result in the development of each worker and result in efficiency & prosperity of the organisation.

C.4. Mental Revolution

Taylor suggests that whatever he has proposed will be of no use unless there is a complete Mental Revolution and the habits of all those engaged in the management, as well as the workmen change. Thus, Mental Revolution implies a revolutionary change in the attitudes of the management and workers towards each other and the work.

Taylor says that this change could be brought about only gradually and through the presentation of many lessons to the workmen, which, together with the teachings which he receives, thoroughly convince him of the superiority of this method.

Mental Revolution calls for change in attitude to imply all the 5 elements which we have discussed.

TEST YOUR GREY MATTER

Q1)   Describe various elements of Scientific Management in detail.

Q2)   'A Mental Revolution is required to achieve Objectives of Scientific management'. Do you agree?

Q3)   How will Scientific Management help in achieving maximum output in place of restricted output according to Taylor?

C.5. Benefits of Scientific Management

1. To workers

i. Provides opportunity to earn more in the form of incentives in higher production.

ii. Better relations with management as both work for common objective.

iii. Training and development facility provides an opportunity to learn and increase skills.

iv. Better working conditions.

v. Most efficient and less fatiguing method is learned which is scientifically developed.

vi. Foreman formation gives them constant guidance for work.

2. To Management/Employer

i. Better relations with workers, so no strikes or lock-outs.

ii. Increase in productivity.

iii. Increase in efficiency i.e. in quality and quantity.

iv. Decrease in wastage of resources.

v. Increase in profit margin.

vi. Proper division of responsibility creates a sense of clarity.

3. To Society

i. Quality of product improves.

ii. Because of increase in efficiency, cost of product goes down.

iii. Prosperity of country increases with increase in productivity of the nation.

iv. Increase in both necessities and luxuries of life of a society.

C.6. Experiments conducted to prove the importance of Scientific Management

Taylor gave examples of the following experiments, which he performed to demonstrate the effects of scientific management:

1. Pig Iron

If workers were moving 12½ tons of pig iron per day and they could be incentivised to try to move 47½ tons per day, left to their own wits they probably would become exhausted after a few hours and fail to reach their goal. However, by first

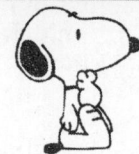

Thinking Time !!

Can you think of the benefits Scientific Management can bring to you, if you apply its principle of 'Standardisation of work in your life?

conducting experiments to determine the amount of resting that was necessary, the worker's manager could determine the optimal timing of lifting and resting so that the worker could move the 47½ tons per days without tiring.

Not all workers were physically capable of moving 47½ tons per day, perhaps only 1/8 of the pig iron handlers were capable of doing so. While these 1/8 were not extraordinary people who were highly prized by the society, their physical capabilities were well-suited to moving pig iron. This showed the importance of 'selection' of worker for the job.

2. The Science of Shovelling

In another study, Taylor ran time studies to determine that the optimal weight that a worker could lift with a shovel was 21 pounds. Since there is a wide range of densities of materials, the shovel should be sized so that it would hold 21 pounds of the substance being shovelled. The firm provided workers with optimum shovels. The result was 2 to 4 times increase in productivity and workers were rewarded with pay increase. Prior to scientific management, workers used their own shovels and rarely had the optimal one for the job.

3. Bricklaying

Gilberth, an engineer and student of Taylor performed experiments that focused on specific motions in bricklaying. The Gilberth husband and wife team used motion picture technology to study the motions of the workers and reduced the movements from 18 motions per brick to 5 and in some cases 2 motions per brick. Thus average worker could lay 350 bricks per hour instead of 120 bricks per hour. This indicated the importance of Scientific Management.

C.7. Critical Evaluation of Scientific Management

Psychologists Viewpoint

i. Workshop Level

It is believed that Scientific Management is focused only on the workshop level and as such has not evaluated the entire organisation. Hence, it conceptualises only half the organisation.

ii. Mechanistic View

It is believed to consider man as merely a 'cog in the machine'. Under time study and work study, it only evaluates how technology can be utilised and rates efficiency on the basis of machine functioning, that too with a stop watch and expects that the worker would contribute in the same manner. This is a mechanistic view, which, the psychologist says, cannot be applied to human beings as it carries emotion and is driven by social and psychological factors too.

iii. Monetary Motivation

According to Taylor, productivity of labour can be increased by increasing rates of incentive and it has no limits. Virtually, it was proved in the Hawthorne experiment by Elton Mayo that though man gets motivation from money, but it works only up to a certain level, beyond which behavioural factors operate.

iv. Excessive Control

Functional foremanship concept no doubt incorporates specialism in functioning, but violates the principle of unity of command and according to Henry Fayol, if unity of command is jeopardised, authority would be undermined.

v. Monotony

Taylor proposed specialisation in job to increase productivity. He did not consider job enlargement for workers. This resulted in monotony and workers felt bored sometimes doing the same job which resulted in decrease in efficiency.

Worker's Viewpoint

i. Use of stopwatches

Use of stopwatches was often a protested issue. It was considered dehumanising, as a result, laws were passed banning the use of stopwatches by civil servants in America and the restriction was lifted in 1949!!

ii. Monotony and Boredom

Workers complained of boredom because of repetitive nature of their jobs.

iii. No initiative

Workers were not happy as there was no room for their initiative. They were to strictly follow what was planned.

iv. Unemployment

There was a belief among workers that increase in efficiency and productivity of each worker will result in requirement of lesser people and thus they would be unemployed. Taylor tried to address this point in his paper convincing that increase in productivity will result in lowering of cost and thus increase in demand for that product which will result in increase in employment.

v. Trade Unions

As Scientific Management increases harmony between workers and management, it weakened the trade unions, which was disliked by some workers.

vi.   Exploitation

Workers believed that they were exploited as they produced much more than the percentage increase in wages which they received.

Employer's viewpoint

i.   Initial Investment

Management was against Scientific Management because of the high initial investment which was required, to standardise the work, train the employees, improve working conditions etc.

ii.   Restructuring

Time involved in introducing Scientific Management to restructure the whole industrial unit would be large and the organisation would have to suffer huge losses due to stopping of work.

iii.   Functional Foremanship

Employer thought that this principle was not practical as one worker reporting to eight foremen may create a problem for the worker to satisfy all of them.

TEST YOUR GREY MATTER

Q1) Briefly describe any 2 experiments which helped Taylor establish his theory of Scientific Management?

Q2) How is the application of Scientific Management useful to (i)Workers (ii) Employee (iii) Society

Q3) "Scientific Management is a clever device for exploitation of labour". Do you agree?

Q4) On what grounds do employers and workers criticise Scientific Management?

Q5) Critically examine psychologist's viewpoint on Scientific Management?

CHAPTER

3

Work Study

By the end of this chapter, you would be able to :

- Understand various studies required to optimise resources.
- Learn about various procedures and techniques used in Method, Motion and Time study.
- Know about science of breaking a set of motions into individual motions.
- Appreciate the advantages derived from these studies and their applications.

The chapter contains :

- Definition and Objectives of Work Study
- Definition and Objectives of Method Study
- Procedure of Method Study
- Techniques used in Recording of Information
- Definition of Motion Study
- Procedure of Motion Study
- Principles of Motion Economy
- Therbligs
- Micromotion Study
- Memomotion Study
- Definition and Objectives of Time Study
- Procedure of Time Study
- Limitations of Time Study

A. THE INSIGHT

- "I have had more in twenty years than any other woman I have known has had in a lifetime", said Lillian Gilbreth, after the death of Frank Gilbreth, her husband.

- Frank and Lillian Gilbreth were one of the great husband-and-wife teams of science and engineering, who, in the early 1900s collaborated on the development of motion study as an engineering and management technique. They even used efficiency methods to raise their 12 children while having busy careers which was the inspiration for the book and movie,' Cheaper by The Dozen'.

B. WORK STUDY

Definition: Work study investigates the work done in an organisation and it aims at finding the best and most efficient way of using available resources i.e. man, material, money and machinery.

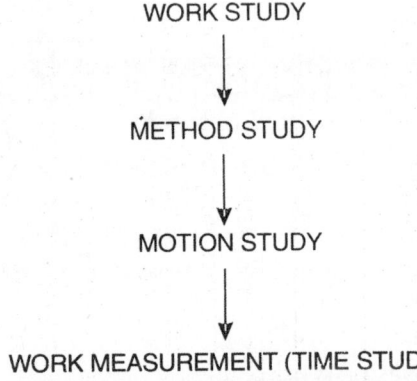

WORK STUDY

↓

METHOD STUDY

↓

MOTION STUDY

↓

WORK MEASUREMENT (TIME STUDY)

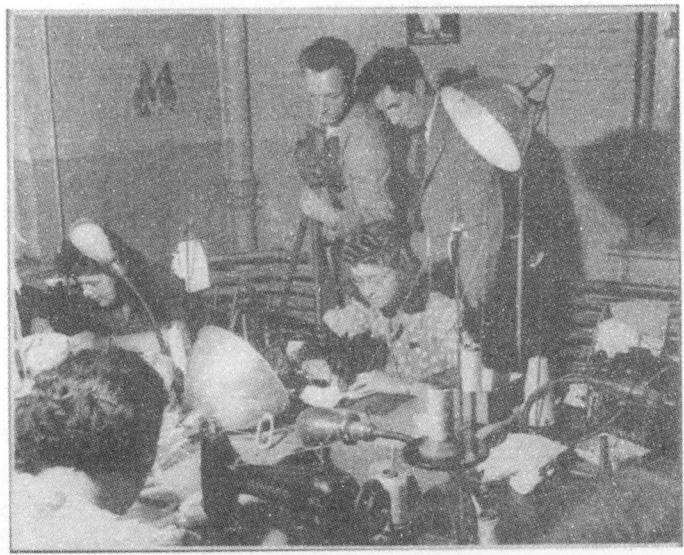

B.1. Advantages/Objectives of Work Study

i.   High production efficiency

ii. Reduced manufacturing costs

iii. Uniform and improved production flow

iv. Fast and accurate delivery dates

v.   Better service to customer

vi. Simplification of operations

vii. Effective use of machines and equipments

viii. Better employee-employer relationship

C. METHOD STUDY

Definition: It is defined as the systematic investigation of the existing method of doing a job in order to develop an easy, efficient, effective and less fatiguing procedure for doing the same job at a lower cost.

C.1. Advantages/Objectives of Method Study

i.   Effective utilisation of men, material and machinery.

ii. Improved working process and standardised procedures.

iii. Efficient and faster material handling.

iv. Better quality.

v.   Reduced fatigue to workers.

C.2. Procedure of Method Study

The following steps are involved in Method Study–

- **Select:** Work to be studied is selected and objectives to be achieved are defined.
- **Record:** All relevant information pertaining to the existing method is recorded.

Techniques used to record are–

i.   Process charts

ii. Diagrams

iii. Motion and Film analysis

iv. Models

- **Critical Analysis:** The data recorded is analysed critically. Questions like, What is done? Who does it? Where? How? When? are asked in it.
- **Develop:** The best method is developed and recorded. It should be practical, safe and economical.
- **Install:** It involves planning, arranging and implementation of the best method. Problems, if any, are resolved and the efficiency of the method is evaluated.
- **Maintain:** Various checks and verifications are done from time to time to ensure proper functioning of the method.

C.3.Techniques Used In Recording Information

1. Process Chart

Definition: A chart representing a process is called a process chart and it records graphically or diagrammatically all the operations connected with a process.

Process charts are of 3 types –

i. Outline Process chart

It records only main operations and events of a process.

ii. Two Handed Process

It records the left hand and right hand activities of an operator as related to each other.

iii. Flow Process Chart

As per A.S.M.E. (American Society of Mechanical Engineers), it is defined as a graphical presentation of the sequence of all operations, transportations, inspections, delays and storages occurring during a process or procedure and also includes information considered desirable for analysis, such as, time required and distance moved.

Symbols which are used to represent the charts –

Event	Symbol	Description
1. Operation	○	A step in procedure
2. Transportation	⇐	Movement of an item from one location to other
3. Inspection	▭	Checking quality or quantity
4. Storage	△	Preservation of an item for some time
5. Delay	D	Temporary halt in a process

There are three types of Flow Process –

i. Man Flow Process Chart

It records the activities or operations performed by an operator or worker.

ii. Equipment Flow Process Chart

It records the way in which a machine or equipment is used.

iii. Material Flow Process Chart

It records all the operations performed on the material i.e. distance moved, storage delay etc.

2. Diagram

Diagram indicates movement whereas process chart indicates only sequence of events.

i. Flow Diagram

A flow diagram is a drawing or a diagram which is drawn to scale. It shows the relative position of production machinery, jigs, fixtures etc. and marks the path followed by men and material.

ii. String Diagram

String Diagram is a model or a scale plan of the shop, in which every machine or equipment is marked and a pin is stuck in the area representing a facility. A continuous coloured thread or string is used to trace the path taken by materials or workers while performing a particular operation. It is used when paths are many and repetitive.

TEST YOUR GREY MATTER

Q1) Define Work Study and state why it is to be done?

Q2) What is Method Study? Briefly describe the steps followed in method study?

Q3) Describe Flow Process Chart in detail after stating what are processes charts?

Q4) How are diagrams different from Process Charts? Explain by comparing the types of Process charts and Diagrams?

D. MOTION STUDY/MOTION ANALYSIS

Definition: It is the study of movement of a machine operator and his machine on the job. The purpose of motion analysis is to design an improved method which eliminates unnecessary motions and uses human effort more productively.

D.1.Procedure of Motion Analysis

Following steps are involved –

i. Operation which is to be studied is chosen.

ii. Motions performed by operator are observed and recorded as list and chart.

iii. Productive and idle motions are identified.

iv. Non-productive motions are eliminated.

v. Principles of Motion Economy are used to redesign the procedure.

vi. Workers are trained to follow the new method.

vii. Standardise the process.

D.2. Principles of Motion Economy

Gilberth designed some principles to develop a better method of doing a job.

They were summarised by Ralph M. Barnes in the 1930s:

Rules to be followed here are

Ref: BARNES, RALPH M., *Motion and Time Study*, Second Edition, John Wiley & Sons, New York, 1940.

a. Use of Human Body

- The **two hands** should begin and end their motions at the same time.
- The two hands should not be **idle at the same time** except during rest periods.
- Motions of the **arms** should be made in opposite and symmetrical directions and should be made simultaneously.
- Hand motions should be confined to the **lowest classification** with which it is possible to perform the work satisfactorily.
- **Momentum** should be employed to assist the worker whenever possible, and it should be reduced to a minimum if it must be overcome by muscular effort.
- **Smooth continuous motions** of the hands are preferable to zigzag motions or straight-line motions involving sudden and sharp changes in direction.
- **Ballistic movements** are faster, easier, and more accurate than restricted (fixation) or "controlled" movements.
- **Rhythm** assists smooth and automatic performance. Arrange the work to permit an easy and natural rhythm.

b. Arrangement of the Work Place and Material Handling

- There should be a **definite and fixed place** for all tools and materials.
- Tools, materials, and controls should be **located close to** and directly in front of the operator.
- **Gravity feed bins** and containers should be used whenever possible.
- **Drop delivers** should be used whenever possible.
- Materials and tools should be **located** to permit the best sequence of motions.

- Provide for adequate **visual perception**. Good illumination is the first requirement.
- Arrange the **height** of the workplace and chair for alternate sitting and standing, when possible.
- Provide a **chair** of the type and height to permit good posture.

c. Design of Tools and Equipment

- Relieve hands of work that can be done more advantageously by a **jig, fixture, or a foot-operated device.**
- **Combine tools** whenever possible.
- **Pre-position tools** and materials.
- Where each finger performs some specific movement, such as in typewriting, the load should be distributed in accordance with the **inherent capacities of the fingers.**
- **Handles** (i.e. cranks and large screwdrivers) should permit as much of the surface of the hand to come in contact with the handle as possible, especially when considerable force is necessary.
- For **light assembly**, a screwdriver handle should be smaller at the bottom.
- **Levers, crossbars, and hand wheels** should be located in such positions that the operator can manipulate them with the least change in body position and with the greatest mechanical advantage.

> **Thinking Time !!**
>
> *Try to Use Method Study and Motion Study to simplify any process which we do in our daily life. E.g. cooking, washing clothes etc.*

D.3. Therbligs

The term **Therblig** was coined by Frank and Lillian Gilbreth for their system of analysing the motions involved in performing a task.

This identification of individual motions, as well as moments of delay in the process, designed to find unnecessary or inefficient motions and to utilise or eliminate even split-seconds of wasted time is called therblig.

> **You should know**
>
> *Gilbreth spelled backwards with 'th treated, as one letter becomes Therblig.*

Every therblig is represented by a symbol, a definite colour and with a word or two to record the same. The list of Therbligs has evolved over the years. Today it is common to use 18 such elements, however; originally the Gilbreths developed a system with 15.

Therblig	Colour	Symbol/Icon	Therblig	Colour	Symbol/Icon
Search	Black		Use	Purple	
Find	Gray		Disassemble	Violet, Light	
Select	Light Gray		Inspect	Burnt Orange	
Grasp	Lake Red		Pre-Position	Sky Blue	
Hold	Gold Ochre		Release Load	Carmine Red	
Transport Loaded	Green		Unavoidable Delay	Yellow Ochre	
Transport Empty	Olive Green		Avoidable Delay	Lemon Yellow	
Position	Blue		Plan	Brown	
Assemble	Violet, Heavy		Rest for overcoming fatigue	Orange	

D.4. Micromotion Study

Micromotion study was also developed by Frank B. Gilbreth.

It is an analysis technique making use of motion pictures (or videotape) taken at a constant and known speed.

Micro motion study uses a motion picture camera and a large clock marked off in hundredths of seconds to analyse the motions of workers. The speed of the camera used was 16 to 20 frames per seconds.

Advantages: The film becomes a permanent record of both the method being used and the time consumed in doing the work.

You should know

There is a famous story concerning Frank Gilbreth himself. He attempted to study the way he shaved in the morning in order to speed the process. Eventually he tried using two razors at once. He reported that this was a "success" in the sense that he saved around 90 seconds shaving time. Unfortunately he then had to spend several minutes patching up the cuts ☺

Disadvantages: Developing the film and analysing the film was a costly affair as it used many frames per minute.

Applications: Micromotion study provides a valuable technique for making minute analysis of those operations that are short in cycle, contain rapid movements, and involve high production over a long period of time. Thus it is very useful in analysing operations such as the sewing of garments, assembly of small parts and similar activities.

D.5. Memomotion Study

It is a special form of micromotion study in which the motion pictures or videotape are taken at slow speeds of about 1 to 2 frames per seconds.

Advantages: In addition to having all of the advantages of micromotion study, it has relatively low film or tape cost (about 6% of the cost at normal camera speeds).

Applications: It is particularly valuable on long-cycle jobs or jobs involving many inter-relationships. Thus it has been used to study the flow and handling of materials, crew activities, multi-person and machine relationships, stockroom activities, department store clerks etc.

E. WORK MEASUREMENT/TIME STUDY

Definition: Work measurement may be defined as the application of different techniques to measure and establish the time required to complete the job by a qualified worker at a defined level of performance, once the best way of doing a job is determined.

E.1. Objectives/Advantages of Work Measurement

i.   Determines a standard time required to do a job.

ii. Used to compare alternative methods and develop a faster method.

iii. Gives information for production, planning and maintenance procedures.

iv. Determines man power requirement.

v.   Provides information on utilisation of equipment.

vi. Helps in predicting exact delivery dates.

vii. Provides a basis of fair incentive scheme.

viii. Results in better employee-employer relationship and effective labour control.

E.2. Procedure of Time Study

i.   Establish the quality of product to be achieved. It should be between low and very high quality.

ii.   Identify the operation which is to be timed.

iii. The best method of performing the operation is determined from method study.

iv.   Select the average worker who is to be studied while performing the work.

v.   Worker and supervisor are taken in confidence and objectives of the project are explained to them.

vi.   Improved working method and the use of equipment, tools, jigs etc. is explained to the worker.

vii. Operation is broken into small elements which are suitable for time study.

viii. Determine the number of operations to be timed, which will depend on the level of confidence needed.

ix.   Record time with the help of stop watch on the time study form.

x.   Performance of worker is also rated.

xi.   After the time values for each element for sufficient number of cycles have been recorded, the mode value is selected. **The mode value** represents the most frequently appearing time value for an element of job.

xii. Mode values of different elements will be added to get the normal time for doing a job. **Normal time** is the time required by an average worker working under normal conditions to perform a job.

xiii. Adding allowances as personal allowances, rest allowances, process allowances, delay allowances etc. to normal time to get standard time.

Standard Time may be defined as the amount of time required to complete a unit of work

i.   under existing working conditions

ii.   using the specified method and machinery

iii. by an operator able to work in a proper manner.

iv.   standard pace.

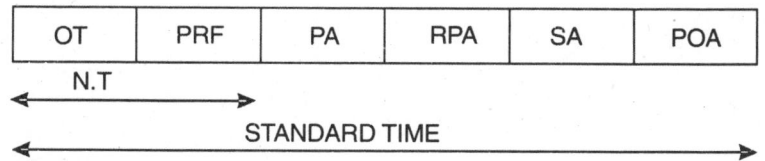

OT	PRF	PA	RPA	SA	POA

OT: Observed Time.

PRF: Performance Rating Factor.

NT: Normal Time.

PA: Process Allowance.

RPA: Rest and Personal Allowance.

SA: Special Allowance.

POA: Policy Allowance

E.3. Stop Watches

Stop watch is accurate time measuring equipment which can run continuously for one hour or half an hour normally and records time by its small hand. One revolution of big hand of the watch records one minute and the scale covering one minute may be calibrated in intervals of $1/300^{th}$ of a minute or $1/100^{th}$ of a minute.

E.4. Limitations of Time Study

i.   It is a very subjective process depending on the accuracy of observer. So, different results are obtained by different observers.

ii. Various inputs required by the procedure as measure of central tendency, personal allowances etc. are also dependent on observer and may vary the results.

iii. Performance rating, if not correct, may affect the Standard time determined.

iv. Workers when observed may not show normal behaviour.

TEST YOUR GREY MATTER

Q1) Define Motion Study and state the steps which are involved in Motion analysis?

Q2) What is 'THERBLIG', explain?

Q3) Differentiate between Micromotion Study and Memomotion Study and state where they are applied?

Q4) What do you understand by work measurement and why is it done?

Q5) Differentiate between Work Improvement and Work Measurement?

Q6) State the steps in Time Study? And define

    (i)   Mode Value

    (ii)   Normal Time

    (iii)   Standard Time

4 Human Relations Approach and Hawthorne Experiments

By the end of this chapter, you would be able to :

- Know where and how Human Relations Approach began.
- Appreciate the reasons which led to different studies and how their conclusions affected the pre-existing notions.
- Know about Elton Mayo and his work at Hawthorne Plant.
- Understand the findings at Hawthorne and their role in the development of the Neo Classical School of thought.

The chapter contains :
- Where these studies began
- Study 1 : Experiments on Illumination
- Study 2 : Relay Assembly Test Room
- Elton Mayo
- Study 3 : Mass Interviewing Program
- Study 4 : Bank Wiring Observation Room
- Study 5 : Personal Counselling
- Findings Of Hawthorne Experiments - Propositions of Neo Classical Theory
- Critical Evaluation of Human Relations Approach

A. THE INSIGHT

- *"Any company controlling many thousand workers.........tends.....to lack any satisfactory criterion of the actual value of its methods of dealing with people"* –

—Elton Mayo, Professor of Industrial Management,
Harvard Business School, 1933

- The above quote clearly gives us the reason as to why Human Relations of Management came into existence.

- Though Scientific Management was very effective, yet it has many drawbacks and industrial experiences indicated that there were more factors responsible, than explained by Scientific Management for improving the performance of an employee in a company.

B. WHERE IT BEGAN

Western Electric Hawthorne Works --

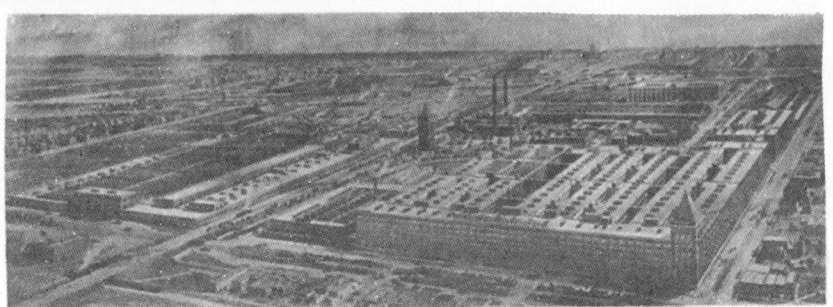

Airplane View of Hawthorne Works, ca. 1925

- Western Electric Hawthorne Works was a manufacturing unit of AT&T Systems. It produced telephones, cables, transmission equipments and switching equipment.
- Employees were assigned to precisely measured tasks in highly specialised departments, from switchboard wiring to punch and die tool making.
- It became one of the forerunners in applying scientific management to its production.
- To better understand worker productivity and job satisfaction, Western Electric became increasingly interested in studies from the social, behavioural and medical sciences.
- Research on productivity at massive manufacturing complex like the Hawthorne works was made possible through partnership among industries, universities and government.
- In 1920, with the support from the National Research Council, the Rockefeller Foundation and eventually Harvard Business School, Western Electric undertook a series of behavioural experiments.
- The Hawthorne studies can be conveniently divided into 5 major parts. Each part was the outgrowth of the preceding one. The 5 studies are referred to as –

You should know

By 1929, more than 40,000 men & women were reporting to work at Western Electric Hawthorne Works.

a. Experiments on Illumination.
b. Relay Assembly Test Room.
    i. Second Relay Assembly Test Room.
    ii. Mica Splitting Test room.
c. Mass Interviewing Program.
d. Bank Wiring Observation Room.
e. Personal counselling.

B.1. Study 1 : Experiments on Illumination

These were conducted between 1924 -1927 and set out to determine the effect of lighting on worker's efficiency.

5 experiments were undertaken in it –

i. Experiment 1

Conducted in 3 separate departments -

(a)   Inspection of small parts

(b)   Assembly of relays.

(c)   Winding coils

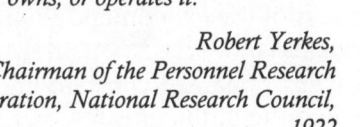

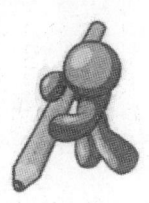

Wisdom Tooth

"We stand on the threshold of a new era in which attention and interest is beginning to shift from…things that are worked with, to the worker; from the machinery of industry, to the man who made, owns, or operates it."

Robert Yerkes,
Chairman of the Personnel Research Federation, National Research Council,
1922

- Light intensity was varied from low to high in 4 levels.
- In the inspection department, production of workers varied without direct relation to illumination.
- In Assembly, production increased but not solely as a result of change in illumination.
- In Winding, production increased with illumination but did not decrease with decrease in illumination.
- It was concluded that the experiment should be more controlled and other factors except illumination must be eliminated.

ii. Experiment 2

- Second experiment was more refined and took place in one department only.
- Two groups, one control group and another test group worked in two different buildings.
- Control group worked under constant illumination and test group under 3 different illumination intensities.
- Both groups increased production to almost same level.

- It was concluded to perform the 3rd experiment to determine what amount of increase in production was due to illumination.

iii. Experiment 3

- In the 3rd experiment only artificial light was used and daylight was eliminated.
- Control group and Test group worked under a constant intensity of 10ft/ candles but intensity of test group was reduced by 1ft/candle per period until it was 3ft/candle.
- Efficiency of employees did not change despite insufficient illumination.

iv. Experiment 4

- In the 4th experiment, 2 volunteer girls worked in a light controlled room.
- Intensity of light was made equal to ordinary moonlight.
- Girls maintained production and reported no eyestrain and less fatigue than working in bright lights.

v. Experiment 5

- The 5th and last illumination experiment was conducted with girls who wound coils.
- First, the light bulbs were changed daily in front of the workers, telling them that its intensity was increased each day and the girls liked it & increased their work rate. Though actually the bulbs were identical to the previous ones.
- In the last part of the experiment, illumination was decreased and the girls found less light unpleasant.
- But if the bulbs remained constant and the electrician reduced the illumination, without telling them, the girls felt that illumination was not changed and felt the same way.

Conclusions

The Hawthorne Effect

This 'anecdote' was a result of this experiment which meant that people change their behaviour when they think somebody is watching them. At the workplace, the efficiency and performance of a worker can change if he is being observed. He may feel motivated or de-motivated by the experiment itself. So he may support the experiment or may even try to fail it.

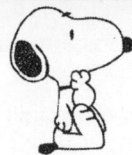

Though the specific problem was not solved, the need to gain more knowledge concerning the problems involving human factors was identified. Thus, it resulted in another study at Hawthorne, called Relay Assembly Test Room

B.2. Study 2 : Relay Assembly Test Room

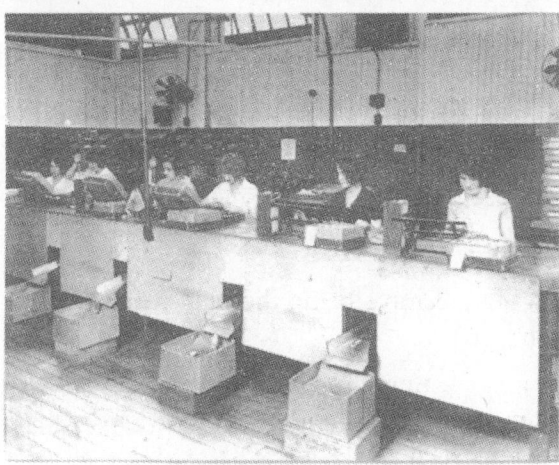

Women in the Relay Assembly Test Room, ca. 1930. Western Electric Company Hawthorne Studies Collection © 2007 President and Fellows of Harvard College; all rights reserved

- 5 relay assembler girls and one layout operator was chosen. One man to keep records and maintain a friendly atmosphere for the experiment was also present.

- Assembly of relay was chosen as it was a simple, repetitive process and so was an accurate measure for production.

- 13 test periods were introduced and several factors such as rest pauses, working time, method of payment etc., were changed to determine their affects on production.

- Production of the girls increased. Each test period has a higher production record than the preceding one.

- 5 tentative explanations suggested were –

    i. Improved material conditions & methods of work

    ii. Shorter hours provided relief from fatigue.

    iii. Shorter work periods provided relief from monotony.

    iv. Wage incentive plan

    v. Change in method of supervision

> ### Wisdom Tooth
>
> *I had no idea there would be so much happening and so many people watching us.*
>
> *Theresa Layman Zajac,*
> *Relay Assembly Test Room Operator,*
> *1976*

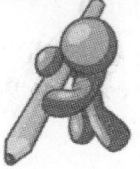

- The First 3 explanations were rejected on close study.
- To know the truth about wage incentive plan, two more experiments were conducted.

a. Second Relay Assembly Test Room

There was no change of environment but only change of payment.

b. Mica Splitting Test Room

Wage payment basis remained same i.e. individual piece rate, but change in working conditions similar to those in test room were made.

Conclusions

i. No evidence of wage incentive being the only reason for continuous production increase was established.

ii. Effect of only wage on output can only be determined if effects of other factors such as interpersonal relations at work and personal situation outside work were also known.

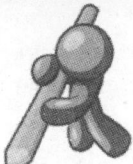

Wisdom Tooth

They say figures don t lie, but we have shown that we can take a set of figures and prove anything we want to.

Donald Chipman,
Supervisor, Western Electric, 1931

Overall Conclusion

Experimenters became aware of sociological and psychological factors which affected the output and this led to study 3.

- The Relay Assembly study began in 1927 and continued till 1932. In the meantime Elton Mayo was called to determine and interpret the Hawthorne experiments.

TEST YOUR GREY MATTER

Q1) Explain the methodology and findings of Illumination Experiments.

Q2) What is Hawthorne Effect?

Q3) Write a short note on Relay Assembly Test Room Experiment.

Elton Mayo

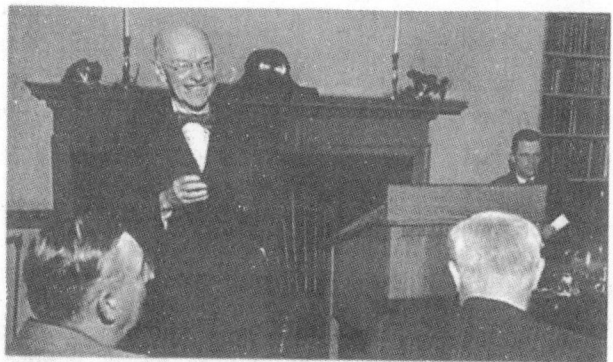

Elton Mayo, ca. 1950

- Born in Adelaide, Australia in 1880.
- He taught mental and moral philosophy at University of Queensland.
- He believed that unlocking the psyche of the worker was key to understanding industrial unrest at home and abroad.
- In 1923, Mayo became a research associate at University of Pennsylvania's Wharton school, studying effect of fatigue on employee attrition.
- Later, he became associate professor in study of human relations at Harvard Business School.

Wisdom Tooth

"So long as commerce specialises in business methods, which take no account of human nature and social motives, so long may we expect strikes and sabotage to be the ordinary accompaniment of industry."

*Elton Mayo,
Professor of Industrial Management,
Harvard Business School, 1920*

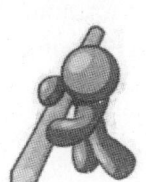

B.3. Study 3 : Mass Interviewing Program

- Mayo and his assistant Roethlisberger began interviewing, conducting about 21,000 interviews.
- Basic aim of this study was to determine the relation between employee morale and supervision and thus to study human relations or attitudes concerning human relations.

Wisdom Tooth

"I think interviewing is a good idea. It helps some people get a lot of things off their chest."

*Western Electric employee, in
Comments and Reactions on
Interviewing Program, ca. 1930*

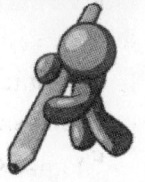

- They discovered that rather than answering direct questions, employees expressed themselves more candidly, if encouraged to speak openly, in what was known as "indirect interviewing".
  - "**Indirect Interview** is defined as a conversation in which the employee is encouraged to express himself freely upon any topic of his own choice."
  - Interview time increased from 30 min to 90 min or even 2 hrs.

Conclusions

i. Company's supervisor training courses were revised as per worker's complaints.

ii. Items such as wages, hours of work and physical conditions were carriers of social values and thus varied according to employee's position in the group and relations with people outside job.

You should know

Mayo was assisted by his research assistant, Fritz Roethlisberger. Unassuming, bookish, and disciplined, Roethlisberger had studied philosophy at Harvard.

iii. Social groups were important and controlled work behaviour of individual members.

iv. Restricted output was a result of pressure of these social groups and there was development of informal personal leadership in those groups.

v. It resulted in the 4th study.

B.4. Study 4: Bank Wiring Observation Room

- Conducted to obtain information about social groups within the company.
- 14 male operators were observed and interviewed in a separate room. There were 9 wiremen, 3 soldermen, and 2 inspectors.
- An observer was stationed in the room to note (i) formal organisation of supervisor and employee (ii) informal groupings of men and (iii) inter-relations of these two types of organisations.
- Interviewer who was not in the room was to gain insight into worker's attitudes, thoughts and feelings.
- It was found that –
  i. Even though they were paid on daily output basis, they did not raise the output.
  ii. Individual production remained fairly constant over a period of time.
  iii. They adjusted the reports and records about the output and working time.

- After studying and analysing, it was concluded that –
  i. They formed a highly organised social structure or Cliques with definite pattern of communication, differentiation and a recognised leader.
  ii. These groups have a set of norms and the whole group followed it. These codes were conflicting to what the management expected from them. Members who did not behave in accordance with the norms were brought back into line or left alone.

Four main determinants of Clique membership are –

a. **Rate Busting:** Don't work too much.

b. **Chiselers:** Don't work too less.

c. **Squealer:** Don't tell supervisor anything that would harm any member of the group.

d. Don't be officious, that is, one should behave as more of a group member socially and not as agents of company. This applied to inspectors, group chiefs, as well as workers.

Reasons for formation of these groups were to protect the group from-

a. **Inside** – controlled through sarcasm, ridicule etc.

b. **Outside** – by constancy of production.

Experiment was closed in 6 months because of a depression.

TEST YOUR GREY MATTER

Q1) Explain briefly the procedure and findings of:
    (i)   Mass Interviewing Program
    (ii) Bank Wiring Observation Room

Q2) What was the methodology adopted to bring back the members who did not behave in accordance with norms of the informal groups?

B.5. Study 5 : Personal Counselling

There were 2 objectives of this study.

i. Have an impartial agency interview for employees, to diagnose their problems and work with supervisors on their methods of supervision.

ii. Improve method of communication within the company in a situation when social organisation conflicted with managerial organisation.

"Personnel Men" were assigned to departments to talk to employees.

It showed improvement in 3 fields –

a. **Personal Adjustments:** Employees showed personality changes and freedom from anxiety etc.

b. **Supervisor – Employee Relations:** Personnel counsellor helped in making supervisors see their problems.

c. **Employee – Management Relations:** Helped in forming policies that resulted in less friction between management and worker.

C. FINDINGS OF HAWTHORNE EXPERIMENTS - PROPOSITIONS OF NEO CLASSICAL THEORY

We can sum up the findings from all the experiments to determine overall conclusions from Hawthorne experiments-

i. **Human Factor:** Human factor acts at workplace and workplace is a social system.

ii. **Sociological and Psychological** factors affected the output of workers.

iii. **Motivation**: Money is not the only motivating factor responsible for the efficiency of worker.

iv. **Social values**: Wages, working hours and working conditions were not entities in themselves but carriers of social values.

v. **Informal Organisation:** Workers formed social groups which had their own norms and codes. The group played an important role in determining the attitude and performance of individual worker.

vi. **Leadership:** The informal groups have their own leaders and workers' behaviour was a result of the norms set and enforced by the leader and group.

vii. **Factors affecting behaviour**: Both factors, inside and outside a workplace affected the behaviour and production of workers.

viii. **Communication:**

Downward communication was necessary to inform about managerial decisions and policies to keep workers informed for proper functioning and upward communication was necessary to transmit feelings and sentiments of workers.

Thinking Time !!

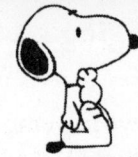

For the teachers - Try both, Scientific Management and Human Relations approach in teaching the students and find out which one gives better results.

And thus, Hawthorne experiments resulted in the formation of Human Relations School or Neo Classical Organisation Theory.

D. CRITICAL EVALUATION OF HUMAN RELATIONS APPROACH

Many thinkers criticise Human Relations approach and Hawthorne experiments on following conditions –

i. **Wrong Interpretations:** It is critically believed that vast difference between the Bank Wiring Observation Room and the Relay Assembly Test Room results was caused by the fact that one group was male and the other female. Evidence from other sources proves this.

ii. **Methodology Used:** Methodology used at Hawthorne is Clinical Insight rather than Scientific Evidence, validity of which is questioned.

iii. **Over-Emphasis on Psychological Aspect:** It is believed that the 'actual work' was ignored by the human relationalists and they were completely people-centric.

iv. **Happiness vs. Productivity:** Neo-classicists considered that happiness of the employees was directly proportional to the productivity, but it was proved later that there is no direct relationship between them.

v. **Constrained Applicability:** The Neo Classical theory is not considered to be universal as practically there are many environmental and work conditions which have not been considered and thus it could not be applied to all organisations.

vi. **Unified approach:** The theory is believed to lack unified approach of Organisational Theory.

TEST YOUR GREY MATTER

Q1) Write short note on Personal Counselling experiment conducted at Hawthorne?

Q2) Examine the contribution of Hawthorne Studies to the development of industrial psychology?

Q3) Comment on the findings of the Hawthorne experiments?

Q4) State and critically evaluate the neo classical theory of organisation?

CHAPTER

5

Motivation

By the end of this chapter, you would be able to :

- Understand the concept of motivation and its use in our personal and professional life.
- Learn about various theories of motivation.
- Appreciate each theory of motivation and learn its practical importance at the workplace.
- Analyse each theory and critically examine each one of them.

The chapter contains :

- Concept of Motivation
- Motivation at Workplace
- Importance of Motivation
- Theories of Motivation
  - ❑ Maslow's Need Hierarchy Theory
  - ❑ Herzberg's Two Factors Theory
  - ❑ ERG Theory
  - ❑ Achievement Motivation Theory/ McClelland Theory
  - ❑ Douglas McGregor - Theory X & Y
  - ❑ Expectancy Theory
  - ❑ Performance-Satisfaction Theory
  - ❑ Equity Theory
  - ❑ Reinforcement Theory

A. THE INSIGHT

- **Age 7:** His family was forced out of their home and he needed to work to support his family.
- **Age 9:** His mother passed away
- **Age 19:** His sister dies
- **Age 22:** A business venture failed
- **Age 23:** He ran for the State Legislature. He lost.

- **Age 23:** In the same year, he also lost his job. He decided he wanted to go to law school but couldn't get in.
- **Age 24:** He borrowed money from a friend to start a business. By the end of the year, he was bankrupt.
- **Age 25:** He ran for the State Legislature again. This time he won.
- **Age 26:** The year was looking better as he was engaged to be married. Unfortunately, his fiancée died and he was grief stricken.
- **Age 27:** This was the year he had a total nervous breakdown and for 6 months was bedridden.
- **Age 29:** He sought to become Speaker of the State Legislature. He was defeated.
- **Age 31:** He sought to become Elector. He was defeated.
- **Age 34:** He ran for Congress. He lost.
- **Age 37:** He ran for Congress again. He won and moved to Washington.
- **Age 39:** He ran for re-election to Congress. He lost.
- **Age 45:** He ran for the Senate of the United states. He lost.
- **Age 47:** He sought the Vice Presidential nomination at a national convention. He got less than 100 votes.
- **Age 49:** He ran for the Senate again. He lost again.
- **Age 51:** Elected President of the United States of America.

He was **ABRAHAM LINCOLN**, one of the greatest Presidents of the United States of America.

He proved what motivation could do and now we are about to study it.

B. MOTIVATION

- **Definition:** Motivation is a term referring to a family of concepts used to explain initiation, direction, maintenance & termination of activities taken up by living organisms.

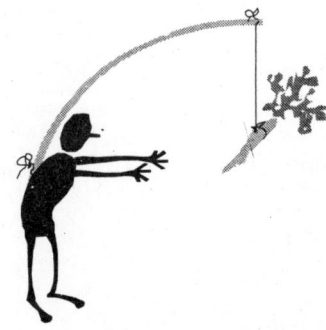

- So there is a series of steps which is to be understood to understand the concept of motivation:

Step 1

- Every action or choice which we make, starts from a point called **Need.**
- **Definition:** Need is a lack or deficit of some necessity.
- Need may be psychological (e.g. need for recognition), physiological (e.g. the need for water, air or food) or social (e.g. need for friendship).

Step 2

- The condition of need leads to drive.
- **Definition:** A drive is a state of tension or arousal produced by a need.

Step 3

- And then we search for ways to reduce or eliminate them. Thus ,motivation becomes goal directed.

Step 4

- The activity we perform may be rewarding or punishing i.e. it may satisfy our need or not satisfy our need.

Step 5

- If the need is satisfied or goal is achieved, it may lead to drive reduction.

Step 6

- If the goal is not achieved, we again reassess our need deficiencies.
- Goal Achieved/Not Achieved is also referred to as **Incentive or Reward/Punishment** i.e. which leads towards goal achievement or away from it.

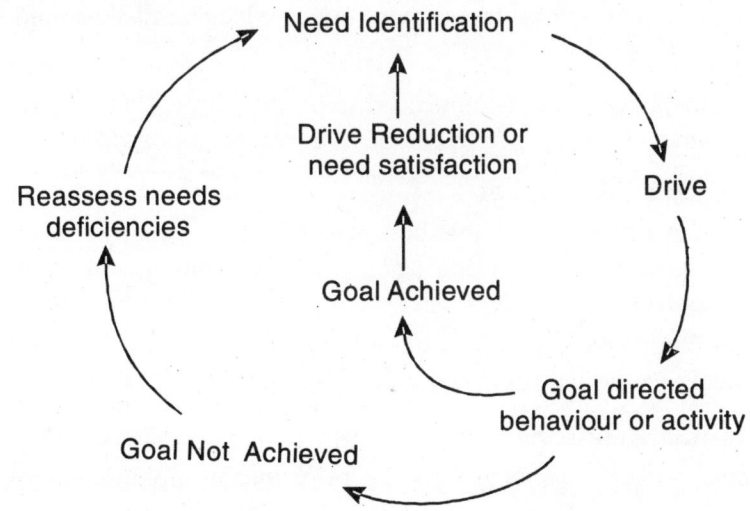

B.1.Motivation at Workplace

- It is found that –
  Performance = f (ability x motivation)
- It means that our performance depends on our ability i.e. skill, competence and clarity of mind to do a job and the desire to accomplish the task i.e. motivation.
- Therefore, if we can understand and apply the concept of motivation, we can increase the performance of an employee for the achievement of organisational objectives.

B.2.Importance of Motivation

If we could apply the concept of 'motivation' at workplace, we could achieve the following results –

i. Quality

- Motivated employee always try to maintain high quality standards, say, he will work little extra to ensure that he made no mistakes in his work.
- A quality criterion is very important issue for organisation to get new work and orders.

ii. Creativity

- A motivated employee uses his creativity to devise a methodology and ways to simplify a job or to find a method to save time.

iii. Efficiency/Productivity

- A motivated worker will improve upon his knowledge and skills and thus result in high productivity.
- It is a fact that fewer workers are needed to produce an automobile in Japan than elsewhere. Motivation is found to be one of the main reasons for that.

iv. Optimisation of Resources

- A motivated worker makes the best use of the company's resources, thus minimising waste and cost, resulting in the maximum use of its physical and financial resources.
- It has been found that a motivated employee even uses less company resources such as telephone, printer for his own personal benefit.

v. Good Human Relations

- A motivated worker is happy and also keeps people around him happy.

- There is less friction or clashes between workers and also between workers and management.

vi. Less Absenteeism and Less Complaints

- As a worker is satisfied, he complains less and works more.
- Even his reasons for being absent decrease and he spends more days working in the organisation.

vii. Less Attrition Rate

- A motivated worker is satisfied and so remains loyal to the company by not leaving it.
- Also, a company with such an employee satisfaction record attracts more competent people applying for the jobs. E.g. - Won't we apply to those companies which give us better salaries?

TEST YOUR GREY MATTER

Q1) Define motivation. Explain it with the help of its relation to human need.

Q2) How is motivation responsible for the performance of an employee? Explain.

Q3) What is the importance of motivation at workplace?

Q4) Discuss the effect of motivation of employees on absenteeism and attrition.

C. THEORIES OF MOTIVATION

- Theories of motivation can be understood by a flow chart:

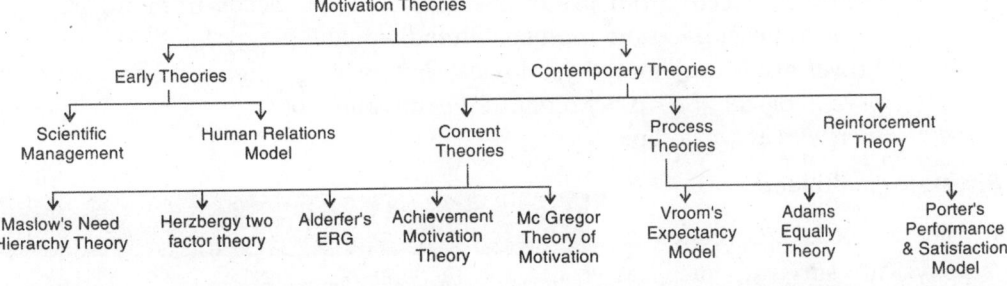

C.1. Earlier Theories

(a) Scientific Management

(b) Human Relations Model

- We have already studied these theories in Unit I and all those who thought that they can escape these theories, please go back and study them!

C.2. Contemporary Theories

C.2.1. Content Theories

- These theories focus on human needs or desires.
- We have already studied how need results in drive and activity. These theories study such needs, their effect on the employee and suggest ways to motivate the employee by satisfying those needs.
- But as each individual has a different value system, beliefs and character, it becomes a very complex process. E.g. Anagha and Purohit feel hungry. Their Manager orders a 'Masala Dosa' for both of them. Both have it and their hunger is quenched but Anagha remains dissatisfied as she wanted to have 'Pizza'.

C.2.1.1. Maslow's Need Hierarchy Theory

- Abraham Harold Maslow (1943) proposed his 'Need Hierarchy Theory'.
- Basic Premise/ Essence of his theory –
    i. It is need which provokes a man to work. Unsatisfied need can influence behaviour but fulfilled need is no-longer a motivator.
    ii. Needs are arranged in the order of their importance (hierarchy) from bottom to top. As we go from the bottom to top, the complexity of need increases.
    iii. The hierarchy is rigid and fixed for every individual, irrespective of societies and culture.
    iv. When the needs from lower level are fulfilled, needs from higher level come to the surface and motivate an individual.
    v. Lower needs are more physiological, but as we go higher it becomes more psychological. So, psychological health and consciousness of a person increases as we go up.

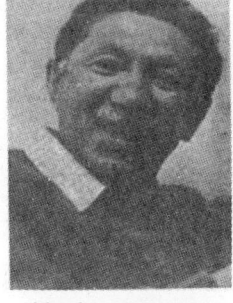

Abraham Maslow

Physiological Need

- These needs are related to physical survival such as food, clothing, shelter (Roti, Kapda aur Makan), air water, sleep and other basic necessities.

Wisdom Tooth

"If you deliberately plan on being less than you are capable of being, then I warn you that you ll be unhappy for the rest of your life."

Abraham Maslow

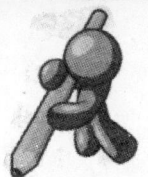

- They are more related to biological maintenance. This is our most important need and we cannot go to the higher ones unless we satisfy them.

Maslow says

"For our chronically and extremely hungry man, utopia can be defined simply as a place where there is plenty of food. He tends to think that, only if he is guaranteed food for the rest of his life, he will be perfectly happy & will never want anything more."

Safety and Security Needs

- These include job security, health security, property, family, social stability, protection against dangers or emergencies such as crime, flood, war etc.

- **Organisational Context-** Job security, salary increase, unionisation, safe working conditions etc.

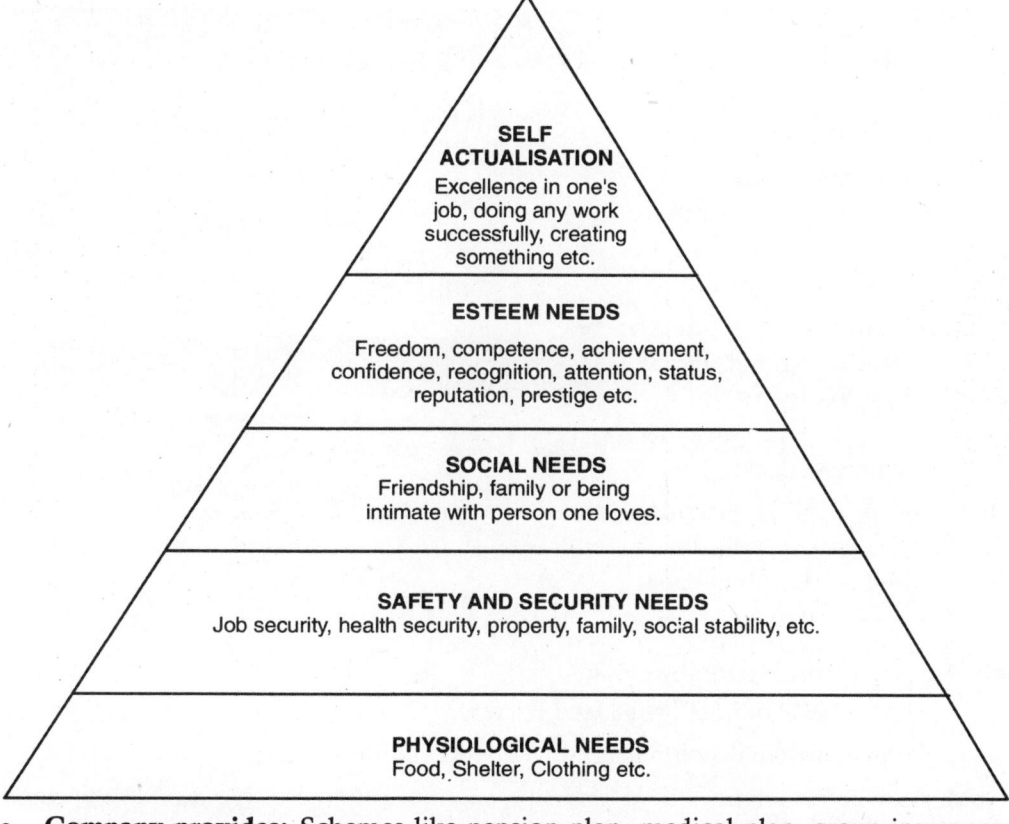

- **Company provides:** Schemes like pension plan, medical plan, group insurance, provident fund, gratuity etc.

Social Needs

- Also called Belonging and Love Needs.
- This arises when physiological and safety needs are satisfied.
- This includes friendship, family or being intimate with the person one loves.
- Maslow said that love involves a healthy relationship between two people, which includes mutual respect, admiration and trust.
- Organisational Context-
  - ❏ Friendly work, environment, compatible peer group, supportive supervision etc.
  - ❏ Company provides schemes like 5 working days a week, LTA etc., so that the person can spend more time with family & friends.

Esteem Needs

Maslow divided this category into two parts –

a. **Self Respect** – Includes freedom, competence, achievement, confidence etc.

b. **Esteem from others** – It includes recognition, attention, status, reputation, prestige and appreciation.

- **Organisational Context:** Job title, merit pay, peer/supervisory recognition, responsibility, challenging work etc.

- **Company provides**: Performance feedback, recognition, encouragement, promotions etc.

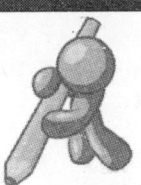

Wisdom Tooth

"A musician must make music, an artist must paint, a poet must write, if he is to be ultimately at peace with himself."

Abraham Maslow

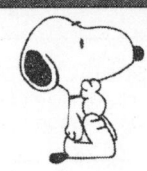

Thinking Time !!

Now, as we have studied Maslow s Need Hierarchy Theory, think and write down what types of needs you have, classify them into different levels and find out where you belong. Discuss it with your friends and family members.

Self Actualisation Needs

- It is the last level of Maslow's Need Hierarchy Theory.
- The term Self Actualisation was coined by Kurt Goldstein.
- **Maslow defines** it as – "This tendency might be phrased as the desire to become more and more what one is, to become everything that one is capable of becoming."

- It is the "full realisation of one's potentials".
- In this one seeks satisfaction from one's own work.
- Organisational Context
  - ❑ Desire for excellence in one's job, doing any work successfully, creating something etc.
  - ❑ Company may provide employees a challenge and opportunity to reach their full career potential.

Critical Evaluation of Need Hierarchy Model

1. **Motivate Employee** – Maslow educated the managers to identify employee needs and answered the questions as to why different people are motivated by different factors.

2. **Dynamic Nature** – The model clarifies that nature of man's need is dynamic in nature. When one need is fulfilled, needs of higher level arises and man is never satisfied.

3. **Different Approach** – Maslow's approach is based on 'Existential Philosophy' which considers man as a healthy, good and creative being who can make his own destiny.

4. **No Hierarchy** – Some critics argue that there is no hierarchy of needs and all the needs exist at some time i.e. they are not closed compartments as suggested by Maslow. To explain this, they say that even though man may be in need of self actualisation, yet he cannot forget his need for food or shelter.

5. **Lack of Universality** – Critics argue that people from different cultures and countries have different priorities of their needs and so it cannot be applied everywhere, as it is.

6. **Individual Differences** - As different cultures have different need hierarchy patterns, so is each individual different from the others in a culture. Therefore, people may have different need- hierarchy patterns.

7. **Practicality** – It has been said that it is not possible for a manager to identify where each of his employee lies in the need hierarchy model and may not be able to apply the principles in actual life.

Wisdom Tooth
"True motivation comes from achievement, personal development, job satisfaction, and recognition" ***Frederick Herzberg***

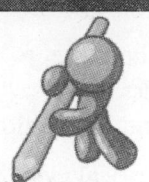

C.2.1.2. Herzberg's Two Factors Theory

- This Theory is based on the research carried out by Herzberg and his associates on a group of employees of a paint company.
- The research team asked 200 employees, consisting of engineers, managers and accountants, to respond to the question "Can you describe, in detail, when you felt exceptionally good about your job and when you felt exceptionally bad?"

The findings can be broadly stated as under

1. The responses received can be grouped within two general categories, motivators and hygiene factors.

2. Motivators consist of factors such as

- Job advancement
- Recognition
- Responsibility
- Achievement

    Hygiene or Maintenance Factors Include

- Supervision
- Pay
- Company Policies
- Working Conditions

3. Satisfaction and dissatisfaction are not two opposite poles of our dimension; rather they are two entirely different dimensions. Satisfaction is affected by motivators and dissatisfaction is affected by hygiene factors.

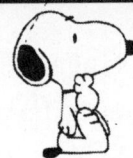

Thinking Time !!

Classify the factors which affect your studies under Motivators and Hygiene Factors and find out whether Herzberg s two factor theory applies to you.

Therefore, to achieve motivation, management should cope with both satisfiers and dissatisfiers. "Improve hygiene factors, dissatisfaction is removed, provide satisfiers, and motivation will take place."

Critical evaluation of 'Herzberg's Two Factor Theory'.

Criticism of the Theory

i. The procedure that Herzberg used is limited by its methodology. When things are going well, people tend to take credit themselves. Contrarily, they blame failure on the extrinsic environment.

ii. No overall measure of satisfaction was utilised. A person may dislike parts of the job, yet think the job is acceptable overall.

iii. Herzberg assumes that there is a relation between satisfaction and productivity. But the research methodology he used looked only at satisfaction, not at productivity. To make such a research relevant, one must assume a high degree of relationship between satisfaction and productivity.

iv. The reliability of Herzberg's methodology is questioned. Raters may contaminate the findings by interpreting one response in one manner while interpreting a similar response differently.

v. The two factors are not actually distinct. Both motivation and hygiene factors contribute to satisfaction as well as dissatisfaction.

Merits of the Theory

Besides the above mentioned short comings, the theory has certain merits. To state a few-

i. One of the most significant contributions of the theory is that it stimulated thought, research and experimentation on the topic of motivation. The previous studies in this direction were largely fragmentary and were largely concerned with laboratory based findings. Herzberg filled this void by calling attention to the need for increased understanding of the role of motivation in organisations.

ii. Herzberg cleared many misconceptions concerning motivation. Most prominent being money, which was earlier viewed as the most potent force on job. He advanced a strong case for content factors which have a considerable bearing on behaviour.

iii. The job design technique of job enrichment is the contribution of Herzberg.

iv. Herzberg double dimensionalised the needs instead of dividing it into five, as done by Maslow.

C.2.1.3. ERG Theory

- Clayton Alderfer in an attempt to rework Maslow's Need Hierarchy and to align it more closely with empirical research devised the ERG Theory.

- He argued that there are three groups of core needs- existence, relatedness and growth. Though similar to Maslow's Hierarchy of Need Theory, ERG theory differs in the following aspects:

1. Instead of five hierarchies of needs, the ERG theory hypothesises only three.

   i) **Existence Needs:** Physiological and safety needs (Such as hunger, thirst etc.)

   ii) **Relatedness Needs:** Social and external esteem (involvement with family, friends, co-workers and employers).

   iii) **Growth Needs:** Internal esteem and self actualisation (desire to be creative, productive and to complete meaningful tasks)

2. The need hierarchy theory postulates a rigid step-like progression. The ERG Theory, instead, hypothesises that more than one need may be operational at the same time.

3. Maslow had stated that a person will stay at a certain level until that need is satisfied. The ERG theory counters this by noting that when a higher level of need is frustrating, the individual's desire to increase low level need takes place.

Evaluation of ERG Theory

Advantages

i. The ERG theory is more consistent with our knowledge of individual differences among people. The variables such as education, family background and cultural environment can alter the importance or driving force that a group of needs holds for a particular individual. The evidence demonstrates that people in other cultures rank the need categories differently.

ii. Although there are some evidences to counter the theory's predictive value, most contemporary analysis of work motivation tends to support Alderfer's theory over Maslow's and Herzberg's theory.

Disadvantages

i. The theory does not offer clear cut guidelines. The ERG model implies that individuals will be motivated to engage in a behaviour which will satisfy one of the three sets of needs postulated by the theory.

ii. ERG theory is newer than the need hierarchy theory and has not yet attained such degree of research interest as has the Need Hierarchy Theory. Thus the empirical nature of this theory is still not proved.

C.2.1.4. Achievement Motivation Theory/ McClelland Theory

- Also known as the **"Three needs Theory"** it was envisaged by **David C. McClelland** and his associates.

- In his theory he pointed out three needs that motivate human behaviour-

Power, Affiliation and Achievement

- The theory states that each person has a need of all three but the magnitude of intensity of a particular need varies from person to person.

- A brief description of the three needs follows:

- **Need for Achievement (nAch)**

  - It is the drive to excel and achieve with respect to a predefined set of standards. Succeeding at a task is important for achievers.

  - Although people with a high need for achievement are often wealthy, their wealth comes from their ability to achieve goals.

  - High achievers prefer immediate feedback on their performance and they generally undertake tasks of moderate difficulty. They neither go for very difficult tasks nor for a very easy one because in the former case they get no achievement satisfaction from accidental successes, and in the latter case there is no challenge for their skills.

  - McClelland believes that the need for achievement can be learned. He has cited numerous instances in which people developed the need to achieve. He believes that the economically backward cultures can be changed if the need to achieve is stimulated.

- **Need for Affiliation (nAff)**

  - It is the desire for friendly and close interpersonal relationships.

  - If asked to choose between working at a task with those who are technically competent and those who are their friends, high nAff individuals will choose their friends.

- **Need for Power (nPow)**

  - It is the need to make others behave in a way in which they would not have behaved otherwise. Actual achievement of goal is less important than the means by which goals are achieved and the satisfaction is derived from being in a position to influence others.

In the figure below, each of the three needs can be over or under-expressed, thereby leaving the leader in a position of potential abuse or insufficiency. In most cases, moderate to high ratings in these areas are desirable rather than excessively high or low ones.

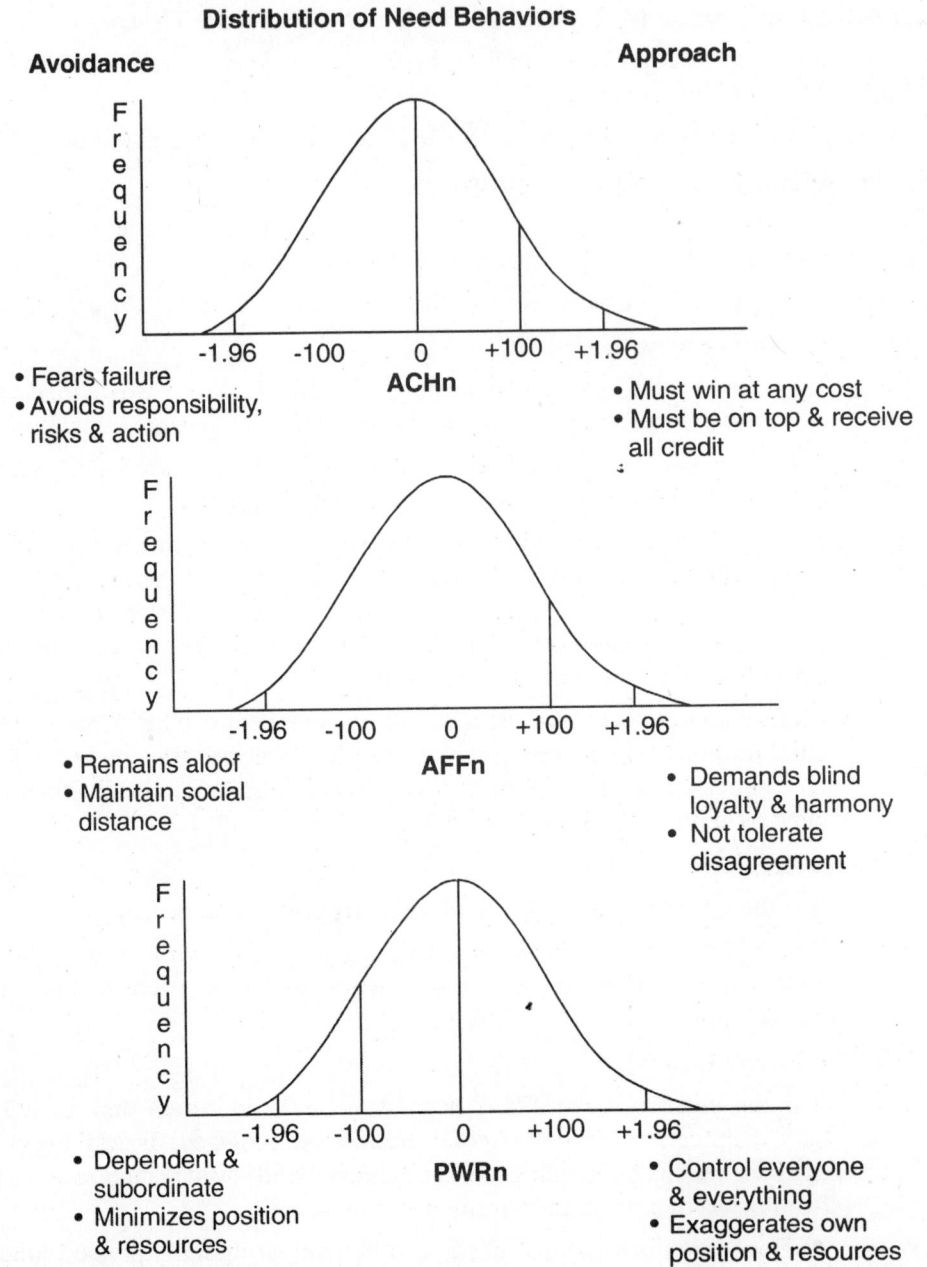

Distribution of Need Behaviors

Avoidance — Approach

ACHn

- Fears failure
- Avoids responsibility, risks & action

- Must win at any cost
- Must be on top & receive all credit

AFFn

- Remains aloof
- Maintain social distance

- Demands blind loyalty & harmony
- Not tolerate disagreement

PWRn

- Dependent & subordinate
- Minimizes position & resources

- Control everyone & everything
- Exaggerates own position & resources

Criticism of the theory

i. Considerable psychological literature indicates that the acquisition of motives normally occurs in childhood and is very difficult to change once it has been established, so it is very difficult in case of adults to change these motives.

ii. McClelland and his associates used the famous Thematic Apperception Test (TAT) of Murray as the basic tool to determine basic needs. While projective techniques such as TAT have many advantages over

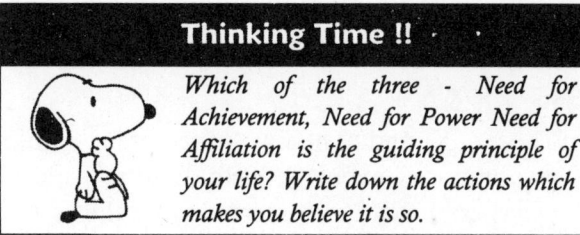

Thinking Time !!

Which of the three - Need for Achievement, Need for Power Need for Affiliation is the guiding principle of your life? Write down the actions which makes you believe it is so.

structured questionnaires, the interpretation of the responses is more subject to researcher's bias.

iii. McClelland argued that the three needs are subconscious- meaning that, we may be high on these needs but may not know it - and measuring them is not easy.

Merits of Theory

On the positive side it may be suggested that

(i) The findings of McClelland highlight the importance of matching the individual and the job. Employees with high achievement needs thrive on work that is challenging, satisfying, stimulating and complex. On the other hand, employees with low achievement needs prefer situations of stability, security and predictability. The theory suggests that managers to some extent raise the achievement needs of subordinates by creating proper work environment.

Relationship between these 4 Content Theories

• As all the 4 theories together becomes a little confusing, we will use following chart to differentiate and understand each of them.

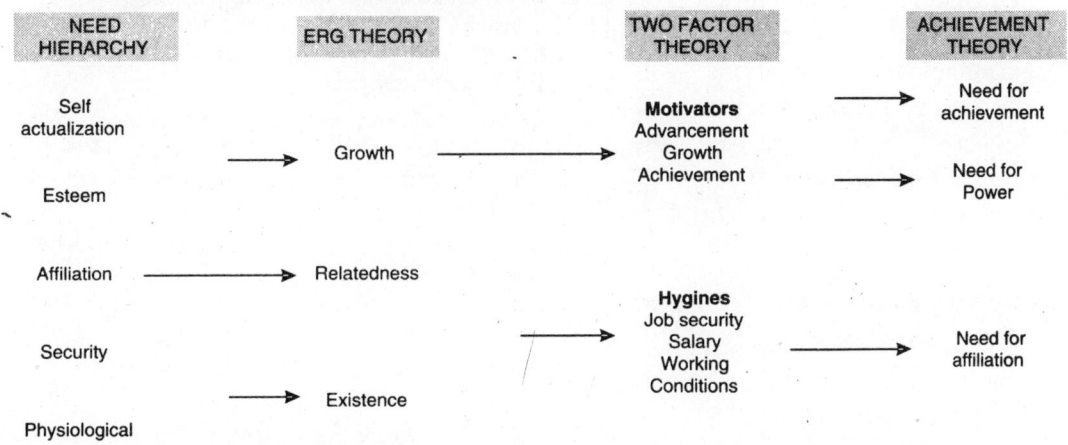

Source: Don Hellriegel, et al, Organisational Behaviour, p.145

C.2.1.5. Douglas McGregor - Theory X & Y

Theory X & Y

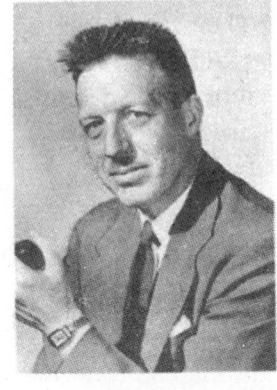

Douglas McGregor

- Theory X and Theory Y represent two sets of assumptions about human nature and human behaviour that are relevant to the practice of management.

- Theory X represents a negative view of human nature that assumes individuals generally dislike work, are irresponsible, and require close supervision to do their jobs.

- Theory Y denotes a positive view of human nature and assumes individuals are generally industrious, creative, and able to assume responsibility and exercise self-control in their jobs.

- One would expect, then, that managers holding assumptions about human nature that are consistent with Theory X might exhibit a managerial style that is quite different than managers who hold assumptions consistent with Theory Y.

The first section explains the development of Theory X and Theory Y. Second, the effect of Theory X and Theory Y on management functions is discussed. Third is a criticism of Theory Y followed by the concluding section, Theory X and Theory Y in the twenty-first century.

Conceptualisation and Development

- In the 1950s, Douglas McGregor (1906-1964), a psychologist who taught at MIT and served as president

You should know

Douglas McGregor

- Born in 1906, in Detroit, and died in 1964, in Massachusetts.

- His grandfather Thomas McGregor founded McGregor Institute in about 1895 to aid Great Lakes sailors and other transient labour. This Institute housed and fed more than 1000 men every year.

- In his youth he worked in his grandfather's institute for transient labourers in Detroit, where he gained insight into the problems faced by labour.

- He worked as a district manager for a retail gasoline merchandising firm. In the course of this job, he learned the concepts of management.

- He was the first full time professor of Psychology at MIT University.

- In 1960, he wrote the book "The Human Side of Enterprise", where he identifies and develops his renowned Theory X and Theory Y.

of Antioch College from 1948-1954, criticised both the classical and human relations schools as inadequate for the realities of the workplace.

- He believed that the assumptions underlying both schools represented a negative view of human nature and that another approach to management based on an entirely different set of assumptions was needed.

- McGregor laid out his ideas in his classic 1957 article "The Human Side of Enterprise" and the 1960 book of the same name, in which he introduced what came to be called the **New Humanism.**

- McGregor argued that the conventional approach to managing was based on three major propositions, which he called Theory X

(i) Management is responsible for organising the elements of productive enterprise-money, materials, equipment, and people - in the interests of economic ends.

> ### Wisdom Tooth
>
> *"Man is a wanting animal - as soon as one of his needs is satisfied, another appears in its place. This process is unending. It continues from birth to death".*
>
> *- Douglas McGregor*

(ii) With respect to people, this is a process of directing their efforts, motivating them, controlling their actions, and modifying their behaviour to fit the needs of the organisation.

(iii) Without this active intervention by management, people would be passive-even resistant-to organisational needs. They must therefore be persuaded, rewarded, punished, and controlled. Their activities must be directed. Management's task was thus simply getting things done through other people.

Assumptions of Theory X

(i) Individuals do not like to work and will avoid it if possible.

(ii) Human beings do not want responsibility and desire explicit direction.

(iii) Individuals are assumed to put their individual concerns above that of the organisation for which they work and to resist change, valuing security more than other considerations at work.

(iv) Human beings are assumed to be easily manipulated and controlled.

- McGregor contended that both the classical and human relations approaches to management depended on this same set of assumptions.

- He called the **Classical style** of management **"hard"** and identified its methods as close supervision, tight controls, and coercion. The hard style of management led to restriction of output, mutual distrust, unionism, and even sabotage.

- McGregor called the **Human Relations** style of management **"soft"** and identified its methods as permissiveness. McGregor suggested that the soft style of management often led to managers' failure to perform their managerial role. He also pointed out that employees often take advantage of an overly permissive manager by demanding more but performing at lower levels.

- McGregor drew upon the work of Abraham Maslow (1908-1970) to explain why Theory X assumptions led to ineffective management. Maslow had proposed that man's needs are arranged in levels, with physical and safety needs at the bottom of the needs hierarchy and social, ego, and self-actualisation needs at upper levels of the hierarchy. Maslow's basic point was that once a need is met, it no longer motivates behaviour; thus, only unmet needs are motivational.

- McGregor argued that most employees already had their physical and safety needs met and that the motivational emphasis had shifted to the social, ego, and self-actualisation needs. Therefore, management had to provide opportunities for these upper-level needs to be met in the workplace, or employees would not be satisfied or motivated in their jobs.

- Such opportunities could be provided by allowing employees to participate in decision making, by redesigning jobs to make them more challenging, or by emphasising good work group relations, among other things.

- According to McGregor, neither the hard style of management based on the classical school nor the soft style of management inspired by the human relations movement were sufficient to motivate employees. Thus, he proposed a different set of assumptions about human nature as it pertains to the workplace.

- McGregor put forth these assumptions, which he believed could lead to more effective management of people in the organisation, under Theory Y.

The major propositions of Theory Y include the following:

(i) Management is responsible for organising the elements of productive enterprise - money, materials, equipment, and people in the interests of economic ends.

(ii) People are not by nature passive or resistant to organisational needs. They have become so as a result of experience in organisations.

(iii) The motivation, potential for development, capacity for assuming responsibility, and readiness to direct behaviour toward organisational goals are all present in people, management does not put them there. It is the responsibility of management to make it possible for people to recognise and develop these human characteristics for themselves.

(iv) The essential task of management is to arrange organisational conditions and methods of operation so that people can achieve their own goals by directing their efforts toward organisational objectives.

Assumptions of Theory Y

(i) Physical and mental effort involved in work is natural and that individuals actively seek to engage in work.

(ii) It also assumes that close supervision and the threat of punishment are not the only means or even the best means for inducing employees to exert productive effort.

(iii) If given the opportunity, employees will display self-motivation to put forth the effort necessary to achieve the organisation's goals.

(iv) Avoiding responsibility is not an inherent quality of human nature; individuals will actually seek it out under the proper conditions.

(v) Ability to be innovative and creative exists among a large, rather than a small segment of the population.

(vi) Rather than valuing security above all other rewards associated with work, individuals desire rewards that satisfy their self-esteem and self-actualisation needs.

Implications of Theory Y

- McGregor identified several approaches to management that he felt were consistent with the precepts of Theory Y. These included decentralisation of decision-making authority, delegation, job enlargement, and participative management. Job enrichment programs that began in the 1960s and 1970s also were consistent with the assumptions of Theory Y.

i. **Decentralisation and Delegation:** If firms decentralise control and reduce the number of levels of management, managers will have more subordinates and consequently will be forced to delegate some responsibility and decision-making to them.

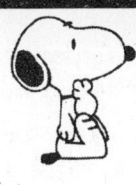

Thinking Time !!

To which theory do you and your friends belong? Theory X or theory Y (Look at the assumptions of both of them to compare it to your personality). Do you think McGregor was correct in assuming that people generally belong to Theory Y.

ii. **Job Enlargement:** Broadening the scope of an employee's job adds variety and opportunities to satisfy ego needs.

iii. **Participative Management:** Consulting employees in the decision making process taps their creative capacity and provides them with some control over their work environment.

iv. **Performance Appraisals:** Having the employee set objectives and participate in the process of evaluating how well they were met.

Details of Some Outcomes of X-Y Theory

Job Enlargement

- Job enlargement means increasing the scope of a job by extending the range of its job duties and responsibilities.

- This contradicts the principles of specialisation and the division of labour whereby work is divided into small units, each of which is performed repetitively by an individual worker.

- Some motivational theories suggest that the boredom and alienation caused by the division of labour can actually cause efficiency to fall. Thus, job enlargement seeks to motivate workers by reversing the process of specialisation.

5 reasons as to why Job Enlargement motivates employees are

i) **Task Variety**: Highly fragmented jobs requiring a limited number of unchanging responses tends to be extremely monotonous. Increase in the number of tasks reduces boredom.

ii) **Meaningful Work Modules:** Frequently jobs are enlarged so that one worker completes a whole unit of work, or at least a major portion of it. This tends to increase satisfaction by allowing workers to appreciate their contribution to the entire project.

iii) **Ability Utilisation:** Jobs that utilise the skills and ability of the worker increase their job satisfaction.

iv) **Worker-Paced Control:** Job enlargement schemes often move a worker from a machine-paced production line to a job in which the worker paces himself/herself. Workers feel less fatigued and are likely to enjoy their work more if they can vary the rhythm and work at their own pace.

v) **Performance Feedback:** Workers performing narrow jobs with short performance cycles repeat the same set of motions endlessly, without a meaningful end point. As a result, it is difficult to count the number of completed performance cycles. Even if they are counted, the feedback tends to be meaningless. Enlarged jobs allow for more meaningful feedback and can be particularly motivating if they are linked to evaluation and organisational rewards.

Disadvantages of Job Enlargement

i) Increase in training cost.

ii) Productivity may fall during introduction of the system.

iii) Unions often demand increase in pay due to increase in workload.

iv) However results have shown that this process can see its effects diminish after a period of time, as even the enlarged job role becomes dull, this in turn can lead to similar levels of de-motivation and job dissatisfaction at the expense of increased training levels and costs. The continual enlargement of a job over time is also known as **'Job Creep,'** which can lead to an unmanageable workload.

Job Enrichment

- Job enrichment is an attempt to motivate employees by giving them the opportunity to use the range of their abilities with challenging and interesting work.

- This idea was developed by Frederick Herzberg in the 1950s.

- It can be contrasted with job enlargement which simply increases the number of tasks without changing the challenge.

- As such, job enrichment has been described as 'vertical loading' of a job, while job enlargement is 'horizontal loading'.

Elements of Enriched Job

(i)   A range of tasks and challenges of varying difficulties (Physical or Mental)

(ii)   A complete unit of work - a meaningful task.

(iii) Feedback, encouragement and communication.

Characteristics of Job Enrichment

i) Direct Feedback: Employees should be able to get immediate knowledge of the results they are achieving. The evaluation of performance can be built into the job or provided by supervisors.

ii) Client Relationship: An employee who serves a client or customer directly has an enriched job. The client can be outside the firm or inside.

iii) New Learning: An enriched job allows its incumbent to feel that he is growing intellectually. An assistant who clips relevant newspaper articles for his boss is therefore doing an enriched job.

iv) Scheduling Own Work: Freedom to schedule one's own work contributes to enrichment. Deciding when to tackle which assignment is an example of self-scheduling. Employees who perform creative work have more opportunity to schedule their assignments than those who perform routine jobs.

v) Unique Experience: An enriched job has some unique qualities or features, such as a quality controller visiting a supplier.

vi) Control Over Resources: Here, the employee has control over his resources and expenses. E.g. He must have authority to order supplies necessary for completing the job.

vii) Direct Communication Authority: An enriched job allows the worker to communicate directly with people who use his or her output, such as quality assurance manager handling a customer's complaint about quality.

viii) Personal Accountability: An enriched job holds the incumbent responsible for the results. He receives praise for good work and blame for poor work.

Advantages of Job Enrichment

i) It increases motivation, performance, satisfaction, job involvement and reduces absenteeism.

ii) Psychological needs of job holder are satisfied.

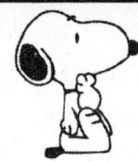

Thinking Time !!

Which of the two would you prefer? Job enlargement or Job Enrichment? How would you implement these two concepts in your studies?

iii) Improvement in the type of work satisfies the job holder.

iv) As the employee gets more authority and responsibility, he becomes more empowered.

Job Rotation

- Job rotation is an approach to management development where an individual is moved through a schedule of assignments designed to give him or her exposure to the entire operation.

- Job rotation is also practiced to allow qualified employees to gain more insights into the processes of a company, and to reduce boredom and increase job satisfaction through job variation.

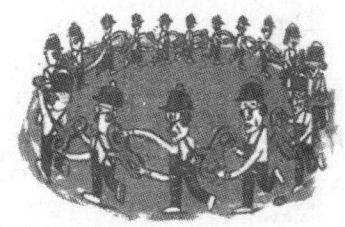

- At senior management levels, job rotation - frequently referred to as management rotation, is tightly linked with succession planning - developing a pool of people capable of stepping into an existing job. Here the goal is to provide learning experiences which facilitate changes in thinking and perspective equivalent to the "horizon" of the level of the succession planning.

- For lower management levels job rotation has normally one of two purposes: **Promotability or Skill Enhancement.**

- In many cases senior managers seem unwilling to risk instability in their units by moving qualified people from jobs where the lower level manager is being successful and reflecting positively on the actions of the senior manager.

- Many military jobs use the job rotation strategy to allow the soldiers to develop a wider range of experiences, and an exposure to the different jobs of an occupation.

TEST YOUR GREY MATTER

Q 1) What are Content theories of Motivation? Name all the Content Theories and explain how they are different from other theories?

Q 2) Describe Maslow's Need Hierarchy Theory and explain each level of the hierarchy?

Q 3) Critically examine Need Hierarchy Theory.

Q 4) Describe Herzberg's Two Factor Theory and critically analyse its importance.

Q 5) What is ERG theory of motivation? Give its advantages and drawbacks.

Q 6) Explain McClelland's Theory of Motivation and mention its advantage as a motivation theory?

Q 7) Why is McClelland's theory of motivation criticised?

Q 8) How do McGregor's Theory X and Theory Y of human behaviour help in motivation of employees?

Q 9) Distinguish between Maslow's need hierarchy and Herzberg's two factor theory?

Q 10) Explain: (i) Job Enlargement (ii) Job Enrichment (iii) Job Rotation.

C.2.2 Process Theories

- There were three assumptions in Content Theories which were practically found to be incorrect and which decreased their usefulness. They were-

  (i) All employees are alike

  (ii) All situations are alike.

  (iii) There is one best way to motivate all employees.

- Therefore, it resulted in the emergence of process theories, which held 'Motivation as an Individual's Decision to Act, so as to put forth some given level of effort'.

C.2.2.1. Expectancy Theory

- The expectancy theory proposed by **Victor Vroom** states that the strength of a tendency to act in a certain way depends on the strength of an expectation that the act will be followed by a given outcome and on the attractiveness of that outcome to the individual.

- This theory is currently the most widely accepted explanations of motivation, although it has its critics but most of the evidence supports the theory.

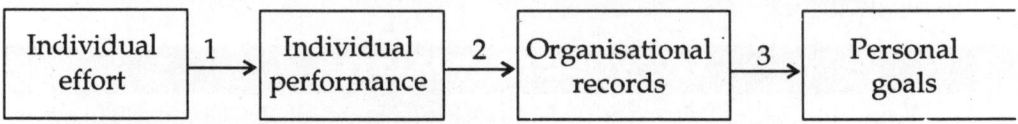

1. Effort-Performance relationship
2. Performance-reward relationship
3. Rewards-personal goals relationship

- Practically speaking, the expectancy theory says that employees will be motivated to exert a high level of effort when they believe that effort will lead to a good appraisal. A good appraisal will lead to organisation rewards which in turn will satisfy employees' personal goals. The theory therefore focuses on three relationships.

1. Effort Performance Relationship
   - ❑ It is the probability that a particular level of effort will be followed by a particular level of performance.
   - ❑ The relationship, also known as expectancy ranges from 0 to 1. This is also known as first level outcome.

2. Performance Reward Relationship
   - ❑ It is the degree perceived by an individual that performing at a particular level will lead to the attainment of a desired outcome.
   - ❑ Also known as instrumentality or second level outcome, it can have value ranging from −1 to +1.
   - ❑ −1 indicates that the attainment of a second level outcome is less likely if a first level outcome has occurred.
   - ❑ +1 suggests that attainment of a second level outcome has occurred.
   - ❑ 0 indicates no relationship between first and second level outcome.

3. Rewards-Personal Goals Relationship

❑ The degree to which organisational rewards satisfy an individual's personal goals or needs and the attractiveness of those potential rewards for the individual.

❑ Also known as valence, it can have values ranging from negative to positive.

❑ An outcome is positive when it is preferred and negative when it is not preferred or is to be avoided.

❑ An outcome has a valence of 0 when an individual is indifferent about receiving it.

• Summary, according to expectancy theory

$$\text{Motivation} = \text{Expectancy} \times \text{Instrumentality} \times \text{Valence}$$

Analysis of Expectancy theory

❑ The expectancy model has been both appreciated as well as criticised. Attempts to validate the theory have been complicated by methodological criterion and measurement problems.

❑ Most of the studies failed to replicate the methodology as it was originally proposed. For example the theory proposes to explain different levels of efforts from the same person under different circumstances, but almost all replication studies have looked at different people.

❑ Some critics suggest that theory has only limited use, arguing that it tends to be more valid for predicting in situations in which effort-performances and performance-reward linkages are clearly perceived by the individual.

❑ On the other hand, there are several arguments in support of the theory. To list a few:

(i) It provides clear guidelines to increase employee motivation by altering the person's expectancy, instrumentality and outcome valence.

(ii) It is a cognitive theory and therefore more realistic.

(iii) It helps managers to see beyond what Maslow and Herzberg showed, that motivation to work can only occur when work can satisfy unsatisfied needs.

C.2.2.2. Performance-Satisfaction Theory

This theory proposed by **Porter and Lawler** suggests that motivation, performance and satisfaction are all separate variables and relate in a way different from what was traditionally assumed.

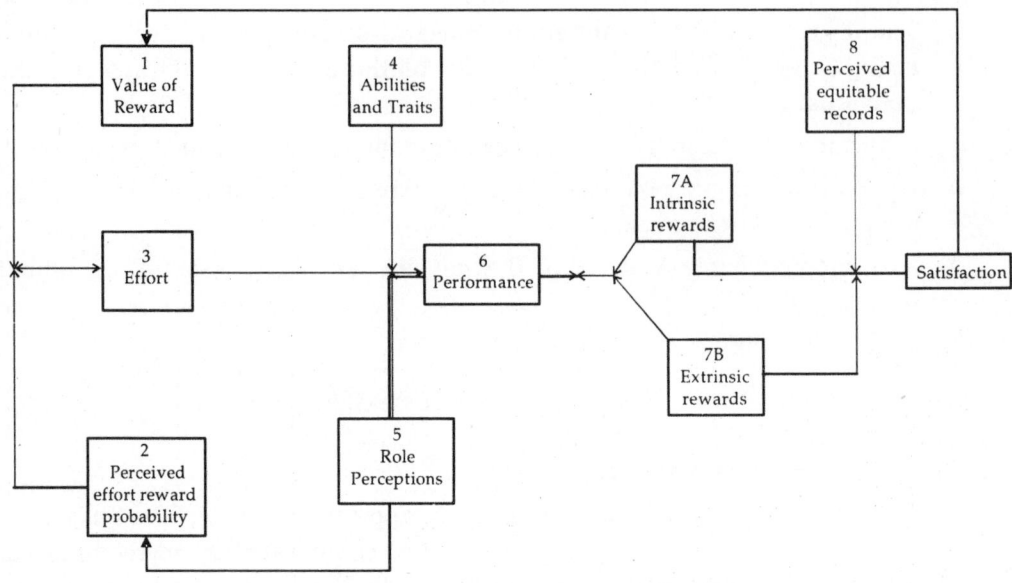

Source: Human Resource Management, K. Aswathappa, p 384

- The figure shows the multivariable model of Porter and Lawler. The model proposes that an effort does not directly lead to performance. It is mediated by abilities, traits and role perceptions. The various elements of the model are discussed below:

(i) Effort: It is the energy that a person invests on a particular job.

(ii) Perceived effort Reward Probability: It is the individual's perception of probability of different rewards with different degrees of efforts. This is closely related to instrumentality proposed in Vroom's Expectancy Theory.

(iii)Performance: It depends on the effort given by the individual and the ability and role perception of the individual.

(iv)Rewards: Rewards may be intrinsic such as sense of self actualisation and extrinsic such as working condition and status. Also perceived equitable rewards vitally affect the performance-satisfaction relationship.

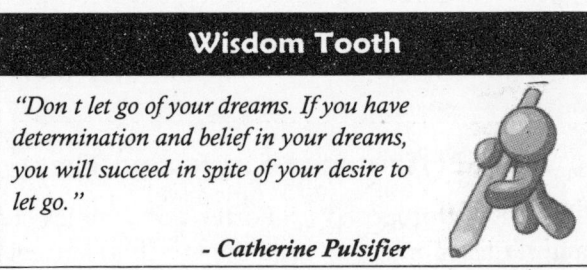

Wisdom Tooth

"Don t let go of your dreams. If you have determination and belief in your dreams, you will succeed in spite of your desire to let go."

- Catherine Pulsifier

(v) Satisfaction: It is the extent to which the actual rewards meet or fall short of the perceived level of equitable reward.

Recommendations of the Theory

(i) Place the right person on the right job.

(ii) Employee must know what is expected from him/her with respect to the role assigned.

(iii) Make sure that the rewards dispersed are valued by employees.

(iv) Link rewards to performance.

C.2.2.3. Equity Theory

- Equity Theory, also known as **'Social Comparison'** theory or **'Inequity Theory'** is based on the assumption that individuals are motivated by their desires to be treated equitably in their work relationships.

- When we see ourselves unrewarded or under rewarded, the tension creates anger; when over-rewarded the tension creates guilt.

- Adams proposed that this state of tension provides motivation to do something to correct it.

- There can be four kind of referents that an employee can select to compare his present state:

    i. **Self inside:** When employee compares with a different position in his own organisation.

    ii. **Self outside:** Employee's experiences at a position outside his own organisation.

    iii. **Other inside:** Another individual or group inside employee's own organisation.

    iv. **Other outside:** Another individual or group outside his own organisation.

- Employees might compare themselves to friends, neighbours, co-workers or colleagues in another organisation.

- They may also compare their present job with previous job. People generally make comparisons with the same sex.

- To reduce the inequality a person may react in any of the following ways:

    (i) Change their input.

    (ii) Change their outcomes.

    (iii) May distort the perception about himself.

    (iv) May distort the perception about others.

    (v) Leave the field.

(vi) May change the referent.

- With respect to the input the following cases may occur to achieve equity:

    (i) Given payment by time, over-rewarded employees will produce more than equitably paid employees.

    (ii) Given payment by quantity of production, over-rewarded employees will produce fewer but higher quality units than equitably paid employees.

    (iii) Given payment by time, under-rewarded employees will produce less or poor quality output.

    (iv) Given payment by quantity of production, under-rewarded employees will produce a large number of low quality units in comparison to equitable paid employees.

Evaluation of Equity Theory

On the positive side, the theory has generated a lot of research and most of the results are supportive. Some of the advantages are listed below:

i. The theory acknowledges the human tendency of comparing oneself to others and these social comparisons influence their output.

i. Compared to Content Theories, equity theory adopts a realistic approach. The theory proposes that major share of motivational behaviour depends on perceived situation rather than actual circumstances.

Despite the above mentioned strengths that equity theory enjoys, some questions still remain unanswered or rather are under-answered. Such as-

(i) What is the relationship between input and outcome?

(ii) Is a given factor an input or an output? The theory doesn't clearly bifurcate the input and output. For example, responsibility can be an input or an output?

(iii) How does the person choose the comparison with other and outside?

(iv) Under what circumstances and how should the inequity resolution method be used?

(v) Though the method is a success in lab experiments, is it practically fair enough on ground?

C.2.3. Reinforcement Theory

- Reinforcement theory is the process of shaping behaviour by controlling the consequences of the behaviour.

- In reinforcement theory a combination of rewards and/or punishments is used to reinforce desired behaviour or extinguish unwanted behaviour.

- Any behaviour that elicits a consequence is called *operant behaviour,* because the individual operates in his or her environment.

- Reinforcement theory concentrates on the relationship between the operant behaviour and the associated consequences and is sometimes referred to as **operant conditioning**.

Background And Development Of Reinforcement Theory

- Behavioural theories of learning and motivation focus on the effect that the consequences of past behaviour have on future behaviour.
- This is in contrast to classical conditioning, which focuses on responses that are triggered by stimuli in an almost automatic fashion.
- Reinforcement theory suggests that individuals can choose from several responses to a given stimulus, and that individuals will generally select the response that has been associated with positive outcomes in the past.
- **E.L. Thorndike** articulated this idea in 1911, in what has come to be known as the **Law of Effect**.

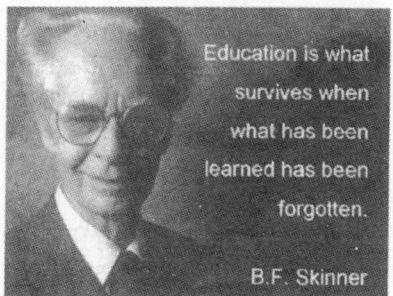

Education is what survives when what has been learned has been forgotten.

B.F. Skinner

- The **Law Of Effect** basically states that, all other things being equal, responses to stimuli that are followed by satisfaction will be strengthened, but responses that are followed by discomfort will be weakened.
- **B.F. Skinner** was a key contributor to the development of modern ideas about reinforcement theory.
- Skinner argued that the internal needs and drives of individuals can be ignored because people learn to exhibit certain behaviours based on what happens to them as a result of their behaviour. This school of thought has been termed the behaviourist or radical behaviourist school.

Reinforcement, Punishment and Extinction

- The most important principle of reinforcement theory is, of course, reinforcement. Generally speaking, there are two types of reinforcement: positive and negative.

Positive Reinforcement

- It results when the occurrence of a valued behavioural consequence has the effect of strengthening the probability of the behaviour being repeated. The specific behavioural consequence is called a **reinforcer.**
- An example of positive reinforcement might be a salesperson that exerts extra effort to meet a sales quota (behaviour) and is then rewarded with a bonus (positive reinforcer).

- The administration of the positive reinforcer should make it more likely that the salesperson will continue to exert the necessary effort in the future.

Negative reinforcement

- It results when an undesirable behavioural consequence is withheld, with the effect of strengthening the probability of the behaviour being repeated.
- Negative reinforcement is often confused with punishment, but they are not the same.
- Punishment attempts to decrease the probability of specific behaviours; negative reinforcement attempts to increase desired behaviour. Thus, both positive and negative reinforcement have the effect of increasing the probability that a particular behaviour will be learned and repeated.
- An example of negative reinforcement might be a salesperson that exerts effort to increase sales in his or her sales territory (behaviour), which is followed by a decision not to reassign the salesperson to an undesirable sales route (negative reinforcer). The administration of the negative reinforcer should make it more likely that the salesperson will continue to exert the necessary effort in the future.

Punishment

- As mentioned above, punishment attempts to decrease the probability of specific behaviours being exhibited.
- Punishment is the administration of an undesirable behavioural consequence in order to reduce the occurrence of the unwanted behaviour.
- Punishment is one of the more commonly used reinforcement-theory strategies, but many learning experts suggest that it should be used only if positive and negative reinforcement cannot be used or have previously failed, because of the potentially negative side effects of punishment.
- An example of punishment might be demoting an employee who does not meet performance goals or suspending an employee without pay for violating work rules.

Extinction

- Extinction is similar to punishment in that its purpose is to reduce unwanted behaviour.
- The process of extinction begins when a valued behavioural consequence is withheld in order to decrease the probability that a learned behaviour will continue. Over time, this is likely to result in the ceasing of that behaviour.
- Extinction may alternately serve to reduce a desired behaviour, such as when a positive reinforcer is no longer offered when a desirable behaviour occurs.

- For example, if an employee is continually praised for the promptness in which he completes his work for several months, but receives no praise in subsequent months for such behaviour, his desirable behaviours may diminish.
- Thus, to avoid unwanted extinction, managers may have to continue to offer positive behavioural consequences.

Schedules Of Reinforcement

- **Reinforcement Schedule:** The timing of the behavioural consequences that follow a given behaviour is called the reinforcement schedule.
- Basically, there are two broad types of reinforcement schedules: continuous and intermittent.

a. Continuous Reinforcement

- If a behaviour is reinforced each time it occurs, it is called continuous reinforcement.
- Research suggests that continuous reinforcement is the fastest way to establish new behaviours or to eliminate undesired behaviours. However, this type of reinforcement is generally not practical in an organisational setting. Therefore, intermittent schedules are usually employed.

b. Intermittent Reinforcement

- It means that each instance of a desired behaviour is not reinforced.
- There are at least four types of intermittent reinforcement schedules: fixed interval, fixed ratio, variable interval and variable ratio.

b.1. Fixed Interval Schedules

- Fixed interval schedules of reinforcement occur when desired behaviours are reinforced after set periods of time.
- The simplest example of a fixed interval schedule is a weekly pay check.
- A fixed interval schedule of reinforcement does not appear to be a particularly strong way to elicit desired behaviour, and behaviour learned in this way may be subject to rapid extinction.

b.2. Fixed Ratio

- The fixed ratio schedule of reinforcement applies the reinforcer after a set number of occurrences of the desired behaviours.
- One organisational example of this schedule is a sales commission based on number of units sold.
- Like the fixed interval schedule, the fixed ratio schedule may not produce consistent, long-lasting, behavioural change.

b.3. Variable Interval

- Variable interval reinforcement schedules are employed when desired behaviours are reinforced after varying periods of time.
- Examples of variable interval schedules are special recognition for successful performance and promotions to higher-level positions.
- This reinforcement schedule appears to elicit desired behavioural change that is resistant to extinction.

b.4. Variable Ratio

- The variable ratio reinforcement schedule applies the reinforcer after a number of desired behaviours have occurred, with the number changing from situation to situation.
- The most common example of this reinforcement schedule is the slot machine in a casino, in which a different and unknown number of desired behaviours (i.e. feeding a quarter into the machine) is required before the reward (i.e. a jackpot) is realised.
- Organisational examples of variable ratio schedules are bonuses or special awards that are applied after varying numbers of desired behaviours occur.
- Variable ratio schedules appear to produce desired behavioural change that is consistent and very resistant to extinction.

Reinforcement Theory Applied To Organisational Settings

- **Behavioural Contingency Management**

  Probably the best-known application of the principles of reinforcement theory to organisational settings is called behavioural modification or behavioural contingency management. Typically, a behavioural modification program consists of four steps:

  i. Specifying the desired behaviour as objectively as possible.
  ii. Measuring the current incidence of desired behaviour.
  iii. Providing behavioural consequences that reinforce desired behaviour.
  iv. Determining the effectiveness of the program by systematically assessing behavioural change.

- Reinforcement theory is an important explanation of how people learn behaviour. It is often applied to organisational settings in the context of a behavioural modification program.

- Although the assumptions of reinforcement theory are often criticised, its principles continue to offer important insights into individual learning and motivation.

TEST YOUR GREY MATTER

Q1) What is the basic concept of process theories? How are they different from content theories and why did they came into existence?

Q2) Describe and analyse Expectancy Theory.

Q3) Explain and give the recommendations of following theories:

(i) Performance-Satisfaction Theory.

(ii) Equity Theory.

Q4) What are Reinforcement theories and how are they applicable to organisational motivation?

Q5) What are major elements of Reinforcement Theory? Explain.

Job Satisfaction

By the end of this chapter, you would be able to

- Understand Job Satisfaction and the reasons for one's commitment to his job.
- Know about the factors which affect Job Satisfaction.
- Evaluate the importance of Job Satisfaction.
- Learn about methods of measuring Job Satisfaction.

The chapter contains :

- Definition of Job Satisfaction
- Job Attitudes
- Organisational Factors related to Job Satisfaction
- Personal Factors related to Job Satisfaction
- Responses of Job Satisfaction
- Importance and Effects of Job Satisfaction
- Measuring Job Satisfaction

A. THE INSIGHT

And you said your job is tough!!!!

Empire State Building Construction Workers

- Akansh and Ashok have same jobs. Akansh loves his job, he works passionately and with full commitment while Ashok looks for situations to pass his time and he is on the lookout for another job.
- Aditya loves his job but is still in search of another job.
- Mayank never liked his job; he is dissatisfied with his company and wants a certain type of job.
- What are the reasons for different attitudes of different people about their jobs and careers? Why is it so? How to control it?
- All these questions are answered when we study 'Job Satisfaction'.

B. JOB ATTITUDES

- **Definition:** Attitudes are statements-either favourable or unfavourable- about objects, people or events. And when it is about Job, it is called Job Attitude.
- There are 3 major Job Attitudes-
  1) Job Satisfaction.
  2) Job Involvement.
  3) Organisational Commitment.

1. Job Satisfaction

- Job satisfaction is a parameter of an attitude towards one's job. It also decides the extent of motivation which one has towards his job.

> **Wisdom Tooth**
>
> *"All paid jobs absorb and degrade the mind."*
>
> *-Aristotle*

- **Definition:** "Job satisfaction is the amount of contentment (or lack of it) arising out of interplay of the employee's positive and negative feelings towards his or her job".
- A person with high level of job satisfaction holds positive feelings about his job while a dissatisfied person holds negative feelings.
- It is the factor which determines employee's behaviour, his productivity and commitment in the organisation.

2. Job Involvement

- **Definition:** Job Involvement measures the degree to which people identify psychologically with their job and consider their perceived performance level important to self-worth.

- People having high level of Job Involvement strongly identify with and really care about the work they do.

3. Organisational Commitment

- **Definition:** Organisational Commitment is a state in which an employee identifies with a particular organisation and its goals and wishes to maintain membership in the organisation.
- While Job involvement is identification with a job; Organisational Commitment is identification with an organisation.
- It is of 3 types-

i. Affective Commitment

It is an emotional attachment with the organisation and a belief in its values. It is good for both the organisation and the employee. Employee wants to work for the organisation, wants to be there and also give extra effort for it. E.g. Sachin Tendulkar wants to be in the Indian Team, wants to perform for his team and always tries to give his best so that India wins.

ii. Continuance Commitment

This is due to the nature of man which fears changes. As employee has worked for some time, he continues to work there. Also, he resists getting out of the safety shell he has built over the years and does not want to take the trouble of finding a new job.

iii. Normative Commitment

It is because the employee feels obliged to the organisation for moral and ethical reasons and wants to work for it. The factors may be, he received special attention or training from the organisation, learned everything from the organisation etc.

Implied example of this can be given by looking at people who work in our country even though they get lucrative offers from abroad because of their love and obligation for the country.

TEST YOUR GREY MATTER

Q1) What is Job Attitude and how does it affect an organisation?

Q2) State different types of Job Attitudes of a person and briefly describe each of them?

Q3) What do you understand by Organisational Commitment and what are its types?

C. FACTORS RELATED TO JOB SATISFACTION

We can classify the factors related to Job satisfaction into two broad categories:

i. Organisational factors.

ii. Personal factors.

i. Organisational Factors / Management Controllable

- As the major amount of time is spent at the work place by all of us. Organisational factors play a very important role. These factors can be controlled by the management

- We will understand this through a chart.

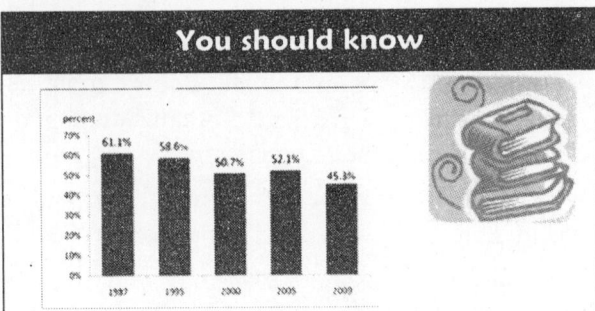

You should know

Declining Job Satisfaction of U.S employees

"While one in 10 Americans is now unemployed, their working compatriots of all ages and incomes continue to grow increasingly unhappy," says Lynn Franco, director of the Consumer Research Center of The Conference Board. "Through both economic boom and bust during the past two decades, our job satisfaction numbers have shown a consistent downward trend."

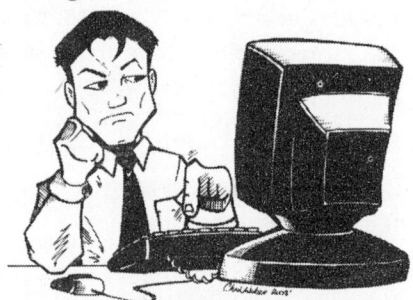

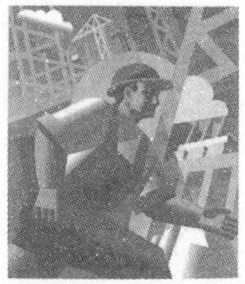

Employee Dissatisfaction	Employee satisfaction
When these conditions are optimal, job dissatisfaction will be eliminated. But these factors do not increase Job Satisfaction. 1. **Salary** – It is most important. 2. **Reward** – Such as annual appraisal, report etc. 3. **Working conditions** – E.g. Proper tools, machines increase safety.	When these factors are optimal, job satisfaction will increase. 1. **Good Leadership practices** – It includes leader/supervisor's behaviour and concern towards employee. 2. **Recognition** – People knowing and recognising one for his work or any special job done is immensely important.

4. **Job security** – It gives stability to employee. 5. **Promotions** – Rising up the organisational ladder prevents employee from getting dissatisfied 6. **Fringe benefits** – These are additional benefits apart from salary, such as housing, children's study facility etc. 7. **Co-Workers** – Friendly relation with people at work.	3. **Advancement/Responsibility** – Getting more important and responsible work from the management. It is a sign of maturity. 4. **Clear direction and objectives** – Expectations from an employee must be clearly conveyed and confusions avoided. 5. **Feedback and support** – Employee must be given feedback about his work from time to time and proper support must be provided if he lacks in some areas. 6. **Work** – Variety of jobs which challenges the worker intellectually satisfies him.

ii. Personal Factors

a. **Intelligence / Education:** More the education or intelligence of the employee, more dissatisfied he becomes if not looked after.

b. **Sex:** As per studies, women workers are more satisfied than men from their jobs.

c. **Marital Status:** Married workers are also more satisfied with their jobs especially if the married couple is working in the same organisation.

d. **Period on Job:** As per a study, the time a person spends on his job and its relation to job satisfaction and dissatisfaction can be represented as.

Job satisfaction	1-3 yrs	7 yrs – onwards
Job dissatisfaction	4-6 yrs	

e. **Age:** Generally, more the age, more the person is satisfied with his job. But it is not always true.

f. **Family members dependent on employee:** More the number of dependents, more are his expectations from job and thus more dissatisfied he becomes.

g. **Interest:** If the nature of the job is of interest to the employee, his satisfaction will increase. E.g. Amitabh Bacchhan will be more satisfied as an actor than as engineer or doctor etc.

h. **Personality Traits**: People having the same traits as required by the job, will be more satisfied. E.g. An introvert person will find it difficult to be in a sales or marketing job.

D. RESPONSES OF JOB SATISFACTION

The consequences of satisfaction and dissatisfaction of an employee can be seen by employees' responses which are theoretically defined as:

Thinking Time !!

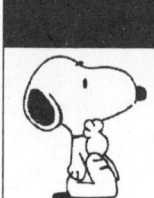

Prepare a list of all the factors, (i)College Management Controlled and

(ii) Personality based, which effects the Education Satisfaction© of a student.

i. **Exit:** This response involves the behaviour of looking for a new position and leaving the organisation.

ii. **Voice:** This response involves the behaviour of actively finding solutions to existing problems and involvement in organisational activities.

iii. **Loyalty:** This response is a passive one and it involves trusting the organisation and waiting for the situation to improve during crisis.

iv. **Neglect:** This is a passive response and involves allowing the situation to get worse and is followed by absenteeism, increase in errors etc.

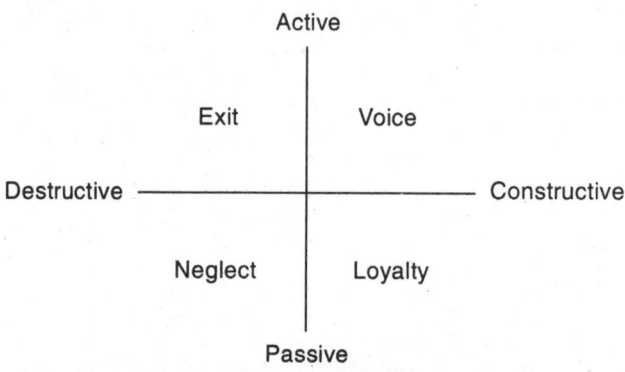

Response to Job Satisfaction

TEST YOUR GREY MATTER

Q 1) Describe the factors which are related to Job Satisfaction.

Q2) What are the four responses of Job Satisfaction?

Q 3) What are the factors which prevents an employee from getting dissatisfied?

E. IMPORTANCE AND EFFECTS OF JOB SATISFACTION

1. Mental health

A person satisfied with the job remains mentally active and happy. Whereas, if a person remains dissatisfied for a long time, tensions and stress may affect him mentally and can also be represented in his behaviour. He becomes unhappy, irritated and troublesome. He may become pessimistic towards life and his personal life also gets affected.

2. Physical Health

If a person is under continuous stress, he may suffer from health problem like headache, heart and digestion related diseases.

3. Absenteeism

There is a negative relationship between the amount of job satisfaction and the degree of work absenteeism. Though dissatisfied workers are more likely to miss work, it is not the only reason for being absent and other factors also affect it.

4. Employee Attrition

Dissatisfaction is one of the prime reasons for employees leaving their jobs. Employees have some needs and expectations from the company e.g. salary, work, responsibility etc. and when they are not met, they become dissatisfied and if it persists for a long time, employees may leave the job.

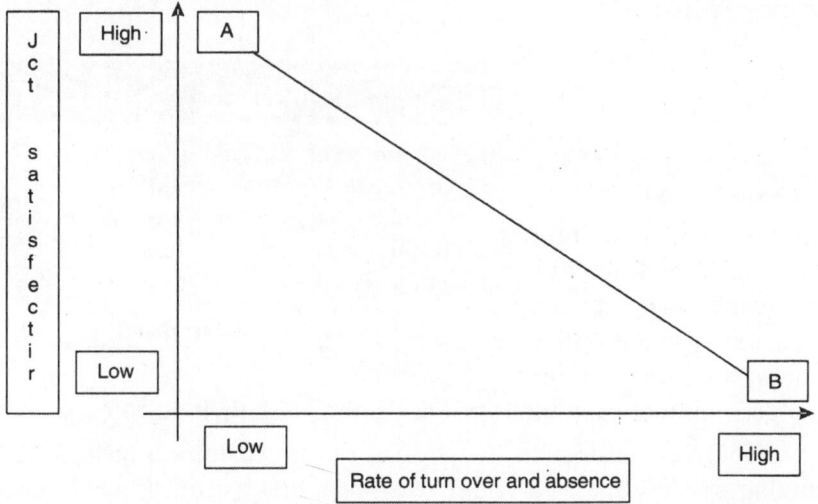

Curve shows relationship between Job satisfaction and Rate of Attrition and Absenteeism

In the above figure line AB shows inverse relationship between job satisfaction and rate of attrition and rate of absenteeism

5. Productivity

"A Happy worker is a productive worker", is NOT an absolutely correct statement and it should not be the foundation of organisational decision making. This relationship is not necessarily straight forward and can be influenced by a number of work-related constructs.

It is finally concluded that for:

- **High complexity jobs,** correlation between satisfaction and performance is **higher.** e.g. for managerial levels or supervisors but is **low** for job with moderate or **less complexity**. Because for lower level jobs, productivity does not depend completely on the workers performance but also on other factors such as machine, material, process adopted etc.

> ### You should know
>
> "A Happy worker is a productive worker" idea was developed in 1930s and 40s due to Hawthorne Experiments, where the full focus was on making the employee happy. But later it was found that the relationship is not very strong, rather it depends on the job. It was also found that vice-versa might also be true, that is: Productive workers are likely to be happy workers. Is it not that if you do a good job, you feel good?

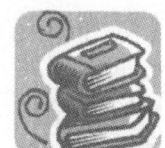

6. Customer Satisfaction

- Satisfied employees increase customer satisfaction.

- In service industries, customer retention is highly dependent on how the employee deals with customers and it has been found that satisfied employees are more energetic, friendly and interested in dealing with their customers.

> ### Wisdom Tooth
>
> "There are countless studies on the negative spillover of job pressures on family life, but few on how job satisfaction enhances the quality of family life."
>
> *Albert Bandura*

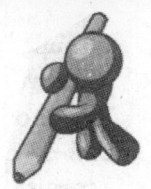

- As employee satisfaction reduces attrition, customers gets services from familiar and experienced employees. This builds a relationship between the organisation and customer.

F. MEASURING JOB SATISFACTION

1. Faces Scale

Carolyn's Job Satisfaction Faces Scale

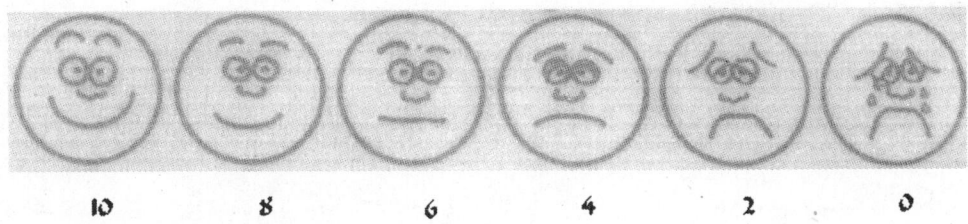

| 10 | 8 | 6 | 4 | 2 | 0 |

- Developed by Kunin (1955).
- It involved only identifying one of the expression which resembled one's Job satisfaction.
- It is easy to use but is not used now because
  i. It lacks construct validity.
  ii. Lacks sufficient details.
  iii. Some employees believe it is so simple that it is demeaning.

2. Job Descriptive Index (JDI)

- Developed by Smith, Kendall and Hulin (1969)
- Job Descriptive Index is a scale used to measure five major factors associated with job satisfaction: the nature of the work itself, compensations and benefits, attitudes towards supervisors, relations with co-workers, and opportunities for promotion.
- It is very easy to use and most commonly used method.
- Its disadvantage is that it does not take into account other than these 5 factors.

Case Study

Job Descriptive Index Example

The data included in the table below was collected from two groups of employees: welders and pipe shop workers. The numbers represent averages for subscales of the JDI , in which the possible range of values is 0 — 3.

JDI Facet	2002 Welders	2002 Pipe Shop	2005 Welders	2005 Pipe Shop
Work itself	1.5	1.8	1.6	1.9
Supervision	2.5	2.2	2.4	1.8
Pay	1	1.2	1.2	1.1
Promotion	0.6	0.8	0.6	0.8
Co-workers	2.5	2.4	2.5	2.3

Consider the following questions with respect to this data:

1. What can you conclude about the overall level of job satisfaction of the employees?
2. What can you conclude about each of the five specific areas of job satisfaction?
3. What, if any, other information would you need in order to plan an intervention that might improve the quality of working life of the employees?
4. Based on this data, what could you do to improve the quality of working life of the employees?

3. Minnesota Satisfaction Questionnaire (MSQ)

- Developed by Weiss, Dawis, England and Lofquist (1967)
- Contains 100 items that yield scores on 20 facets i.e. 5 questions on each facet.
- It is an easy and reliable method which is applicable to all organisations and all managers, supervisors, and employees.
- Its disadvantage is that it is very long.

You should know

MSQ measures job satisfaction on 20, five-item scales:

Ability Utilization	Co-workers	Moral Values
Achievement	Creativity	Recognition
Activity	Independence	Responsibility
Advancement	Security	Supervision--HumanRelations
Authority	Social Service	Supervision--Technical
Company Policies	Social Status	Variety
Compensation		Working Conditions

5 Response choices are: Very Satisfied; Satisfied; "N" (Neither Satisfied nor Dissatisfied); Dissatisfied; Very Dissatisfied

TEST YOUR GREY MATTER

Q1) Write a short note on the relation of Job satisfaction with:

(i) Absenteeism (ii) Attrition (iii) Productivity

Q2) What are the various methods of measuring Job Satisfaction? Briefly explain each of them.

Q3) What is the difference between Job Descriptive Index and Minnesota Satisfaction Questionnaire?

CHAPTER 7

Stress Management

By the end of this chapter, you would be able to

- Know about the nature and various levels of stress.
- Learn about different types of stress and will be able to recognise them by their symptoms.
- Understand the effects of stress on the employee and the organisation.
- Determine various causes of stress and will also learn to counteract them by applying methods of stress management.

The chapter contains :

- Concept of Stress
- Stages of Stress
- Types of Stress.
- Symptoms of Stress
- Job Stress
- Causes of Stress
- Consequences/Effects of Stress
- Stress Management

A. THE INSIGHT

- It is estimated that over 1,00,000 people die by suicide in India every year. Be it farmers from Vidarbha or a boy hanging himself due to failure in an examination.
- It has been found that 60-80% of industrial accidents are due to stress. Some, like Exxon Valdez oil spill and Three Mile Island nuclear disaster have direct cleanup costs of billions of dollars and also cause large scale of environmental damage.
- The International Labour Organisation (branch of the UN) reports that 1 in 10 workers are affected on the job by anxiety, depression, and stress. The increase in job-related stress is "alarming" according to the 2000 survey, and costs to governments are as high as 4% of their GNP. In the US, 200 million working days are lost annually due to mental health problems.

- Japanese office workers frequently work 3000 hours a year, an average of more than 8 hours a day, every day of the year – and 3500 hours is not uncommon among bank workers. (The average North American worker puts in 1700 hours per year at the office or factory.) Just as it is common to work long hours, it is not uncommon for 40-yr old men to literally drop dead of strokes or heart attacks caused by excessive stress.

- These are some effects which result from stress and it becomes mandatory for us to understand it.

B. CONCEPT OF STRESS

- **Definition:** "Stress is a person's adaptive response to a stimulus that places excessive psychological and physical demands on him or her."

- According to this definition, stress is induced by a physical or psychological stimulus known as *stressor*.

- Stressor create stress when

$$S = P > R$$

i.e. Stress occurs when Pressure is greater than resource or when the demand exceeds the person's ability to respond.

C. STAGES OF STRESS (GENERAL ADAPTATION SYNDROME)

There are three stages of stress

i. Alarm Reaction

- It is the immediate reaction to a stressor.

- **Fight or Flight**: Humans exhibit a "fight or flight" response. When a person experiences a shock or perceives a threat, he quickly releases hormones that help him to survive.

- These hormones help us to run faster and fight harder. They increase heart rate and blood pressure, delivering more oxygen and blood sugar to power important muscles. They increase sweating in an effort to cool these muscles, and help them stay efficient. They divert blood away from the skin to the core of our bodies, reducing blood loss if we are damaged.

You should know

Forbes magazine estimates that the American industry will lose $300 billion per annum due to absenteeism, health costs, and stress management programs.

- Also, these hormones focus our attention on the threat, to the exclusion of everything else. All of this significantly improves our ability to survive in such conditions.
- But there is a decrease in the effectiveness of the immune system, thus making persons more susceptible to illness.

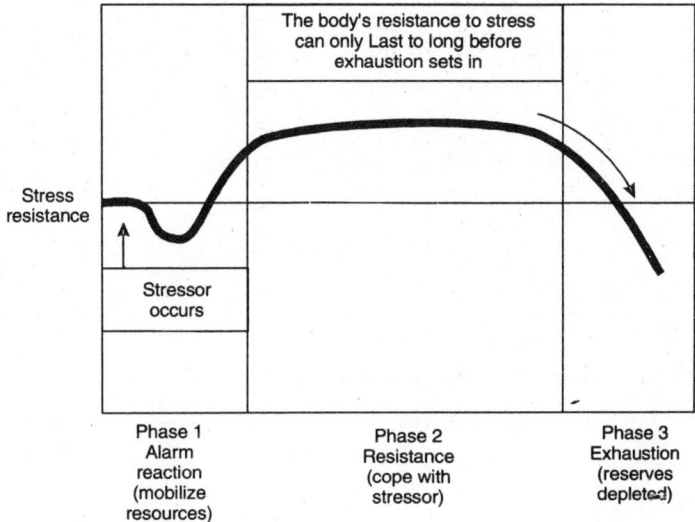

ii. Stage of Resistance

- It is a stage of maximum adaptation.
- Body adapts to the stressors it is exposed to.
- Changes at many levels take place in order to reduce the effect of the stressor.
- E.g. The person will devise a plan to complete the task assigned to him. If he opts to flee from the stressor, he will delegate the task to someone else.
- This phase lasts for as long as the person can support this heightened resistance.

iii. Stage of Exhaustion

- If the stress has continued for some time, body's resistance to the stress may gradually be reduced or may collapse quickly.
- The immune system and the body's ability to resist disease may be almost totally eliminated.

> ## You should know
>
> - **Myths about stress**
> *Myth 1 I must be stressed to succeed...*
> *Myth 2 All Stress is bad...*
> *Myth 3 If only I could move/change my job/ leave my spouse/get rid of my boss, then my stress would go away...*
>
> *Myth 4 There is nothing I can do about stress...*
>
>

- People who experience long-term stress may succumb to heart attacks or severe infection due to their reduced immunity.

D. TYPES OF STRESS

Based on its nature, stress can be classified into two types:

i. Eustress or Positive Stress

- *Eustress* is a word consisting of two parts. The prefix is derived from the Greek *eu* meaning either "well" or "good". When attached to the word "stress", it literally means "good stress".
- Eustress accompanies achievement and exhilaration.
- Examples of eustress can be-
  1. Meeting or engaging in a challenge.
  2. Coming first in a race.
  3. Getting a promotion at your job.
  4. Watching a suspense or horror movie.
  5. Love, marriage, or childbirth.
  6. Riding a roller-coaster.
  7. The holidays.
  8. Purchasing something, such as a new car.

ii. Distress or Negative Stress

- It is the negative stress which results when a person is unable to completely adapt to stressors and results in various inappropriate behaviours such as aggression, passivity, insecurity, helplessness, desperation etc.

- People under constant distress are more likely to become sick, mentally or physically.

- Example of distress are:
  - Difficult work environment
  - Overwhelming sights and sounds.

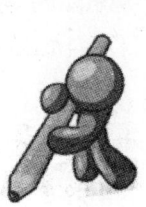

Wisdom Tooth

"When you find yourself stressed, ask yourself one question:

Will this matter in 5 years from now?

If yes, then do something about the situation.

If no, then let it go."

Catherine Pulsifer

- ❑ Threat of personal injury.
- ❑ Work under constant pressure.

E. SYMPTOMS OF STRESS

There are four types of symptoms:

i. Physical symptoms

ii. Mental symptoms

iii. Behavioural symptoms

iv. Emotional symptoms

i. Physical Symptoms

Following physical symptoms are observed when a person is under prolonged stress:

- Sleep pattern changes
- Fatigue
- Headaches
- Aches and pains
- Indigestion
- Dizziness
- Fainting
- Sweating & trembling
- Tingling hands & feet
- Breathlessness
- Palpitations

ii. Mental symptoms

Following mental symptoms are observed when a person is under stress:

- Lack of concentration
- Memory lapses
- Difficulty in making decisions
- Confusion
- Disorientation
- Panic attacks
- Tension
- Anxiety
- Boredom
- Job Dissatisfaction

iii. Behavioural Symptoms

Following behavioural symptoms are observed due to stress:

- Change in productivity.
- Absence
- Attrition
- Appetite changes - too much or too little
- Eating disorders - anorexia, bulimia
- Increased intake of alcohol & other drugs
- Increased smoking
- Restlessness
- Nail biting

iv. Emotional Symptoms

Following emotional symptoms indicates that a person is under stress:

- Depression
- Impatience
- Fits of rage
- Tearfulness
- Deterioration of personal hygiene and appearance

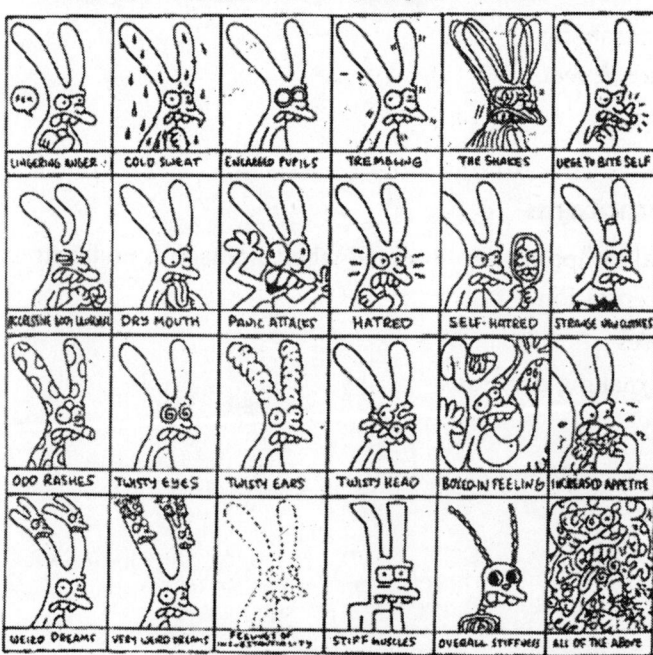

The 24 Warning Signs of Stress

F. JOB STRESS

Definition: Job stress can be defined as the harmful physical and emotional responses that occur when the requirements of the job do not match the capabilities, resources or needs of the worker.

- Job stress is often confused with challenge, but these concepts are not the same. Challenge energises us psychologically and physically, and it motivates us to learn new skills and master our jobs. When a challenge is met, we feel relaxed and satisfied.

- But job stress is different - the challenge has turned into job demands that cannot be met, relaxation has turned to exhaustion, and a sense of satisfaction has turned into feelings of stress.

G. CAUSES OF STRESS

Various causes of stress are shown below:

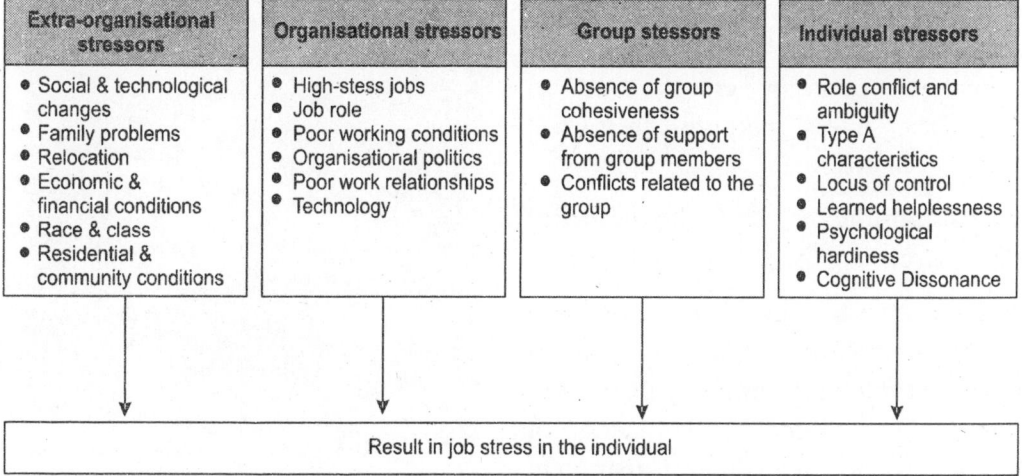

Extra-organisational stressors	Organisational stressors	Group stessors	Individual stressors
• Social & technological changes • Family problems • Relocation • Economic & financial conditions • Race & class • Residential & community conditions	• High-stess jobs • Job role • Poor working conditions • Organisational politics • Poor work relationships • Technology	• Absence of group cohesiveness • Absence of support from group members • Conflicts related to the group	• Role conflict and ambiguity • Type A characteristics • Locus of control • Learned helplessness • Psychological hardiness • Cognitive Dissonance

Result in job stress in the individual

1. Extra-Organisational Stressors

Since organisations are open systems, an employee is affected not only by the things happening within the organisation but also by those which occur outside.

i. Social & Technological Changes

Societal Patterns and technological changes have influenced the lifestyles of people. The advances in medical science have reduced the threat of many illnesses, increased the life span of individuals and improved the quality of life in general. However, increase in urbanisation, along with accompanying elements such as time pressure, overcrowding and fast lifestyles have reduced the well-being of individuals and increased their chances of experiencing stress.

ii. Family Problems

Research states that stress levels are higher in families in which both, husband and wife work.

iii. Relocation

Relocating to a new place can also act as a potential stressor

iv. Economic & Financial Conditions

Adverse financial conditions may also cause stress amongst employees.

v. Race & Class

Certain sociological variables such as race, sex, and class also tend to induce stress in employees. Employees who belong to minority groups tend to experience stress because they feel socially isolated.

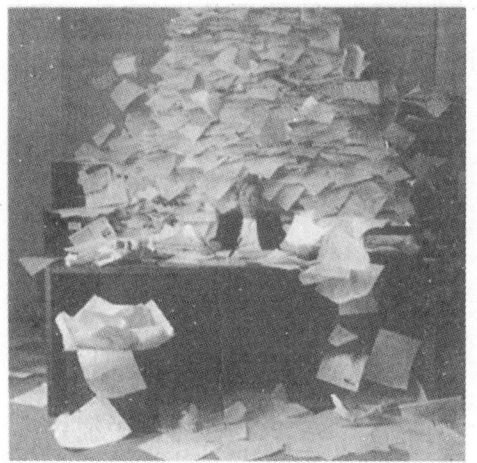

vi. Residential & Community Conditions

The social level, region and community to which employees belong also play an important role in determining their stress levels. For example, the lack of neighbourliness in huge apartment complexes.

2. Organisational Stressors

i. High – Stress Jobs

High stress jobs are those in which people have hectic work schedules and major job responsibilities. Such employees are constantly under pressure to perform well and if they are unable to do so, they may have to face dire consequences. For e.g. sales managers, foremen etc.

ii. Job Role

A person may also feel stressed if his job role has certain unpleasant characteristics such as work overload, insufficient amount of work, role ambiguity, role conflict, and responsibility for the work of others. People also feel disgruntled when they do not have enough tasks to keep them busy, or if their skills and talents are underutilised.

iii. Poor Working Conditions

Working conditions also act as potential stressors. Extreme heat, noise and overcrowding can result in stress amongst employees.

iv. Organisational Politics

Organisational politics may increase competition among various groups of employees and lead to power struggles between them.

v. Poor Work Relationships

How are your relationships with your manager or a team-member? You don't trust your co-workers, don't feel respected or feel that people don't listen to you? All these amount to stresses that seriously affect your performance. Many studies carried out across different organisations revealed that approximately 60 percent of the workforce felt that the most stressful aspect of their job was their poor relationship with their immediate superior.

vi. Technology

The expansion of technology—computers, pagers, cell phones, fax machines and the Internet—has resulted in heightened expectations for productivity, speed and efficiency, increasing pressure on the individual worker to constantly operate at peak performance levels. Workers working with heavy machinery are under constant stress to remain alert. There is also the constant pressure to keep up with technological breakthroughs and
improvisations.

3. Group Stressors

Groups tend to have a great impact on the behaviour of their members and others who come in contact with them.

i. Absence of group cohesiveness

It is very important for an employee to feel that he is a part of the group. He may feel stressed out if the task execution is designed in such a way that it does not encourage group cohesiveness. Likewise, lack of cohesiveness may also occur if the other group members exclude an employee or if the manager prohibits an employee from being a participant in group activities.

ii. Absence of support from other members

Group members count on the support of others within the group. In the absence of such support, they have no one to share their problems. Consequently, they may bottle up their feelings and experience high levels of stress.

iii. Conflicts related to the group

A group member may experience a conflict between his personal goals and those of the group. These conflicts can result in high levels of stress for individual members of the group.

4. Individual stressors

i. Role conflict and ambiguity

An individual is generally a member of various groups such as work, family, community; recreational club etc. He plays a variety of roles in different groups as well as balances the various roles he plays. Sometimes, these roles place conflicting demands on the individual. For instance, a person might not be able to devote enough time to his family because of work pressures.

ii. Type A characteristics

As per the category

- **Type A** are people who have high level of commitment, are competitive, aggressive, impatient, time-conscious, concerned about their status. They desire to achieve. Such personalities are more prone to chances of stress and incompatibility.

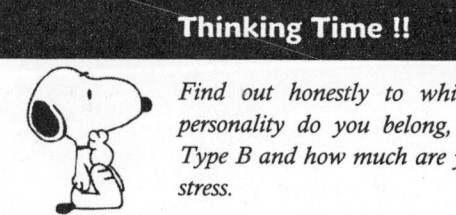

Thinking Time !!

Find out honestly to which Type of personality do you belong, Type A or Type B and how much are you prone to stress.

- **Type B** are those who have a relaxed and balanced approach and are more confident in their approach towards work. They are less competitive and have weaker sense of time urgency. They are less susceptible to stress.

iii. Psychological Hardiness

It decides the level and capacity of a person to handle stress since it varies from individual to individual. Thus, people having high level of hardiness in handling stress are persons who know how to handle the situation better and in a planned way so as to reduce the level of stress

You should know

Personality Type A and B

TYPE A	TYPE B
Always moving, walking, and eating rapidly	Never suffer from a sense of time urgency with its accompanying impatience
Feel impatient with the rate at which most events take place	Feel no need to display or discuss either their achievements or accomplishments unless such exposure is demanded by the situation
Strive to think or do two or more things at once.	Play for fun & relaxation, instead of exhibit their superiority at any cost
Cannot cope with leisure time.	Can relax without guilt.
Are obsessed with numbers, measuring their success in terms of how many or how much of everything they acquire.	Is mild mannered and has no pressing deadlines.

iv. Locus of control

The degree of control that an individual exercises over his work is known as the locus of control. Individuals who possess an internal locus of control believe that they have control over their environment. Conversely, individuals who possess an external locus of control believe that they have no control over their environment. In other words, if an individual feels that he has no control over his job (external locus of control); he is more likely to feel stressed out.

v. Learned helplessness

It explains the behaviour of certain individuals who become helpless in a stressful situation and do not attempt to change things. They learn to accept certain stressors as a part of their work life, and believe that they can do nothing to change or alter these stressors

vi. Cognitive dissonance

- When there is a gap between what we do and what we think, then we experience cognitive dissonance, which is felt as stress.

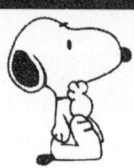

Thinking Time !!

Make a list of stressors in your student life and also the steps you should take to counteract them so that so can stay focused on your goal.

- Thus, if I think that I am a nice person and then do something that hurts someone else, I will experience dissonance and stress.

- Dissonance also occurs when we cannot meet our commitments. We believe we are honest and committed, but when circumstances prevent us from meeting our promises we are faced with the possibility of being perceived as dishonest or incapable (i.e. a social threat).

TEST YOUR GREY MATTER

Q1) What is Stress? Explain.

Q2) Describe General Adaptation Syndrome explaining all three stages?

Q3) Explain Eustress and Distress and differentiate between them.

Q4) What are the behavioural symptoms of stress?

Q5) Define Job Stress.

Q6) Define 'Stressors'. Enlist various categories of Stressors.

Q7) What are the organisational factors which are responsible for causing stress?

Q8) Explain Type A and Type B personalities. Describe them in relation to stress.

Q9) What are Group Stressors? How are they responsible for stress?

H. CONSEQUENCES/EFFECTS OF STRESS

H.1. Effects of Stress on Individual

a. Physical problems

- Studies revealed that the early symptoms of stress are
  - Headaches
  - Increase in Blood Pressure and Sweating
  - Hot flushes
  - Loss of Appetite
  - Gastrointestinal Disorders
  - Fatigue

- Prolonged exposure to high stress levels can often result in severe physiological disorder which may seriously affect the health of employees, such as
  - ❑ High Blood Pressure
  - ❑ High Level of Cholesterol
  - ❑ Ulcers
  - ❑ Heart Disease
- Therefore, organisations should try to bring down the stress levels of employees because the physiological problems related to stress can affect the financial health of organisations in the long run.

b. Psychological problems

- High levels of stress can make a person feel
  - ❑ Angry
  - ❑ Anxious
  - ❑ Bored
  - ❑ Depressed
  - ❑ Dissatisfied
  - ❑ Tense
  - ❑ Irritated
  - ❑ Unable to relax and concentrate
- This can result in poor performance at the workplace because the individual may not be able to take decisions or focus on the tasks at hand.

c. Behavioural problems

- High levels of stress may change the behaviour patterns of individuals. They may display any of the following symptoms –
  - ❑ Sleep disorders
  - ❑ Over-eating
  - ❑ Loss of appetite
  - ❑ Increased smoking
  - ❑ Alcohol consumption
  - ❑ Use of addictive drugs
  - ❑ Rude behaviour
  - ❑ Nervousness in social interactions such as Rapid Speech and Fidgeting
  - ❑ Feeling of job insecurity
  - ❑ Feeling of incompetence

> ### You should know
>
> *In the United States, the average duration of leave due to stress is four times greater than the amount of leave resulting from occupational injuries and industrial disease.*

d. Effect on Performance

- The relationship between stress and performance is depicted in the form of an inverted U-curve.

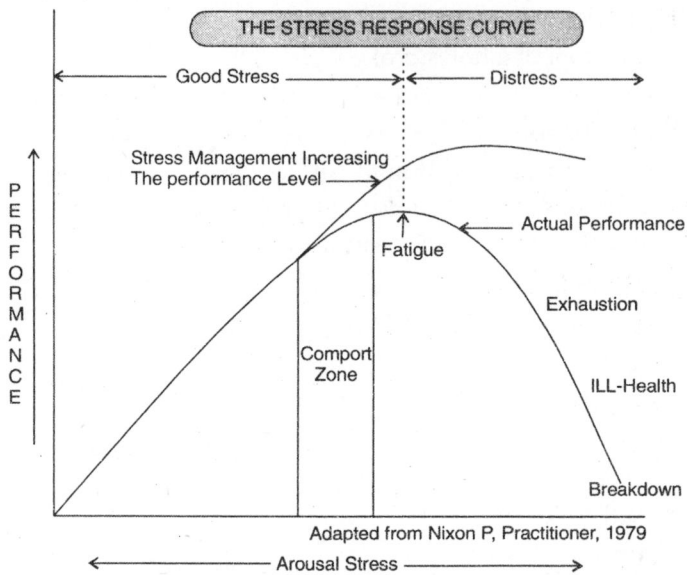

THE STRESS RESPONSE CURVE

Adapted from Nixon P, Practitioner, 1979

- Our ability to perform increases up to a certain level of stress arousal. This is healthy tension or eustress. But if this stress continues uncontrolled and a fatigue point is reached, any further stress arousal will take the performance level down, ultimately leading to exhaustion, ill-health and finally breakdown.

- If stress management is applied daily and regularly before the fatigue point is reached, the stress performance curve can be straightened up dramatically and the performance level can be improved.

Thinking Time !!

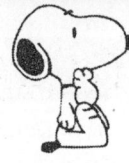

Look at the stress performance curve again and mark out where your position is now. If it is above the danger level, take immediate steps to bring it to normal. Take a printout of this graph and keep it with you. If your teacher is pushing you too hard without providing a break, show him / her the graph ☺

H.2. Effects of Stress on Organisation

Following effects are observed on the organisation due to stress:
- Increase in Absenteeism
- Increase in attrition

- Decrease in productivity
- Increase in unsafe working practices and accidents
- Increase in liability to legal claims and actions by stressed workers
- Damages the organisation's image both among its workers and externally
- In the long term it affects staff recruitment of the organisation

You should know

Measuring Stress- What Is Your Annual Stress Level?

Stress Level varies according to the type of stress you face. As described earlier, stress can occur during positsive changes as well as negative occurrences in your life.

To measure your annual stress level, take a printout of the following form and fill it out. Keep the score as a record for comparison after 1 year.

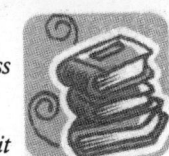

The Holmes and Rahe Stress Scale

S. No	Stress Event	Stress Points	No of Times/year	Score
1	Death Of Spouse/child	100	X	=
2	Divorce	73	X	=
3	Marital Separation	65	X	=
4	Detention in Jail	63	X	=
5	Death of Close Family Member	63	X	=
6	Major personal injury/ illness	63	X	=
7	Marriage	50	X	=
8	Marital reconciliation	45	X	=
9	Fired From Work	47	X	=
10	Retirement from Work	45	X	=
11	Major Health Problems In Family	44	X	=
12	Pregnancy	40	X	=
13	Sexual Difficulties	39	X	=
14	Gaining a new family member	39	X	=
15	Major Business Adjustments	39	X	=
16	Major Change In Financial State	38	X	=
17	Death Of A Close Friend	37	X	=
18	Changing To A Different Work	36	X	=
19	Major Arguments with spouse	35	X	=
20	Taking a Mortgage more than $5000	31	X	=
21	Foreclosure on a Mortgage/Loan	30	X	=
22	Major Change in Responsibility at Work	29	X	=
23	Son/Daughter leaving Home	29	X	=
24	In-Law Troubles	29	X	=
25	Outstanding Personal Achievement	28	X	=
26	Wife Beginning/Ceasing Work outside	26	X	=
27	Beginning or Ceasing formal school	26	X	=

28	Major Changes In Living Conditions	25	X	=
29	Revision Of Personal Habits	24	X	=
30	Troubles With The Boss	23	X	=
31	Major Change In Working Hours	20	X	=
32	Change In Residence	20	X	=
33	Changing To A New School	20	X	=
34	Major Change In Usual Type Of Recreation	19	X	=
35	Major Change In Religious Activities	19	X	=
36	Major Change In Social Activities	18	X	=
37	Taking A Mortgage less than $5000	17	X	=
38	Major Change In Sleeping Habits	16	X	=
39	Major change in family get-togethers	15	X	=
40	Major Change In Eating Habits	15	X	=
41	Vacation	13	X	=
42	Festival Celebrations	12	X	=
43	Minor Violations Of The Law	11	X	=
	GRAND TOTAL			=

SCORE KEY

Total Score	Comments
Below 50	Are you bored with life? Take action!
50-200	Congratulations! You are managing well.
200-300	Watch out! You need to slow down! Start Stress Management Program
Above 300	**You are above the board**

CAUTION: The above scale is only a guideline. Stress values may change according to individual responses to specific incidents in life.

I. STRESS MANAGEMENT

I.1. Individual Strategies to Cope with Stress

i. Problem-focused strategies

- These strategies help an individual cope with stress by identifying the source of stress and determining the course of action that will reduce the stress levels. For example, suppose an employee is assigned a task which he is not very clear about and he has to do it within a short span of time. Consequently, he is bound to feel stressed out.

- However, feeling tense or panicking will not help him. Instead, he can discuss his problem with his superior and request for help in the form of time, resources etc. By doing so, the employee feels relieved and is able to perform his job in a more effective manner.

The most commonly used problem-focused strategies are

a) Time management.

b) Requesting others for help.

c) Shifting to another job.

a. Time Management

A major reason for stress among individuals is poor time management. People become anxious, frustrated, and even panicky when they are not able to manage their time effectively. Therefore, people learn how to manage their time well so that they can complete their task and meet their deadlines. Some basic principles of time management are:

- Deciding on a daily basis the activities to be carried out along with the time frame for completing them.
- Prioritising the activities on the basis of their urgency and importance.
- Carrying out important activities first.
- Taking care of demanding tasks during that part of the day when one is very energetic and alert.

b. Requesting Others for Help

- A person can ask his colleagues or superior for help in dealing with certain work-related problems.
- Such support from peers and superior goes a long way in reducing the stress levels of employees.
- Alternatively, he could request the human resources department to provide him with additional training. This will help to update his knowledge and skills, thereby enabling him to deal with the stressors effectively.

c. Shifting to Another Job

- At times, employees may not be able to bring down their stress levels despite their best efforts.
- In such cases, it may be in the best interests of the individual to either change the nature of his job or seek employment in another organisation.
- However, before taking this extreme step, the employee should ask the management to change his job role if the stress is caused by various job- related problems.

ii. Emotion – Focused Strategies

a. Relaxation

Individuals can reduce their tension by means of certain relaxation techniques like meditation, hypnosis, and massage therapy.

b. Exercise

It has been medically proven that physical exercise such as walking, aerobics, jogging, swimming, cycling, tennis etc. are very effective in bringing down stress levels.

c. Psychological strategies

Certain psychological strategies, such as increased self-awareness and perceptual adaptation are used to control the effect of stress on an individual.

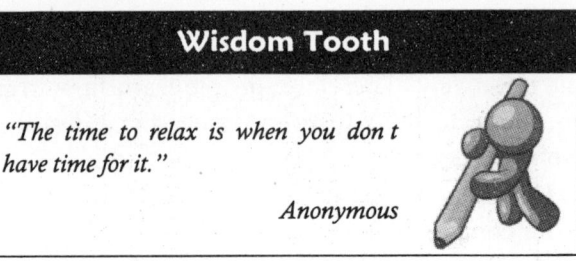

> **Wisdom Tooth**
>
> *"The time to relax is when you don t have time for it."*
>
> *Anonymous*

- Increased self-awareness makes a person perceptive to early signs of stress and thus helps him to manage stress effectively.

- Perceptual adaptation is a strategy that helps an individual to deal effectively with those stressors on which he either has no control or is unable to eliminate totally.

d. Recreation

If people work incessantly without respite, they are likely to feel stressed out. Everyone needs hobbies and recreation to take their minds off work and help them relax and enjoy themselves.

e. Companionship

Loneliness tends to make people stressed out. In general, people who have close and supportive relationships with their families and friends tend to experience lower levels of stress.

1.2. Organisational Strategies to Cope With Stress

i. Problem Focused Strategies

a. Redesigning the job

- Organisations can carry out a job analysis to determine the reasons for stress and the problems caused by it.

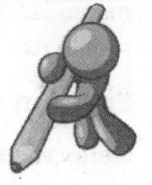

> **Wisdom Tooth**
>
> *"Stress is not what happens to us. It s our response to what happens.*
>
> *And response is something we can choose."*
>
> *Maureen Killoran*

- Job analysis can also help in determining, if there is role ambiguity or conflict, if employees are overloaded with work or have too little work, and whether the working conditions are good or not.

b. Proper selection and placement

The recruitment and selection policies of an organisation should clearly specify the educational qualifications, experience, skills and abilities that an employee should possess to handle a particular job. This will ensure employee- job compatibility.

c. Training

Proper training reduces work related stress among employees. It ensures that employees develop the necessary skills to perform their job effectively.

d. Team building

The rigid and impersonal work environment prevalent in many organisations is a major cause of high levels of stress among employees. Organisations can use the team based approach to help employees cope with stress related problems.

e. Providing various day care facilities

Employee's preoccupation with family problems increases the chances of errors and accidents and causes stress among employees. Therefore, many organisations provide in- house facilities in which employees can take care of their children and their elderly parents or relatives.

ii. Emotion Focused Strategies

a. Promoting open communication within the organisation

- Employees are likely to feel more stressed out when they are unsure about what is happening within the organisation.
- Ambiguity leads to percolation of rumours within the organisation and this may cause anxiety and tension among the employees.
- Therefore, employees should be kept informed about changes taking place within the organisation and how they are likely to be affected by these changes.

b. Employee assistance programs

This program helps employees by offering free counselling within the organisation or by referring them to specialists, who can help them cope with their problems.

c. Mentoring

Many organisations adopt a mentoring program in which employees with less experience are placed under the guidance and care of senior and experienced employees. Mentors reduce the stress levels of new employees as they clarify matters and guide them on task performance.

d. Wellness program and personal time off

Wellness programs are designed by the organisation to improve physical and mental condition of the employees. For example, workshops conducted by organisations to make their employees quit smoking.

e. Psychological Counselling

It is the discussion of any emotional problem with an employee in order to decrease it. It helps in reducing stress by allowing the employee to let out his feelings and emotions and gives him emotional support to find the solution to his problems.

TEST YOUR GREY MATTER

Q1)   What are the effects of stress on the individual and the organisation?

Q2)   What are the behavioural problems caused by stress?

Q3)   Stress and Performance are inversely related to each other. Do you agree? Explain.

Q4)   Discuss the strategies of coping with stress among workers in modern organisation.

Q5)   What are the steps taken by the management to combat stress among employees?

Q6)   Can redesigning the job be of any help to prevent stress? If yes, how?

Q7)   Time management is stress management. Comment.

CHAPTER

8 | Organisational Culture

By the end of this chapter, you would be able to

- Understand the concept and importance of Organisational Culture.
- Learn about different aspects of Organisational Culture.
- Know about Organisational Climate and its significance to the organisation.
- Identify various elements and factors that build Organisational Climate.
- Appreciate the concept of Morale.
- Know about the importance of morale and learn about different aspects of morale which affect the organisation.

The chapter contains :

- Concept of organisational culture
- Nature of organisational culture
- Elements of organisation culture
- Characteristics of organisational culture
- Role and significance of organisational culture
- Levels of organisational culture
- Components of culture
- Types of organisational culture
- Creation of culture
- Maintenance of culture
- Signs of organisational culture
- Concept of organisational climate
- Characteristics of organisational climate
- Elements of organisation climate
- Steps to build positive and employee centred climate
- Meaning of morale
- Nature of morale
- Factors influencing morale
- Importance of morale
- Measurement or evaluation of morale
- Building of high morale
- Types of morale
- Morale vs. Motivation

A. THE INSIGHT

What is the difference between?

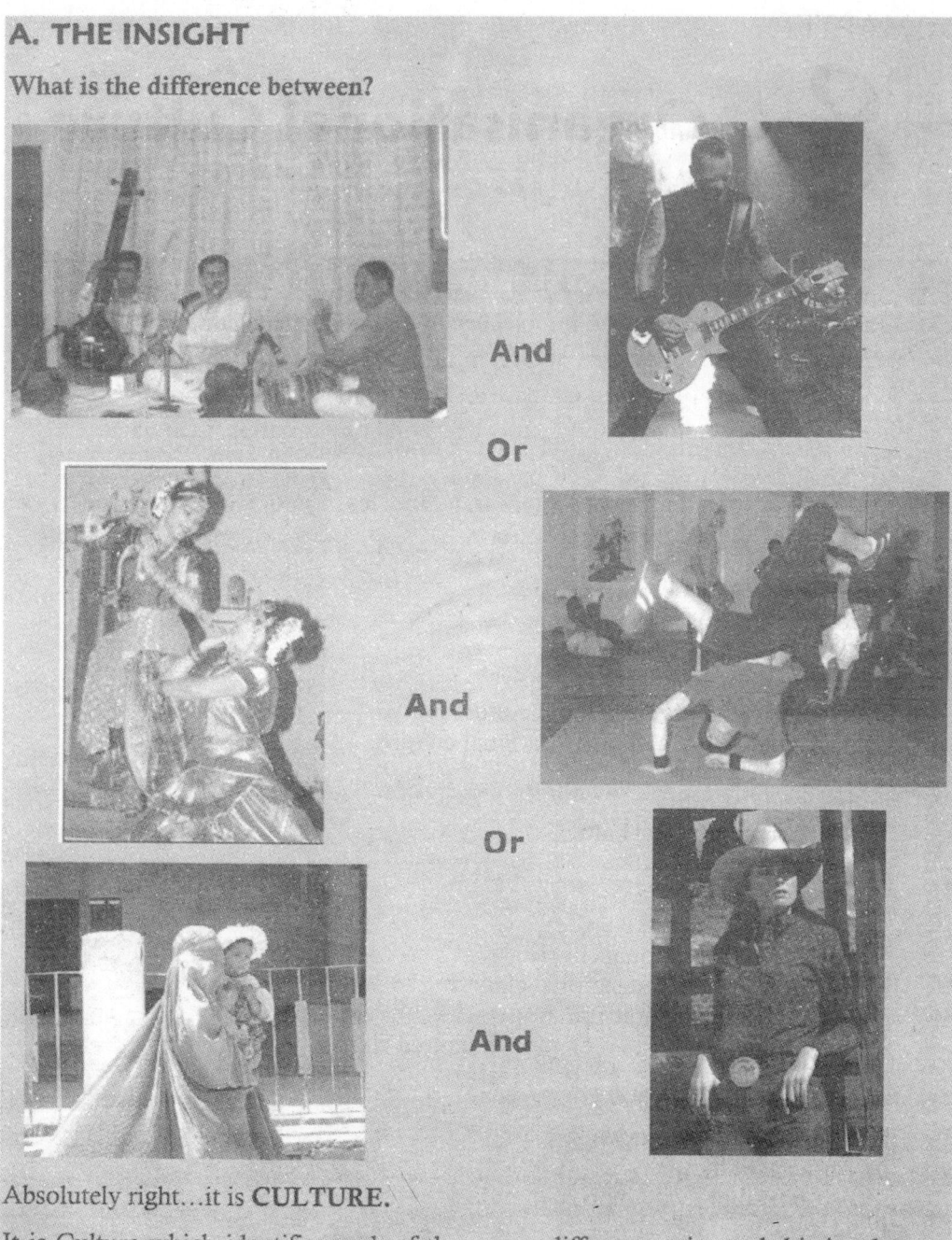

And

Or

And

Or

And

Absolutely right…it is **CULTURE.**

It is Culture which identifies each of them as a different entity and this is what we will study, but in the organisational context.

B. CONCEPT OF ORGANISATIONAL CULTURE

Organisational culture is an idea in the field of Organisational studies and management which describes the psychology, attitudes, experiences, beliefs and values of an organisation.

Definition: "Organisation Culture is the specific collection of values and norms that are shared by people and groups in an organisation and that control the way they interact with each other and with stakeholders outside the organisation."

C. NATURE OF ORGANISATIONAL CULTURE

- The culture of an organisation may reflect in various forms adopted by the organisation. These could be:

  i.   The physical infrastructure.

  ii.   Routine behaviour, language, ceremonies.

  iii. Gender equality, equity in payment.

  iv.   Dominant values such as quality, efficiency etc.

  v.   Philosophy that guides the organisation's policies towards its employees and customers like 'Customer first' and the manner in which employees deal with customers.

Together, they reflect organisational culture.

- In large organisations it is found that there is a dominant culture and a number of sub–cultures.

Dominant Culture: The core values shared by the majority of the organisational members constitute the dominant culture. Therefore, whenever one refers to the culture of an organisation, one actually talks about the dominant culture of an organisation.

Subculture: Subcultures within an organisation are a set of shared understandings among members of one group, department etc. For example, the human resource department of an organisation may have a sub–culture, unique and different from the production department.

This means that this department will not only have the core values of the organisation's dominant culture but also some unique values.

- Existence of dominant culture is mandatory to maintain consistency of behaviour and judge the effectiveness of various departments. Hence, the aspect of common or shared understanding is an essential component of organisational culture.

D. ELEMENTS OF ORGANISATIONAL CULTURE

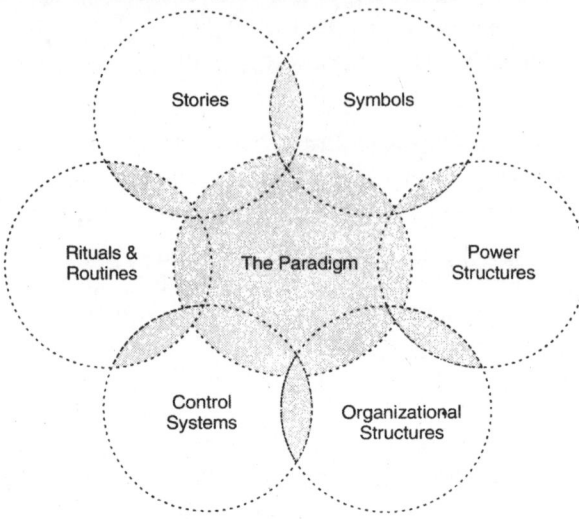

Johnson (1988) described a cultural web, identifying a number of elements that can be used to describe or influence Organisational Culture:

i. **The Paradigm**: What the organisation is about; what it does; its mission; its values.

ii. **Control Systems**: The processes in place to monitor what is going on.

iii. **Organisational Structures**: Reporting lines, hierarchies and the way that work flows through the organisation.

iv. **Power Structures**: Who makes the decisions, how widely spread is power, and on what is power based?

v. **Symbols**: These include organisational logos and designs, but also extend to symbols of power such as parking spaces and executive washrooms.

vi. **Rituals and Routines**: Management meetings, board reports etc.

vii. **Stories and Myths**: Build up about people and events, message about what is valued within the organisation.

E. CHARACTERISTICS OF ORGANISATIONAL CULTURE

i. **Innovation and Risk-Taking:** The degree to which employees are encouraged to be innovative and take risks.

ii. **Attention to Detail:** The degree to which employees are expected to exhibit precision, analysis, and attention to detail.

iii. **Outcome Orientation**: The degree to which management focuses on results or outcomes rather than on technique and process.

iv. **People Orientation**: The degree to which management decisions take into consideration the effect of outcomes on people within the organisation.

v. **Team Orientation**: The degree to which work activities are organised around teams rather than individuals.

vi. **Aggressiveness**: The degree to which people are aggressive and competitive rather than easygoing.

vii. **Stability**: The degree to which organisational activities emphasise maintaining the status quo in contrast to growth.

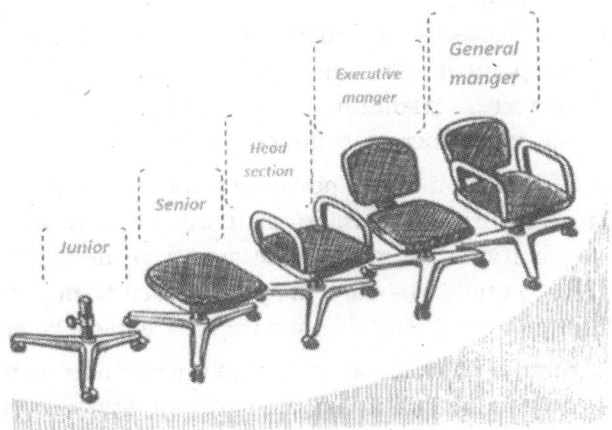

F. ROLE AND SIGNIFICANCE OF ORGANISATIONAL CULTURE

In a survey conducted by the management consulting firm Bain & Company in 2007, worldwide business leaders identified corporate culture to be as important as corporate strategy for business success. It has been found that Organisational Culture serves the following role which makes it an important asset to the organisation:

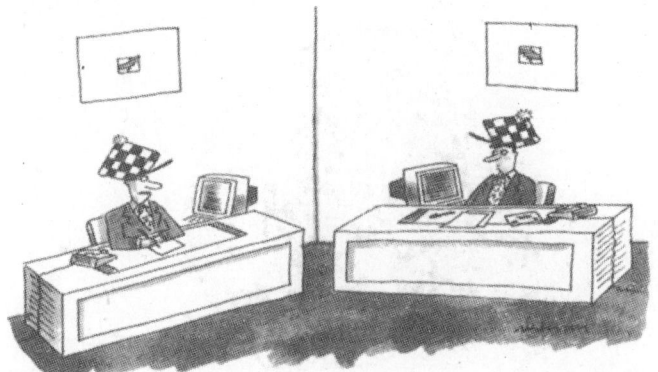

"I don't know how it started, either. All I know is that it's part of our corporate culture."

i. Culture, or shared values within the organisation, may be related to increased performance. Researchers found a relationship between organisational cultures and company performance, with respect to success indicators such as revenues, sales volume, market share and stock prices.

ii. Having the "right" culture may be a competitive advantage for an organisation and having the "wrong" culture may lead to performance difficulties, may be responsible for organisational failure, and may act as a barrier, preventing the company from changing and taking risks.

    For example, if a company is in the high-tech industry, having a culture that encourages innovativeness and adaptability will support its performance. However, if a company in the same industry has a culture characterised by stability, a high respect for tradition, and a strong preference for upholding rules and procedures, the company may suffer because of its culture.

iii. Organisational Culture is a more powerful way of controlling and managing employee behaviours than organisational rules and regulations. For example, when a company is trying to improve the quality of its customer service, rules may not be helpful, particularly when the problems customers present are unique. Instead, creating a culture of customer service may achieve better results.

iv. Culture creates sustainability for an organisation and acts as the most powerful force for cohesion. Organisations require stability in order to survive. Organisational culture can provide the stability by allowing people to communicate with each other, coordinate efforts, and differentiate members from non-members.

v. Organisation develops and grows because of the social recognition it gets due to its culture.

G. LEVELS OF ORGANISATIONAL CULTURE

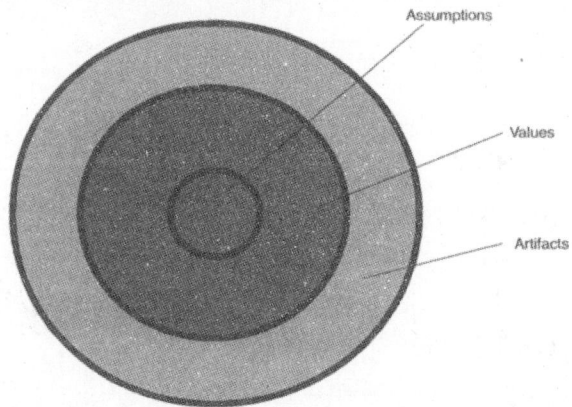

Organisational culture consists of some aspects that are relatively more visible, as well as aspects that may lie below one's conscious awareness. **Schein** divides organisational culture into three levels:

i. Basic Assumptions

- At the deepest level, below our awareness, lie basic assumptions.
- These assumptions are taken for granted and reflect beliefs about human nature and reality.

ii. Values

- At the second level, values exist; they are the heart of organisational culture.
- Values are shared principles, standards, and goals.
- Shared value helps turn routine activities into valuable, important actions that may provide a very distinctive source of competitive advantage.
- Values should be linked with work. Employees should be taken into confidence and good work done by them should be recognised so that other workers are motivated to work harder for the organisation.
- Organisations should therefore develop a "dominant and coherent set of shared values" so that individuals behave in line with the organisational philosophy.

iii. Artefacts

- Finally, at the surface, we have artefacts, or visible aspects of organisational culture.
- They include organisational heroes, rites and rituals, cultural symbols, saga, physical environment, employee interactions, company policies, reward systems and other observable characteristics.

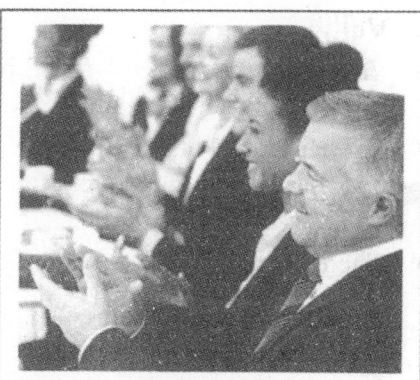

  □ **Organisational Heroes:** Organisational culture originates from the top management and their leadership styles. These leaders become the role model. Employees would like to copy their behaviour, work ethics and represent what an organisation stands for. Thus, the modelled behaviour helps in instilling organisational values.

  □ **Rites and Rituals:** These activities are also used to influence the behaviour and understanding of organisational members, like departmental song, colours and company picnic or retirement dinners.

- ❑ **Cultural symbols:** "Cultural symbols are the objects, acts, or events that serve to transmit a cultural meaning". Corporate uniform, tie, buttons etc. are examples of this.
- ❑ **Saga:** Saga is a heroic account of accomplishments. Sagas are important because they are used to tell new members the real mission of the organisation, how the organisation operates, and how an individual can fit into the organisational settings.
- ❑ Physical Environment, Employee Interactions include how people dress, where they relax, where they work, how they talk to others etc.

Now, we will look at all three together with an example.

In an organisation, a **basic assumption** employees and managers share might be that happy employees benefit their organisations. This might be translated into **values** such as equality, high-quality relationships and having fun. The **artefacts** reflecting such values might be an office layout that includes open spaces and gathering areas equipped with pool tables and frequent company picnics.

H. COMPONENTS OF CULTURE

Culture can be divided into five components: Values, Beliefs, Myths, Traditions and Norms.

i. Values

- Values are the ways in which individuals assess certain traits, qualities, activities or behaviours as good or bad, productive or wasteful.
- E.g. High level of service to the customer might be a core value of an organisation and this value might be reflected in such things as the organisation's motto, actual quality performance etc.
- There are two kinds of values:

    a) **Instrumental Values:** They represent the "means" an individual prefers to achieve important "ends."

    b) **Terminal Values:** They are preferences concerning the "ends" to be achieved.

ii. Beliefs

- Beliefs reflect individuals' understanding of the way the organisation works and the probable consequences of the action they take.
- In some organisation, people may have the belief that innovation is the way to get ahead while in other organisations, people may have the belief that controlling is the way to get ahead.

iii. Myths

- Myths are the stories or legends that persist within the organisation.
- For example, there can be a myth surrounding the danger of taking initiative in presenting new ideas.
- They are not written but are passed on to new members by signs or clues telling him what is to be done or what is not to be done.

iv. Traditions

- Traditions are repetitive significant events such as celebrations, special awards, retirement parties and holiday dinners.
- These events are a basic means of perpetuating culture values and highlight what is held in high esteem in the organisation.

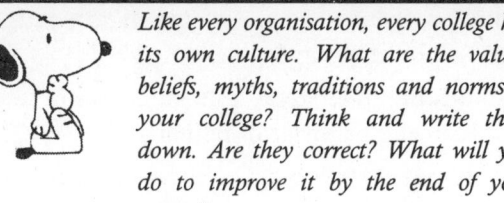

Thinking Time !!

Like every organisation, every college has its own culture. What are the values, beliefs, myths, traditions and norms of your college? Think and write them down. Are they correct? What will you do to improve it by the end of your course?

v. Norms

- Norms are organisational, informal rules regarding communication process, dress code, work habits, work hours, and implicit codes of interpersonal behaviour.
- These "rules of conduct" are not written down in any employee handbook.

I. TYPES OF ORGANISATIONAL CULTURE

Organisational culture can vary in a number of ways. Some of the bases of differentiation are presented below:

Strong and Weak Culture

- Organisational culture can be strong or weak based on the sharing of the core values among organisational members and the degree of commitment the members have to these core values.
- The higher the sharing and commitment, the stronger the culture and it increases the possibility of consistency of behaviour amongst its members. While in a weak culture, each one of the members shows behaviour unique to them.

Power Culture

- A power culture emanates from centralised power in a charismatic leader. This leader acts decisively and unilaterally, but always with the best intentions for the organisation.

- Power cultures are demanding of the people within the organisation. In a dysfunctional stage, power cultures can produce inefficient organisations where everyone waits for approval before moving forward on an idea.

- This is seen in organisations that have become too large for one person to maintain all the control and authority. Employees may also spend too much time playing political games and trying to curry favour with the boss instead of actually working.

- Members of this type of culture often become burnt out, and disloyal employees face a hostile and oppressive environment.

Role Culture

- A role culture is a highly structured environment where clear objectives, goals and procedures exist. An employee is judged almost solely on how well they meet these objectives and goals.

- In a functional stage, role cultures operate highly efficiently and include built-in checks and balances of power.

- This culture rewards dependability and consistency and due to its well articulated procedures, produces little stress.

- However, taken to extremes, role cultures can create an organisation of automatons that simply follow the rules and have very little concern for that which is not in their prescribed area. This mentality creates an environment where cooperation and collaboration are non-existent and a person's talent may go unused. Change comes very slowly in role cultures and those within the culture, especially a dysfunctional one, may become afraid to take risks.

Achievement Culture

- An achievement culture is one where people work hard to achieve goals and better the group as a whole.

- This culture generally consists of highly motivated people who need little or no supervision. Rules and procedures are limited as they may interfere with the accomplishment of work.

- When a rule gets in the way of achieving a goal, the rule is simply ignored. The best tools and methods for producing results are utilised, and when one goal is met, everyone quickly moves on to another.

- Because of this environment and mindset, achievement cultures tend to be highly adaptive.

- Unfortunately, members of achievement cultures tend to burn out on their work. It may be difficult to establish control if the need arises as the culture cultivates individuals.

- Members may also become highly competitive with each other and the mindset of "whatever it takes" can lead to dishonest and illegal behaviour.

Support Culture

- A support culture acts like a tiny community where people support and trust each other.

- Members of this culture will co-operate, make sure everyone is together on an idea, and do all that they can to resolve conflict. Support cultures consist of good communication and excellent service, both internal and external.

- This culture creates a nurturing environment where members like to spend time together and sometimes personal and professional lives can become blurred. When a support culture becomes dysfunctional, the needs of the individuals are placed over the needs of the organisation. Due to a commitment to consensus, decisions come slowly.

- Support cultures tend not to be very task-oriented. And too much time spent together fosters personal differences that often hinder work and ruin the excellent service that is a hallmark of support cultures.

Organisational culture can also be classified in the basis of **forms of attention and control orientation i.e. on the value matrix:**

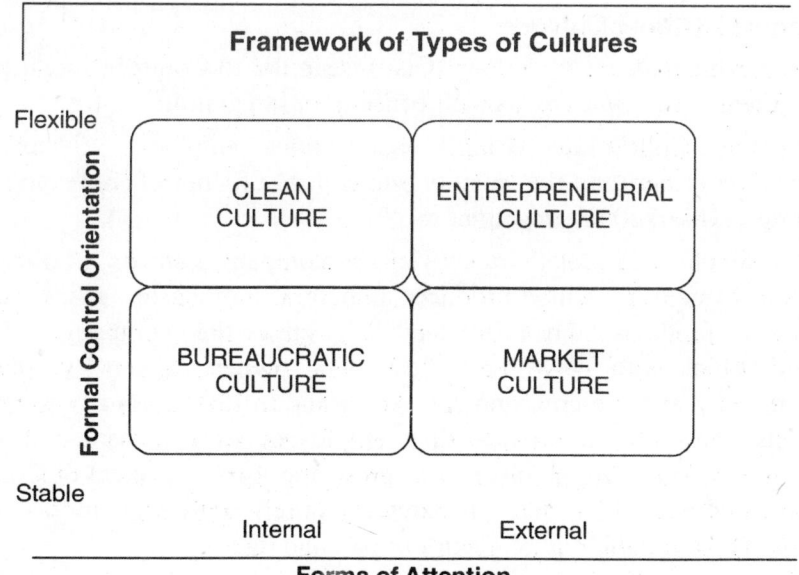

Framework of Types of Cultures

i. Control (Bureaucratic) Culture

- Bureaucratic cultures are defined by stability and control as well as internal focus and integration.
- They value standardisation, control and a well-defined structure for authority and decision making.
- Effective leaders in hierarchical cultures are those that can organise, coordinate and monitor people and processes.
- Good examples of companies with hierarchical cultures are McDonald's (they value standardisation and efficiency) and government agencies (they value rules and bureaucracy).

ii. Compete (Market) Culture

- In the value matrix Compete (Market) culture is similar to Control (Bureaucratic) in that they value stability and control; however, instead of an inward focus they have an external orientation and they value differentiation over integration.
- While most major American companies throughout the 19th and much of the 20th centuries believed a hierarchical organisation was most effective, the late 1960s gave rise to Compete (Market) organisations.

iii. Collaborate (Clan) Culture

- In the value matrix Collaborate (Clan) is similar to Control (Bureaucratic) in that there is an inward focus with concern for integration.
- However, Collaborate (Clan) organisations emphasise flexibility and discretion rather than the stability and control of Control (Bureaucratic) and Compete (Market) organisations.
- An example of a Collaborate (Clan) is company named 'X' owned by a person named 'Y', which produces all-natural toothpastes, soaps, and other hygiene products. The founder, 'Y', grew the company to respect relationships with co-workers, customers, owners, agents, suppliers, the community and the environment. According to their company statement of beliefs, they aim to provide their employees with "a safe and fulfilling environment and an opportunity to grow and learn." Typical of Collaborate (clan) cultures, 'X' is like an extended family with high morale and 'Y' himself takes on the role of mentor or parental figure.

iv. Create (Entrepreneurial/Adhocracy) Culture

- In the value matrix Create (Entrepreneurial) are similar to Collaborate (Clan) in that they emphasise flexibility and discretion; however, they do not share the same inward focus. Instead, they are like Compete (Market) in their external focus and concern for differentiation.

- Entrepreneurial or Adhocratic organisations value flexibility, adaptability, and thrive in what would have earlier been viewed as unmanageable chaos.
- High-tech companies like Google are prototypical Create (Entrepreneurial). Google develops innovative web tools, taking advantage of entrepreneurial software engineers and cutting-edge processes and technologies. Their ability to quickly develop new services and capture market share has made them leaders in the marketplace.

J. CREATION OF CULTURE

Creation of cultures provides understanding of how they can be changed and the factors that are most important in the creation of an organisation's culture include

- Founders' values and preferences
- Industry demands

i. Founder Values

- A company's culture, particularly during its early years, is tied to the personality, background and values of its founder(s), as well as their vision for the future of the organisation.
- When entrepreneurs establish their own businesses, the way they want to do business determines the organisation's rules, the structure set up in the company and the people they hire to work with them.
- Founder values become part of the corporate culture to the degree to which they help the company become successful.
- For example, the TATA Group still has commitment towards social services and charity as was established by Jamshedji Tata, the founder of TATA group and these values helped distinguish their brand from larger corporate brands and attracted a loyal customer base.

ii. Industry Demands

- While founders undoubtedly exert a powerful influence over corporate cultures, the industry characteristics also play a role.
- Companies within the same industry can sometimes have widely differing cultures.
- At the same time, industry characteristics and demands act as a force to create similarities among organisational cultures.
- For example, despite some differences, many companies in the insurance and banking industries are stable and rule-oriented, many companies in the high-

tech industry have innovative cultures, and those in the non-profit industry may be people-oriented. If the industry is one with a large number of regulatory requirements—for example, banking, health care, and high-reliability (such as nuclear power plant) industries—then we might expect the presence of a large number of rules and regulations, a bureaucratic company structure, and a stable culture.

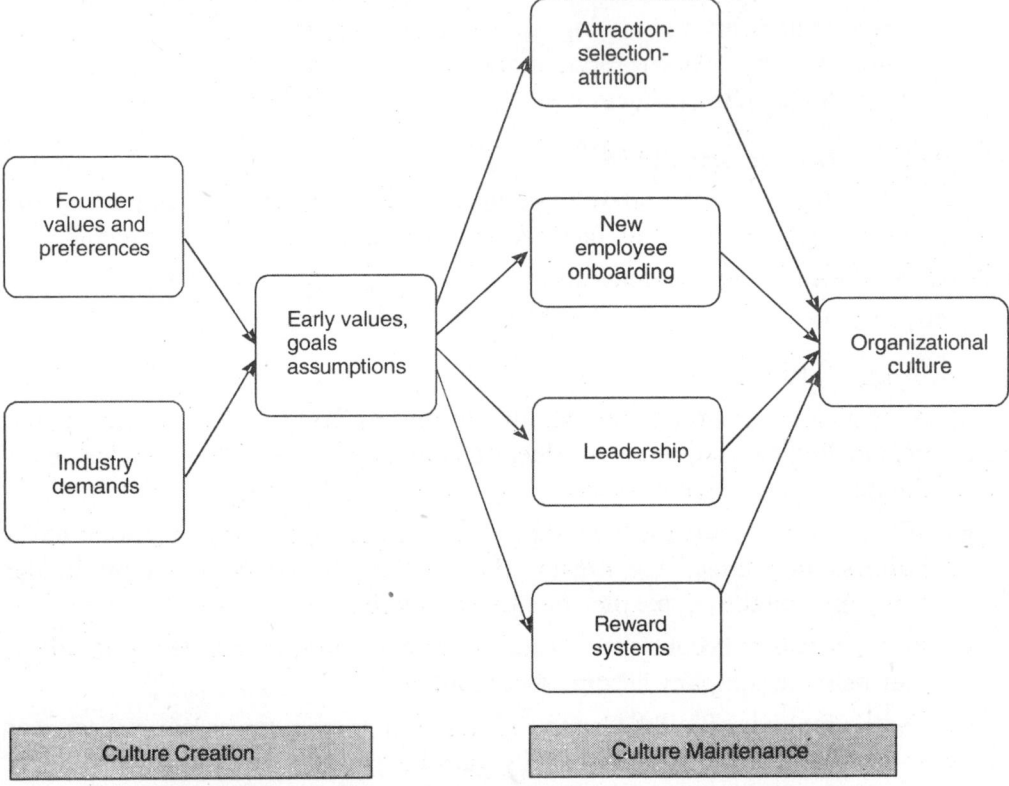

Figure: Model Describing How Cultures Are Created and Maintained

K. MAINTENANCE OF CULTURE

- As a company matures, its cultural values are refined and strengthened. The early values of a company's culture exert influence over its future values.

- Organisational culture determines what types of people are hired by an organisation and what types of people are left out.

- Moreover, once new employees are hired, the company assimilates new employees and teaches them the way things are done in the organisation. This process is called attraction-selection-attrition and on-boarding processes.

i. Attraction-Selection-Attrition

- Organisational culture is maintained through a process known as **attraction-selection-attrition (ASA).**

- First, employees are attracted to organisations. Someone who has a competitive nature may feel comfortable in and may prefer to work in a company where interpersonal competition is the norm. Others may prefer to work in a team-oriented workplace. Research shows that employees with different personality traits find different cultures attractive.

- At this point in the process, the second component of the ASA framework prevents them from getting in: **Selection.**

- Just as candidates are looking for places where they will fit in, companies are also looking for people who will fit into their current corporate culture. Many companies hire people who fit in their culture, as opposed to fit in a certain job.

- Even after a company selects people for person-organisation fit, there may be new employees who do not fit in. This results in the process of **Attrition.**

- Attrition refers to the natural process where the candidates who do not fit in leave the company.

ii. New Employee On-Boarding

- Another way in which an organisation's values, norms, and behavioural patterns are transmitted to employees is through on-boarding (also referred to as the **Organisational Socialisation Process**).

- On-boarding refers to the process through which new employees learn the attitudes, knowledge, skills, and behaviour required to function effectively within an organisation.

- If an organisation can successfully socialise new employees into becoming organisational insiders, new employees will feel accepted by their peers and confident regarding their ability to perform; they will also understand and share the assumptions, norms and values that are part of the organisation's culture.

- This understanding and confidence in turn translate into more effective new employees who perform better and have higher job satisfaction, stronger organisational commitment and longer tenure within the company.

- Organisations engage in different activities to facilitate On-boarding, such as implementing orientation programs or matching new employees with mentors.

iii. Leadership

- Leaders are instrumental in creating and changing an organisation's culture. There is a direct correspondence between the leader's style and an organisation's culture.

- For example, when leaders motivate employees through inspiration, corporate culture tends to be more supportive and people-oriented. When leaders motivate by making rewards contingent on performance, the corporate culture tended to be more performance-oriented and competitive. In these and many other ways, what leaders do directly influences the cultures of their organisations.

- Part of the leader's influence over culture is through role modelling. Many studies have suggested that leader behaviour, consistency between organisational policy and leader actions, and leader role modelling determine the degree to which the organisation's culture emphasises ethics. The leader's own behaviour will signal to individuals, what is acceptable behaviour and what is unacceptable.

- Leaders also shape culture by their reactions to the actions of others around them. For example, do they praise a job well done or do they praise a favoured employee regardless of what was accomplished? How do they react when someone admits to making an honest mistake? What are their priorities?

iv. Reward Systems

- Finally, the company culture is shaped by the type of reward systems used in the organisation and the kinds of behaviours and outcomes it chooses to reward and punish.

- One relevant element of the reward system is whether the organisation rewards **"behaviours"** or **"results"**.

- Some companies' supervisors and peers may evaluate an employee's performance by assessing the person's behaviour as well as the results. In such companies, we may expect a culture that is relatively people - or team - oriented, and employees act as part of a family.

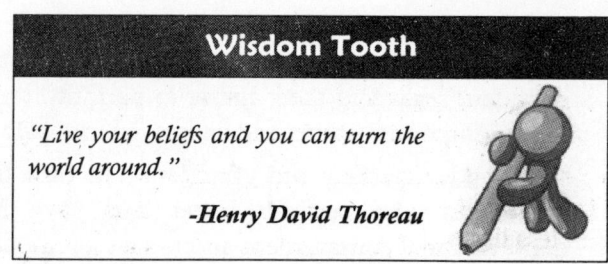

> **Wisdom Tooth**
>
> *"Live your beliefs and you can turn the world around."*
>
> *-Henry David Thoreau*

- However, in companies in which goal achievement is the sole criterion for reward, there is a focus on measuring only the results without much regard to the process. In these companies, we might observe outcome-oriented and competitive cultures.

- Whether the organisation rewards **"performance"** or **"seniority"** would also make a difference in culture. When promotions are based on seniority, it would be difficult to establish a culture of outcome orientation.

- Finally, the types of behaviours that are **"rewarded"** or **"ignored"** set the tone for the culture. Which behaviours are rewarded, which ones are punished, and which are ignored will determine how a company's culture evolves.

L. SIGNS OF ORGANISATIONAL CULTURE

- Culture influences the way members of the organisation think, behave, and interact with one another but how do you find out about a company's culture?

- There are many ways of finding out about a company's culture like observing employees or interviewing them and in this section we discuss five ways in which culture shows itself to observers and employees.

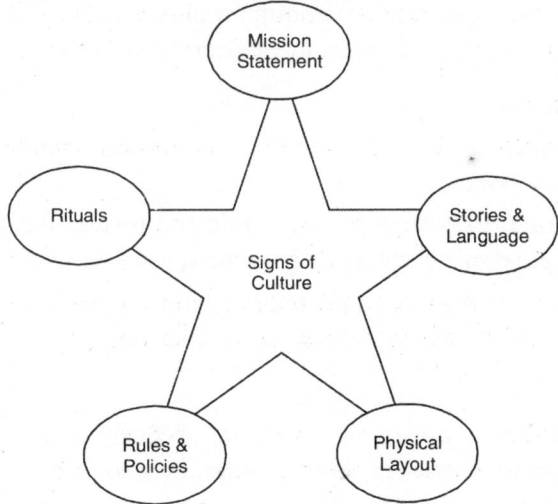

Figure: Visual Elements of Culture

i. Mission Statement

- A mission statement is a statement of purpose, describing who the company is and what it does. Though many companies have mission statements, they do not always reflect the company's values and its purpose.

- An effective mission statement is well known to the employees, is transmitted to all employees starting from their first day at work and influences employee behaviour.

- Some mission statements reflect who the company wants to be as opposed to who they actually are. If the mission statement does not affect employee behaviour on a day-to-day basis, it has little usefulness as a tool for understanding the company's culture.

- A mission statement that is taken seriously and widely communicated may provide insights into the corporate culture.

- For example, the Mayo Clinic's mission statement is "The needs of the patient come first." This mission statement evolved from the founders who are quoted as saying, "The best interest of the patient is the only interest to be considered." Mayo Clinics have a corporate culture that puts patients first.

ii. Rituals

- Rituals refer to repetitive activities within an organisation that have symbolic meaning.

- Usually, rituals have their roots in the history of a company's culture. They create friendship and a sense of belonging among employees. They also serve to teach employees corporate values and create identification with the organisation.

iii. Rules and Policies

- Another way in which an observer may find out about a company's culture is to examine its rules and policies.

- Companies create rules to determine acceptable and unacceptable behaviour and, thus, the rules that exist in a company signal the type of values it has.

- Policies about issues such as decision making, human resources, and employee privacy reveal what the company values and emphasises.

iv. Physical Layout

- A company's building, layout of employee offices and other workspaces communicate important messages about a company's culture.

- For example, the Nike campus in Beaverton is set on 74 acres and boasts an artificial lake, walking trails, soccer fields, and cutting-edge fitness centres. The campus functions as a symbol of Nike's values such as energy, physical fitness, an emphasis on quality and a competitive orientation. In addition, at fitness centres at the Nike headquarters, only those using Nike shoes and apparel are allowed in. This sends a strong signal that loyalty is expected.

- The layout of the office space also is a strong indicator of a company's culture. A company that has an open layout where high-level managers interact with employees may have a culture of team orientation and egalitarianism, whereas a company where most high-level managers have their own floor may indicate a higher level of hierarchy.

v. Stories and Language

- Perhaps the most colourful and effective way in which organisations communicate their culture to new employees and organisational members is through the skilful use of stories.

- A story can highlight a critical event an organisation faced and the organisation's response to it, or a heroic effort of a single employee illustrating the company's values. Stories usually engage employee emotions and generate employee identification with the company or the heroes of the tale.

- A compelling story may be a key mechanism through which managers motivate employees by giving their behaviour direction and by energising them towards a certain goal.

- Moreover, stories shared with new employees communicate the company's history, its values and priorities, and create a bond between the new employee and the organisation.

- Language is another way to identify an organisation's culture.

- Companies often have their own acronyms and buzzwords that are clear to them and help set apart organisational insiders from outsiders. In business, this code is known as jargon.

- **Jargon** is the language of specialised terms used by a group or profession. Every profession, trade, and organisation has its own specialized terms.

TEST YOUR GREY MATTER

Q1) What do you understand by Organisational Culture?

Q2) List out major Elements and Characteristics of Organisational Culture?

Q3) Differentiate between Dominant Culture and Sub-Culture?

Q4) What is the importance of Organisational Culture to the organisation?

Q5) Explain what are: (i) Basic Assumptions (ii) Values (iii) Artefacts

Q6) List out major components of Organisational Culture. Explain each of them.

Q7) How are 'Myths' and 'Beliefs' an important part of organisational culture?

Q8) What are the different types of cultures? Explain each of them briefly.

Q9) Differentiate between:

Control culture, Compete culture, Collaborate culture and Create culture

Q10) What is the influence of company founders on the company culture? Give examples based on your personal knowledge.

Q11) What is the role of physical layout as an indicator of company culture?

What type of a physical layout would you expect from a company that is people-oriented? Team-oriented? Stable?

Q12) Give the various factors of maintenance of organisational culture?

Explain (i) Attraction-Selection-Attrition.

(ii) New Employee On-boarding.

Q13) What are the methods of finding out the types of culture followed by any organisation?

M. CONCEPT OF ORGANISATIONAL CLIMATE

According to Bowditch and Buono "Organisational culture is the nature of beliefs and expectations about organisational life, while climate is an indicator of whether those beliefs and expectations are being fulfilled."

- Typical climates correspond to human feelings or moods: excitement, depression, anger, fear, optimism or anxiety.

- Like human mood, an organisation's climate can be caused by internal and external factors. If the CEO or other prominent leaders are in a certain mood, they can infect the entire organisation. Leaders whose moods are highly variable could lead to teams with wildly fluctuating climates.

- Just as most people won't be in the same mood all the time, an organisation's climate is also changing.

- Shifting emotions are good as it makes the organisation seem more human. It would be mechanical if the climate of the workplace never altered.

- An emotionally variable climate is, like a similarly expressive person, more open, transparent and understandable.

You should know

FUNNY TERMINOLOGY USED IN ORGANISATION AS A PART OF ITS CULTURE

- **Good Communication Skills:** *Spends lot of time on phone.*
- **Quick Thinking:** *Offers good excuses.*
- **Loyal:** *Cannot get a job anywhere.*
- **Outgoing Personality:** *Always going out of office.*
- **Active Socially:** *Drinks a lot.*
- **Independent worker:** *Nobody knows what he/she does.*
- **Careful Thinker:** *Won't make a decision.*
- **Uses Logic:** *Get someone else to do his job.*
- **Relaxed Attitude:** *Sleeps at desk.*
- **Work is First Priority:** *Too ugly to get a date.*

- We feel comfortable when we can read another person's feelings. The same applies to our workplace. It's unhealthy to suppress emotion in organisations or people.

N. CHARACTERISTICS OF ORGANISATIONAL CLIMATE

The nature of organisational climate will be clear from its following characteristics:

i. General Perception

Organisational climate is a general expression of what an organisation is. It represents the summary perception which people have about an organisation.

ii. Quality Concept

It is an abstract and intangible concept. It is difficult to explain the components of organisational climate in quantifiable units.

iii. Distinct Identity

It reflects how an organisation is different from another organisation. It gives a distinct identity to the organisation.

iv. Enduring Quality

It is built up over a period of time. It represents a relative quality of the internal environment that is experienced by the organisational members.

v. Multi-Dimensional Concept

There are several dimensions of the concept of organisational climate such as individual autonomy, authority structure, leadership style, pattern of communication, degree of conflict and cooperation etc.

O. ELEMENTS OF ORGANISATIONAL CLIMATE

i. **Flexibility** – how free the employees are to innovate

ii. **Responsibility** – degree to which the employees feel free to work without asking for the permission of and guidance from the manager

iii. **Standards** – the sign that the organisation emphasises excellence, that the goals for the employees are really high but attainable

iv. **Rewards** – the employees receive regular feedback and that they are rewarded accordingly

v. **Clarity** – the employees know, what is expected from them and how their efforts relate to the organisational goals

vi. Team Commitment – the employees know they belong to the winning team or the winning organisation and that all of the employees work towards the same goals or objectives.

P. STEPS TO BUILD POSITIVE AND EMPLOYEE-CENTRED CLIMATE

- Organisational climate clearly influences the success of an organisation. Many organisations, however, struggle to cultivate the climate they need to succeed and retain their most highly effective employees.
- Hellriegel and Slocum (2006) explain that organisations can take steps to build a more positive and employee-centred climate through:

    i.   **Communication** – how often and the means by which information is communicated in the organisation.

    ii. **Values** – the guiding principles of the organisation and whether or not they are modelled by all employees, including leaders.

    iii. **Expectations** – types of expectations with regard to how managers and employee behave and make decisions.

    iv. **Norms** – the normal, routine ways of behaving and treating one another in the organisation.

    v.   **Policies and rules** – these convey the degree of flexibility and restriction in the organisation.

    vi. **Programmes** – programming and formal initiatives help support and emphasise a workplace climate.

    vii. **Leadership** – leaders who consistently support the climate are desired.

Q. MEANING OF MORALE

Definition: "Morale is defined as the possession of a feeling, on the part of the employee, of being accepted and belonging to a group of employees through adherence to common goals and confidence in the desirability of these goals."

- The definition reveals three aspects

    (i)   Feeling of being accepted by one's work group.

    (ii) Sharing common goals with one's work group.

    (iii) Having confidence in the desirability of these goals.

- This definition also reveals that morale is the degree of enthusiasm and willingness with which the members of a group work to perform their assignments.

- Morale represents a composite of feelings, attitudes and sentiments that contribute to general feelings of satisfaction. It is a state of mind and spirit affecting the willingness to work, which in turn, affects organisational and individual objectives. It shapes the climate of an organisation.

R. NATURE OF MORALE

- Morale represents the collective attitudes of the workers.

- High morale represents an attitude of satisfaction with desire to continue and willingness to strive for the goals of the group. It is a manifestation of satisfaction, sense of contentment and need fulfilment through work.

- Morale is both an **individual** and a **group** phenomenon. In the group case, high morale is reflected in good team work and team spirit. Under conditions of high morale, workers have few grievances, frustrations and complaints; they are clear about the goals.

- Morale is multi-dimensional in nature, in the sense that it is a complex mixture of several elements. It recognises the influences of job situation on the attitudes of individuals and also includes the role of human needs as motivational forces.

> **Wisdom Tooth**
>
> *"The best morale exists when you never hear the word mentioned. When you hear a lot of talk about it, it is usually lousy."*
>
> *Dwight D. Eisenhower*

- Morale is mostly regarded as a long term phenomenon. Raising morale to a high level and maintaining it is a long-run and continuous process which can't be achieved through short-run measures such as gimmicks, contests or one-shot actions.

S. FACTORS INFLUENCING MORALE

Following factors affect morale within the workplace:

- Job security
- Management style
- Staff feeling that their contribution is valued by their employer
- Realistic opportunities for merit-based promotion
- The perceived social or economic value of the work being done by the organisation as a whole
- The perceived status of the work being done by the organisation as a whole
- Team composition

- The work culture

T. IMPORTANCE OF MORALE

- Employee Morale plays a vital role in the organisation's success. High Morale leads to success and Low Morale brings defeat in its wake. The success or failure of the organisation depends much upon the Morale of its employees.
- Morale of employees must be kept high to achieve the following benefits:
  i. Willing cooperation towards objectives of the organisation.
  ii. Loyalty to the organisation and its leadership or management.
  iii. Good discipline i.e. voluntary conformity to rules and regulations.
  iv. High degree of employees' interest in their jobs and organisation.
  v. Pride in the organisation.
  vi. Reduction of rates of absenteeism and labour attrition.

U. MEASUREMENT OR EVALUATION OF MORALE

- The indicators of morale are the various attitudes and behaviour patterns of employees, which have to be properly and correctly interpreted to determine the kind of organisational climate and morale which prevail at a given time.
- The statistical measurement of morale is not possible because it relates to the inner feelings of human beings. We can say that morale is increasing or decreasing, but cannot measure how much it has increased or decreased.
- Below are given some methods of measurement of the employee's morale which present only the tendencies or the attitude of the employee morale:
  i. Observation
  ii. Attitude or morale surveys
  iii. Company records
  iv. Counselling

i. Observation

- By this method, executives observe the behaviour of their employees, listen to them while they talk, and note their actions e.g. shrugging of shoulders, a change in facial expression, a shuffling of feet, a nervous fluttering of hands, a change in work habits or avoidance of company.
- Any departure or deviation from the normal is likely to tell them that something is wrong and needs to be set right.

ii. Attitude or Morale Surveys

- This method is generally used to discover the feelings of employees about their jobs, their supervisors, company policies or the organisation as a whole.
- It is classified into two categories – the interview method and the questionnaire method.

(a) The Interview Method

- In this method, employees are interviewed so that a judgement may be arrived at about their feelings and opinions about the different aspects of their jobs and the company for which they work.
- An interview may be a face to face affair or it may be oral or it may be in the form of an evaluation that is put down in writing.

(b) The Questionnaire Method

- This method is generally used to collect employee opinions about the factors which affect morale and their effect on personnel objectives.

iii. Company Records and Reports

- These are usually prepared by the personnel department at regular intervals with the assistance of supervisors and department heads.

iv. Counselling

- This method is used to find out the causes of the dissatisfaction of the employees and to take remedial action, and offer advice on personal matters.

V. BUILDING OF HIGH MORALE

Following factors are responsible for building high morale:

i. Fair Remuneration

- Considering the nature of the job, cost of living and pay scales of other companies, the wage structures should be properly evaluated, since this is the most important factor affecting employee morale.
- The basic and incentive pay plans should not only be fair, but should also bear fair relationship among them.

ii. Incentive System

- There should be a proper incentive system in the organisation to ensure monetary and non-monetary rewards to the employees to motivate them.

iii. Congenial Working Environment

- The conditions under which workers are made to work should be congenial for their mental and physical well-being.

- Adequate provision of light, air, safety, sanitation and cleanliness, noise prevention, smoke and fumes clearance, should be made for physical and mental comfort and satisfaction.

- The rest rooms, recreation facilities, canteen and cafeteria, gardening, medical, first aid and other such facilities may help in boosting the employee morale.

iv. Job Satisfaction

- The employees should be properly placed in the jobs according to their merits, aptitudes, interests and capabilities.

- A well placed employee takes pride and interest in his work and feels satisfied.

v. Two-Way Communication

- There should be two-way communication between the management and the workers as it exercises a profound influence on morale.

- The workers should be kept informed about the organisation policies and programmes through conferences, bulletins and informal discussion with the workers.

- Workers should be allowed to ask questions and satisfy themselves about their doubts.

vi. Training

- There should be proper training of the employees so that they may do their work efficiently and avoid frustration.

- When the workers are given training, they get psychological satisfaction as they feel that the management is taking interest in them.

vii. Workers' Participation

- There should be industrial democracy in the organisation. Management should allow workers' participation in management.

- Whenever a change is to be introduced which affects the workers, they must be consulted and taken into confidence.

- Workers must be allowed to put forward their suggestions and grievances to the top management

viii. Social Activities

- Management should encourage social group activities by the workers.

- This will help to develop greater group cohesiveness which can be used by the management for building high morale.

ix. Counselling

- Large organisations may appoint trained psychologists to act as counsellors for employees.
- The employees who do not wish to go to their supervisors for their problems can go to the counsellor, who is considered a man outside the chain of command and who enjoys staff position in management.

W. TYPES OF MORALE

There are broadly two types of Morale:

i. High Morale

- High morale represents enthusiasm among the workers for better performance.
- High Morale represents employee's strength, dependability, pride, confidence and devotion.
- Some of the advantages of high morale are:
  a) Willing cooperation towards objectives of the organisation.
  b) Loyalty to the organisation and its leadership.
  c) Good Leadership.
  d) Sound superior-subordinate relations.
  e) High degree of employee's interest in their job and organisation.
  f) Pride in the organisation.
  g) Reduction in absenteeism and labour attrition.
  h) Reduction in grievance.
  i) Reduction in industrial conflict.
  j) Team building.
  k) Employee empowerment.

ii. Low Morale

- Low morale indicates the presence of mental unrest. Mental unrest not only hampers production but also leads to dissatisfaction of the employees.
- Low morale exists when doubt and suspicion are common and when individuals are depressed and discouraged i.e. there is a lot of mental tension.
- Such a situation will have the following adverse consequences:
  a) High rates of absenteeism and labour attrition.

b) Excessive complaints and grievances.

c) Frustration among the workers.

d) Friction among the workers and their groups.

e) Antagonism towards leadership of the organisation.

f) Lack of discipline.

g) Decreased quality.

h) Decreased productivity.

X. MORALE AND PRODUCTIVITY

The relationship between Morale and Productivity is very complex and is not uniform. It varies with organisations and individuals, but generally there may be four possible combinations of morale and productivity:

i. High Morale And High Productivity

- This is the best state and a good manager should aim for it.
- It represents the best management techniques and best possible use of all the available resources.
- Thus, it occurs when all the conditions are optimum, such as - workers are motivated, they are properly trained and management is capable and concerned.

ii. Low Morale And Low Productivity

- It is the worst of all states.
- It occurs when workers are highly de-motivated and management is incapable of either increasing the morale or the productivity by any technique.
- It results in wastage of resources.

iii. High Morale And Low Productivity

- High morale with low productivity might occur due to several reasons. In this case though the workers are pleased, they are not motivated towards their work.
- It may also occur that workers might be motivated and give their best, yet productivity might decrease due to faulty materials and technology, wrong supervision, low degree of skills and weak management and planning.
- This situation mostly occurs in informal groups when morale of the individual is high due to fulfilment of social needs for belonging and affiliation, but the productivity is low because of restriction of output in accordance with informal group norms.

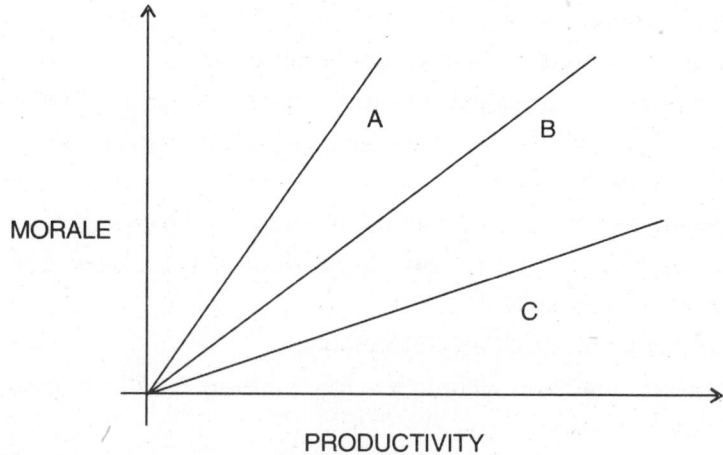

A = HIGH MORALE AND LOW PRODUCTIVITY

B = HIGH MORALE AND HIGH PRODUCTIVITY

C = LOW MORALE AND HIGH PRODUCTIVITY

iv. Low Morale And High Productivity

- High productivity with low morale occurs when management uses strict supervision, discipline and punishments.
- It is generally observed with low or semi-skilled workers.
- But this type of system does not work in the long run and may collapse suddenly.

Y. MORALE VS. MOTIVATION

- **Morale** encompasses employees' attitudes toward their work, their co-workers, their customers, and even themselves.

  In workplaces where morale is high, employees approach their work with energy, enthusiasm and willingness. They want to come to work and are enthusiastic about work once they get there. On the other hand, when morale is low, employees can become bored, discouraged and lethargic.

- **Motivation,** on the other hand, refers to employees' drive to get the job done. Highly motivated employees tend to be high producers, but that does not necessarily mean their morale is high. People are often motivated by "negative incentives" such as a fear of losing their job, an excessive need for rewards or an overly competitive need to outperform a colleague.

- Best results come when a workplace has both high morale and high motivation. Following are some ways to accomplish this:
  i. Reward employees for exceeding expectations

ii. Ask for employees' input when creating incentives

iii. Hold employees accountable for their performance

iv. Ask employees for their feedback on your performance and management style

v. Ask employees for their opinions and feelings on issues and decisions that impact the work environment

vi. Give employees all the information they need to do a great job

vii. Talk to employees about the overall mission of the business and about how their efforts contribute to it

viii. Provide regular feedback on performance

ix. Use proven, effective techniques for praising and correcting employee performance

x. Involve employees in decisions that affect their jobs

xi. Establish effective and user-friendly channels of communication

xii. Use "we" language

xiii. Always celebrate success

TEST YOUR GREY MATTER

Q1) Define (i) Organisational Climate and (ii) Morale.

Q2) What are the characteristics of Organisational Climate?

Q3) List out the elements of Organisational Climate.

Q4) How will you build a positive And Employee-Centred Climate if you are the head of an organisation?

Q5) Why is Morale important to an organisation? Explain.

Q6) How will you measure the Morale of an organisation?

Q7) Give the difference between High and Low Morale?

Q8) What factors are important for building the morale of employees?

CHAPTER

9

Leadership

By the end of this chapter, you would be able to :

- Understand about Leadership, its nature and features.
- Appreciate the importance of leadership in an organisation
- Learn about different types of leaders and their traits.
- Know about different theories and will be able to judge what factors are important for being a good leader.

The chapter contains :

- Leadership concept
- Features/Nature of Leadership
- Leadership skills
- Leadership vs. Management
- Role of leadership
- Functions of leadership
- Traits of a Good Leader
- Factors of Leadership
- Types of Leaders
- Leadership Styles
- Likert's four systems of management
- Leadership Theories
- Trait Approach to Leadership
- Behavioural Theories
- Situational Approaches to Leadership
- Successful versus Effective Leadership

A. THE INSIGHT

Following is the Story of one of the greatest leaders of all times

Alexander the Great

Alexander the Great was the son of a Macedonian general named Philip. His mother was Olympias. She told Alexander he was the son of a Greek god, and he seemed to think of himself as divine.

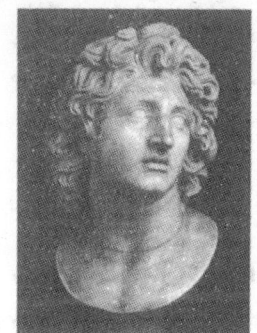

He was a pupil of Aristotle, one of the foremost philosophers of his time. He studied literature and learned to play the lyre. He was fearless and strong.

When he was 12 years old, he saw a fine horse he wanted. No one had been able to ride the horse. He determined the horse was terrified of his shadow and that's why he wouldn't let anyone near. He turned the horse so he was facing the sun. In this way he could not see his shadow. He got on the horse and was able to ride him.

His father bought the horse and Alexander named him Bucephalus. His father said to him, *"You must find a kingdom worthy of you, my son. Macedon is too small for you."*

He later built a city and named it after his horse, the city of Bucephala.

Alexander became one of the greatest generals in history. When he conquered the Persians, he honoured their soldiers and commander who had died in battle. When he won a battle, he combined the remaining soldiers of the enemy with his army to form a greater army. He usually did not allow his soldiers to mistreat the conquered people.

He suffered along with his soldiers when they were at war. If they didn't have water or food, he would not accept food or drink either. When the soldiers were walking, he walked also and refused to ride or be carried. He set an example for his troops.

He is still known to be one of the greatest leaders of the world. He conquered the whole world by his power of leadership.

B. LEADERSHIP CONCEPT

Definition: Leadership is a process of social influence in which one person can enlist the aid and support of others in the accomplishment of a common task.

- Thus, leadership is a quality in which one person influences the behaviour of others to attain certain objectives.

- Similarly, in an organisational context a leader tries to influence his subordinates to shape the goal of an organisation and motivates their behaviour towards the attainment of organisational objectives.

C. FEATURES/NATURE OF LEADERSHIP

- Leadership is not a single activity; rather it is a continuous process.
- Basic purpose of a leader is to influence the behaviour of others or followers.
- It is a relationship between the leader and his followers.
- Objective of leadership is attainment of common objectives of both leader and his followers.
- Leadership is a situation-related activity. It is at a particular point of time and in a given set of circumstances.

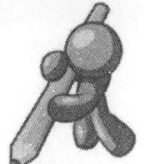

Wisdom Tooth

"Leadership is the art of influencing and directing people in such a way that will win their obedience, confidence, respect and loyal cooperation in achieving common objectives."

U. S. Air Force

D. LEADERSHIP SKILLS

A behavioural expert, Robert Katz, had identified that leaders broadly use three skills- technical, human and conceptual skills.

i. Technical Skills

- A person's knowledge and ability to make effective use of any process or technique constitutes his technical skills.
- Employees at operational and professional levels are required to have certain technical skills (for e.g. an engineer, an accountant).

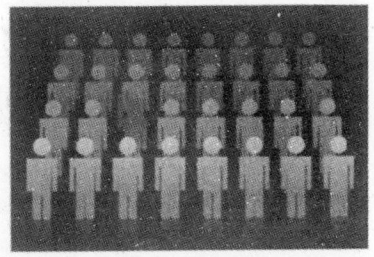

- However, as employees are promoted to managerial positions, these technical skills become less relevant, while other skills become more important. (See Fig. 1)

ii. Human Skills

- An individual's ability to cooperate with other members of the organisation and work effectively in teams is referred to as human skills.
- Human skills also involve developing positive interpersonal relationships, solving people's problems and gaining acceptance of other employees.

- Effective human skills are an essential requirement at all levels of the organisational hierarchy and especially for people in leadership positions.

iii. Conceptual Skills

- Conceptual skills refer to the ability of an individual to analyse complex situations and to rationally process and interpret available information.
- It also encompasses an ability to foresee the future consequences of his present day actions from the organisational point of view.
- Conceptual skills are of least importance to employees at the operational level and are of utmost importance to managers at higher levels.

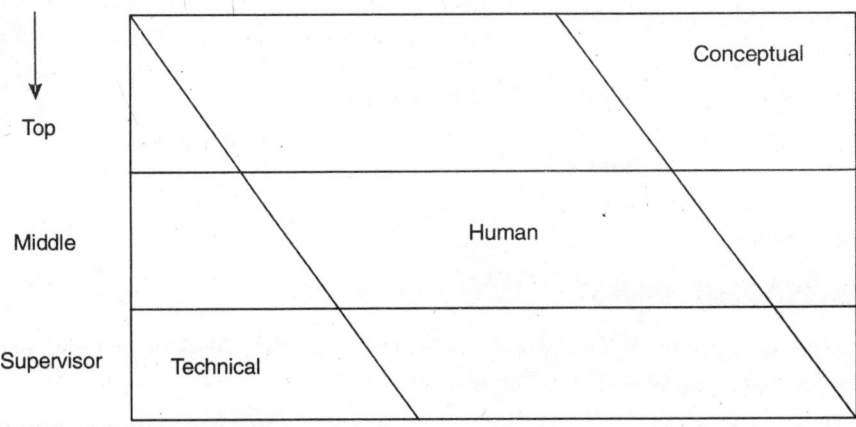

Fig.1 Knowledge and skills required

E. LEADERSHIP VS. MANAGEMENT

"Leaders manage and managers lead, but the two activities are not synonymous.... Management functions can potentially provide leadership; leadership activities can contribute to managing. Nevertheless, some managers do not lead, and some leaders do not manage". This is **Bernard Bass's** assessment in his 1,200 page opus, *"Bass and Stogdill s Handbook of Leadership"* (page 383).

- **Warren Bennis** – popular writer of leadership resources and business professor at the University of Southern California – shares the same view.
    - "There is a profound difference between management and leadership, and both are important. To manage means to bring about, to accomplish, to have charge of or responsibility for, to conduct. Leading is influencing, guiding in a direction, course, action, opinion. The distinction is crucial".

❑ He says, "Managers are people who do things right and leaders are people who do the right thing".

- Bennis further defines the difference using the following paired contrasts *(taken from, "Learning to Lead: A Workbook on Becoming a Leader", p. 9. Perseus Books / Addison Wesley, 1997):*

i. The manager administers; the leader innovates.

ii. The manager maintains; the leader develops.

iii. The manager accepts reality; the leader investigates it.

iv. The manager focuses on systems and structures; the leader focuses on people.

v. The manager relies on control; the leader inspires trust.

vi. The manager has a short-range view; the leader has a long-range perspective.

vii. The manager asks how and when; the leader asks what and why.

> ### Wisdom Tooth
>
> *"A manager takes people where they want to go. A great leader takes people where they don t necessarily want to go but ought to."*
>
> ***Rosalyn Carter***

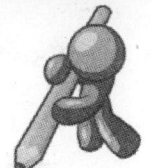

viii. The manager has his or her eye always on the bottom line; the leader has his or her eye on the horizon.

ix. The manager imitates; the leader originates.

x. The manager accepts the status quo; the leader challenges it.

xi. The manager is the classic good soldier; the leader is his or her own person.

F. ROLE OF A LEADER

1. **Initiates Action:** Leader is a person who starts the work by communicating the policies and plans to the subordinates from where the work actually starts.

2. **Motivation:** He motivates the employees with economic and non-economic rewards and thereby gets work done by the subordinates.

3. **Providing Guidance:** A leader has to not only supervise but also play a guiding role for the subordinates. Guidance here means instructing the subordinates in the way they have to perform their work effectively and efficiently.

4. **Creating Confidence:** Confidence is an important factor which can be achieved through expressing the work efforts to the subordinates, explaining them their role clearly and giving them guidelines to achieve the goals effectively. It is also important to hear the employees with regards to their complaints and problems.

5. **Building Morale:** Morale denotes willing co-operation of the employees towards their work and getting them into confidence and winning their trust. A leader can be a morale booster by achieving full co-operation so that they perform to the best of their abilities as they work to achieve goals.

6. **Builds Work Environment:** An efficient work environment helps in sound and stable growth. Therefore, human relations should be kept in mind by a leader. He should have personal contacts with employees and should listen to their problems and solve them. He should treat employees on humanitarian terms.

7. **Co-ordination:** Co-ordination can be achieved through reconciling personal interests with organisational goals. This synchronisation can be achieved through proper and effective co-ordination which should be the primary motive of a leader.

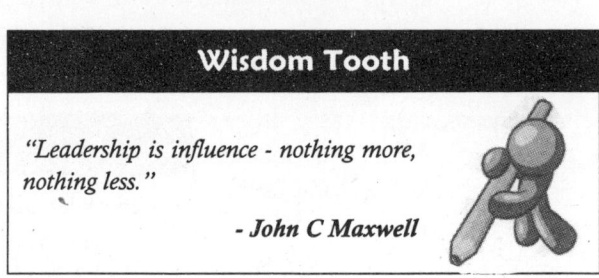

Wisdom Tooth

"Leadership is influence - nothing more, nothing less."

- John C Maxwell

G. FUNCTIONS OF LEADERSHIP

1) To Develop Team Work

The first basic function of the leader is to develop his work-group as a team. The responsibility of a leader is to create a friendly work-environment by keeping a close view of his subordinates' competence, needs and potential abilities.

2) To Act as a Representative of the Work-Group

The leader of a work-group is expected to act as a link between the group and the top management. The leader is expected to communicate the problems and grievances of his subordinates to top management in desired circumstances.

3) To Act as a Counsellor of the People at Work

The leader is expected to guide and advise the concerned subordinate when he is facing problems in connection with his performance at work.

4) Time Management

The leader's function is to check the timely completion at different stages of work and also ensure quality and efficiency of work performed by the group.

5) Proper Use of Power

The leader should be intelligent and observant enough to exercise his power in relation to his subordinates in different ways as per the needs of the situation. The leader can use powers like reward power, coercive power, expert power, formal or informal power to stimulate positive response from his subordinates.

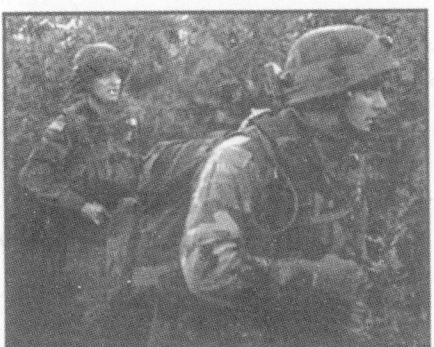

Soldiers patrol during a training exercise in the final phase of the Primary Leadership Development Course. The course allows junior enlisted soldiers deployed to receive the professional development training they need to become better leaders. - U.S. Army photo by Spc. Jorge Lozada.

H. TRAITS OF A GOOD LEADER

Source: Compiled by the Santa Clara University and the Tom Peters Group:

- **Honest:** They display sincerity, integrity, and honesty in all actions. Deceptive behaviour does not inspire trust.
- **Competent:** Their actions are based on reason and moral principles; they do not make decisions based on childlike emotional desires or feelings.
- **Forward-looking:** They set goals and have a vision of the future. The vision must be owned throughout the organisation. Effective leaders envision what they want and how to get it. They habitually pick priorities stemming from their basic values.
- **Inspiring:** They display confidence in all that they do. By showing endurance in mental, physical, and spiritual stamina, they inspire others to reach for new heights.
- **Intelligent:** They read, study, and seek challenging assignments.
- **Fair-minded:** They show fair treatment to all people. Prejudice is the enemy of justice. They display empathy by being sensitive to the feelings, values, interests and well-being of others.

- **Broad-minded:** They seek out diversity.

- **Courageous:** They have the perseverance to accomplish a goal, regardless of the seemingly insurmountable obstacles. They display a confident calmness when under stress.

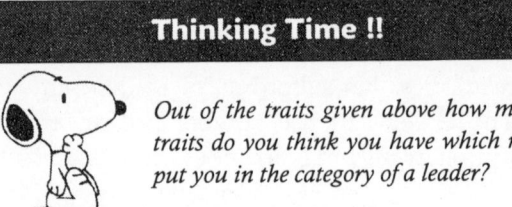
- **Straightforward:** They use sound judgment to make good decisions at the right time.

- **Imaginative:** They make timely and appropriate changes in thinking, plans, and methods. They show creativity by thinking of new and better goals, ideas, and solutions to problems. They are innovative.

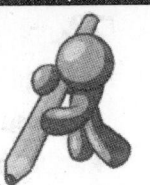
I. FACTORS OF LEADERSHIP

There are four major factors in leadership:

i. Follower

- Different people require different styles of leadership. For example, a new hire requires more supervision than an experienced employee.

- A person who lacks motivation requires a different approach than one with a high degree of motivation.

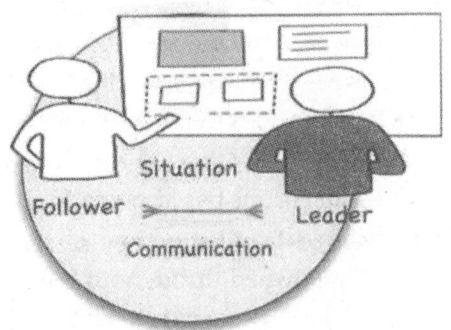

- The fundamental starting point is having a good understanding of human nature, such as needs, emotions and motivation.

ii. Leader

- Leader must have an honest understanding of himself, what he knows, and what he can do.

- It is the followers, not the leader who determine if a leader is successful. If they do not trust or lack confidence in their leader, then they will be uninspired. To be successful, a leader has to convince his followers that he is worthy of being followed.

iii. Communication

- Leaders lead through two-way communication. Much of it is non-verbal.
- What and how a leader communicates either builds or harms the relationship between him and his employees.

iv. Situation

- All situations are different. What one does in one situation may not always work in another. Leaders use their judgment to decide the best course of action and the leadership style needed for each situation

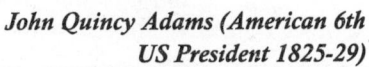
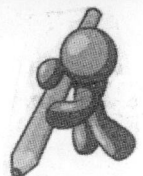

Wisdom Tooth

"If your actions inspire others to dream more, learn more, do more and become more, you are a leader."

John Quincy Adams (American 6th US President 1825-29)

- For example, a leader may need to confront an employee for inappropriate behaviour, but if the confrontation is too late or too early, too harsh or too weak, then the result may prove ineffective.
- Various forces affect these factors. Examples of the forces are leader's relationship with his seniors, the skill of his people, the informal leaders within the organisation, and how the company is organised.

J. DISTINGUISHING BETWEEN TYPES OF LEADERS AND STYLES OF LEADERSHIP

- There seems to be no standard academic way of distinguishing between "types" of Leaders and "styles" of Leadership. But, in this course, the terms have specific meanings and there is an important distinction between them.
  - □ A **"type" of Leader** is determined and identified by the "personality" displayed by the leader in terms of the core trait that is emphasised and by the combination of other core traits and personal qualities that are displayed and used to gain the trust of the people and lead them to commit to undertaking the major task facing the organisation.
  - □ A **"style" of Leadership** is defined and identified by the competencies and skills that the leader "applies" to guide, facilitate and support the people of the organisation in their efforts to accomplish the task.

K. TYPES OF LEADERS

There are three generally accepted types of leaders—Charismatic, Transactional, Transformational.

K.1.Charismatic Leader

- A leader has some charisma which acts as a influencer.
- Charisma is a God-gifted attribute in a person which makes him a leader irrespective of the situation in which he works.
- Charismatic leaders are those who inspire followers and have a major impact on their organisations through their personal vision and energy.
- According to **Robert House** *"Charismatic leader has extremely high levels of self confidence, dominance, and strong conviction in the normal righteousness of his/her beliefs, or at least the ability to convince the followers that he/she possesses such confidence or conviction."*
- Examples of charismatic leaders: 1. Mahatma Gandhi 2. Swami Vivekananda

- **Characteristic of charismatic leaders are –**
  - ❑ Followers accept the leader unquestioningly.
  - ❑ Followers obey the leader willingly.
  - ❑ Followers' beliefs are similar to the leader's beliefs.
  - ❑ Followers trust the correctness of the leader's belief.

Charismatic leadership

- Max Weber, a sociologist, was the first scholar to discuss Charismatic Leadership.
- He defined **Charisma** (from Greek for "gift") as a certain quality of an individual personality, by virtue of which he or she is set apart from ordinary people and treated as endowed with supernatural, superhuman, or at least specifically exceptional powers or qualities.
- According to Robert House's **Charismatic Leadership Theory**, followers make attributions of heroic or extraordinary leadership abilities when they observe certain behaviours.

Key Characteristics of a Charismatic leader

i. **Vision and Articulation**: Has a vision expressed as an idealised goal-that proposes future better than the status quo; and is able to clarify the importance of the vision in terms that are understandable to others.

ii. **Personal risk**: Willing to take on high personal risk, incur high costs, and engage in self sacrifice to achieve the vision.

iii. **Sensitivity to followers' needs**: Perceptive of others' abilities and responsive to their needs and feelings.

iv. **Unconventional Behaviour**: Engages in behaviours that are perceived as novel and counter to norms.

K.2. & K.3. Transactional and Transformational leaders

- In general, a relationship between two people is based on the level of exchange they have. Exchange need not be money or material; it can be anything. The more exchange they have the stronger the relation. A manager expects more productivity from employee in order to give good rewards. In this way, if something is done to anyone based on the return, then that relation is called as **'Transactional'**.

- In politics, a leader announces benefits in their agenda in exchange for the vote of the citizens. In business, a leader announces rewards in return for productivity. These relations are all about requirements, conditions and rewards (or punishment). Leaders who show this kind of relationship are called *'Transactional Leaders'*.

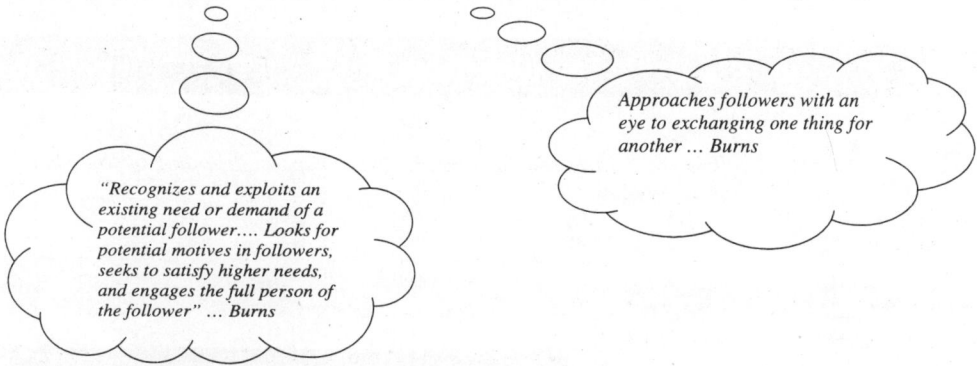

"Recognizes and exploits an existing need or demand of a potential follower.... Looks for potential motives in followers, seeks to satisfy higher needs, and engages the full person of the follower" ... Burns

Approaches followers with an eye to exchanging one thing for another ... Burns

- In life, at one point of time, things happen without expectation from the other side. For example, a mother's dedicated service to her kid. A mother does not expect anything from the child and the service she provides in raising the child is unconditional, dedicated, committed. Mother plays a major role in shaping the kid's life. This type of relation is called as **'Transformational'**.

- Leaders do exist in this world with these behaviours. Transformational leaders work towards a common goal with followers; put followers in front and develop them; take followers' to next level; inspire followers to transcend their own self-interests in achieving superior results.

Transactional Leadership	Transformational Leadership
<ul><li>Leaders are aware of the link between the effort and reward</li><li>Leadership is responsive and its basic orientation is dealing with present issues</li><li>Leaders rely on standard forms of inducement, reward, punishment and sanction to control followers</li><li>Leaders motivate followers by setting goals and promising rewards for desired performance</li><li>Leadership depends on the leader's power to reinforce subordinates for their successful completion of the bargain.</li></ul>	<ul><li>Leaders arouse emotions in their followers which motivates them to act beyond the framework of what may be described as exchange relations</li><li>Leadership is proactive and forms new expectations in followers</li><li>Leaders are distinguished by their capacity to inspire and provide individualised consideration, intellectual stimulation and idealised influence to their followers</li><li>Leaders create learning opportunities for their followers and stimulate followers to solve problems</li><li>Leaders possess good visioning, rhetorical and management skills, develop strong emotional bonds with followers</li><li>Leaders motivate followers to work for goals that go beyond self-interest.</li></ul>

Thinking Time !!

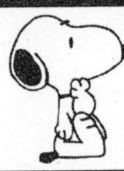

We talked about Alexander at the start of our chapter. According to you what type of leader is he? Why?

L. LEADERSHIP STYLES

- The way in which leaders influence their followers is referred to as leadership style.

- The leadership style of an individual is determined by the extent of control he exercises over his followers and the way he behaves with them.

Wisdom Tooth

"Transactional leaders work within the organisational culture as it exists; the transformational leader changes the organisational culture".

Bass

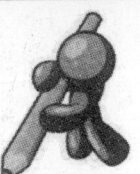

- It also depends on the types of duties the leader performs and the types of duties and responsibilities he gives to his followers.

- Following are the leadership styles:

L.1.Autocratic Leadership Style

Leaders who adopt this style retain all the authority and decision making power. They do not consider employee's suggestions, opinions or views. They believe that they are more competent and intelligent than their subordinates.

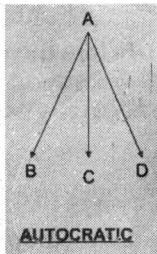

Characteristics of Autocratic Leadership Style

- The classical approach.
- Staff expected to obey orders without receiving any explanations.
- Structured set of rewards and punishments.
- Rely on threats and punishment to influence staff.
- Do not trust staff.
- Communication flows from the leader to the followers.

Should be used when	Should not be used when
o *New, untrained staff do not know which tasks to perform or which procedures to follow* o *Effective supervision provided only through detailed orders and instructions* o *Staff do not respond to any other leadership style* o *Limited time in which to make a decision* o *A manager s power challenged by staff* o *Work needs to be coordinated with another department or organisation*	o *Staff become tense, fearful, or resentful.* o *Staff expects their opinions to be heard.* o *Staff depends on their manager to make all their decisions.* o *Low staff morale, high attrition and absenteeism and work stoppage.*

There Are Three Categories of Autocratic Leadership Styles:-

i. **Strict Autocrat:** He follows autocratic styles in a very strict sense. His method of influencing subordinates' behaviour is through negative motivation, that is, by criticising subordinates, imposing penalty etc.

ii. **Benevolent Autocrat:** He also has centralised decision-making power in him, but his motivation style is positive. Some people like to work under strong authority and they derive satisfaction from this leadership.

iii. Incompetent Autocrat: Sometimes, superiors may adopt autocratic leadership style just to hide their incompetence because in other styles they may be exposed before their subordinates. However, this cannot be used for a long time.

Advantages

i.   Managers provide strong motivation and reward to the workers.

ii. Quick decisions as they are made by only one person.

iii. Less competent subordinates also have scope to work in the organisation under this style as they do negligible planning, organising, and decision making.

Limitations of Autocratic Leadership

i.   People in the organisation dislike it, especially when it is strict and the motivation style is negative.

ii. Employees lack motivation as frustration, low morale, and conflict developed in the organisation affects the organisational efficiency.

iii. There is more dependence and less individuality in the organisation. As such, future leaders in the organisation do not develop.

L.2.Participative Leadership Style

Definition: Participation is defined as mental and emotional involvement of a person in a group situation which encourages him to contribute to group goals and share responsibility in them.

* **Characteristics of this leadership style are:**

    ❑ Participative leaders encourage employees to participate in decision making. The leader listens to subordinates' ideas and opinions, but takes the final decision himself.

    ❑ They keep the staff informed about everything that affects their work and shares decision making and problem solving responsibilities

    ❑ It is also known as **Consultative, Democratic or Ideographic Style.**

PARTICIPATIVE

Should be used when	Should not be used when
o *Wants to keep staff informed about matters that affect them.* o *Wants to provide opportunities for staff to develop a high sense of personal growth and job satisfaction.*	o *If security is an issue, this style may be inappropriate because many people are involved from an early stage* o *If there is a time constraint, this style should not be used because it is slow*

o *A large or complex problem that requires lots of input to solve* o *Want to encourage team building and participation.*	*and time consuming.*

Advantages

i. Highly motivating technique for employee.

ii. Employee's productivity is high because of active participation of employees in decision-making.

iii. They share the responsibility with the superiors and try to safeguard him also.

iv. It provides organisational stability by raising morale and attitude of employees.

Disadvantage

i. Complex nature of organisation requires a thorough understanding of its problems which lower level employees may not be able to do. As such, participative does not remain meaningful.

ii. Some people in the organisation want minimum interaction with their superiors or associates. For them, participative technique is discouraging instead encouraging.

iii. Participation can be used covertly to manipulate employees.

L.3.Laissez-Faire Leadership Style

• The leader completely delegates the responsibilities, and decision making power to the subordinates.

• Typically this happens when the team is highly capable and motivated, and it doesn't need close monitoring or supervision.

• **Characteristics of this leadership style are:**

❑ It is also known as the "hands-off" style.

❑ The manager provides little or no direction and gives staff as much freedom as possible.

❑ All authority or power is given to the staff and they determine goals, make decisions, and resolve problems on their own.

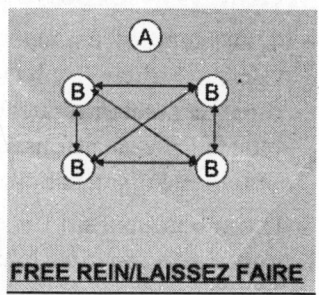

FREE REIN/LAISSEZ FAIRE

Should be used when	Should not be used when
• *Staff highly skilled, experienced, and educated*	• *Staff feel insecure at the unavailability of a manager*
• *Staff have pride in their work and the drive to do it successfully on their own*	• *The manager cannot provide regular feedback to staff on how well they are doing*

• Outside experts, such as staff specialists or consultants used • Staff trustworthy and experienced	• Managers unable to thank staff for their good work • The manager doesn t understand his or her responsibilities and hoping the staff cover for him or her

Advantages

- It makes an environment of friendliness, individuality as well as team spirit.
- It helps subordinates to develop independent personality.
- Highly motivated and achievement oriented employees are suitable for this environment.

Disadvantages

- It provides poor management and makes the employees lose their sense of direction and focus.

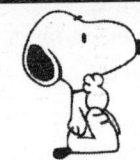

Thinking Time !!

Classify your teachers on the basis of the styles of leadership and the method they use to control the class. Which teacher s style do you like the most and whose style helps you to learn the most?

- The disinterest of the management and leadership causes the employees to become less interested in their job and their dissatisfaction increases with time.

M. LIKERT'S FOUR SYSTEMS OF MANAGEMENT

Dr Rensis Likert studied human behaviour within many organisations. After extensive research, Dr. Rensis Likert concluded that there are four systems of management.

System (1) - Exploitive Authoritative

- In this type of management system the job of employees/subordinates is to abide by the decisions made by managers and those with a higher status than them in the organisation.
- The subordinates do not participate in the decision making. The organisation is concerned simply about completing the work.
- The organisation will use fear and threats to make sure employees complete the work set. There is no teamwork involved.

System (2) - Benevolent Authoritative

- Just as in an exploitive authoritative system, decisions are made by those at the top of the organisation and management.
- However employees are motivated through rewards (for their contribution) rather than fear and threats.
- Information may flow from subordinates to managers but it is restricted to "what management wants to hear".

System (3) - Consultative

- In this type of management system, subordinates are motivated by rewards and a degree of involvement in the decision making process.
- Management will constructively use their subordinates' ideas and opinions. However involvement is incomplete and major decisions are still made by senior management.
- There is a greater flow of information (than in a benevolent authoritative system) from subordinates to management; although, the information from subordinate to manager is incomplete and euphemistic.

System (4) - Participative (Group)

- Management has complete confidence in their subordinates/employees.
- There is lot of communication and subordinates are fully involved in the decision making process. Subordinates comfortably express opinions and there is lot of of teamwork.
- Teams are linked together by people, who are members of more than one team. Likert calls people in more than one group as **"linking pins"**.
- Employees throughout the organisation feel responsible for achieving the organisation's objectives. This responsibility is motivational especially as subordinates are offered economic rewards for achieving organisational goals which they have participated in setting.

TEST YOUR GREY MATTER

Q1) Define leadership. Name the important features of leadership?

Q2) What are the various skills required for leadership?

Q3) "A good leader is not necessarily a good manager". Discuss this statement and compare leadership with management.

Q4) Name the various functions of Leadership in an organisation?

Q5) Write short notes on:

a) Charismatic Leader

b) Transactional Leader.

Q6) Differentiate between Transactional and Transformational Leadership.

Q7) What are the types of leadership styles? Describe each of them briefly.

Q8) Give both Advantages and Disadvantages of

a) Autocratic Leadership Style

b) Participative leadership style

c) Laissez-Faire Leadership Style

Q9) Explain Likert's Four Systems of Management

N. LEADERSHIP THEORIES

- A review of the leadership literature reveals an evolving series of 'schools of thought' from "Great Man" and "Trait" theories to "Transformational" leadership (see table).

- While early theories tend to focus upon the characteristics and behaviours of successful leaders, later theories begin to consider the role of followers and the contextual nature of Leadership.

Trait Theories	The lists of traits or qualities associated with leadership exist in abundance and continue to be produced. They draw on virtually all the adjectives in the dictionary which describe some positive or virtuous human attribute, from ambition to zest for life.
Behaviourist Theories 1. McGregor's Theory X & Theory Y Managers 2. Blake and Mouton's Managerial Grid 3. Ohio and Michigan state studies	These concentrate on what leaders actually do rather than on their qualities. Different patterns of behaviour are observed and categorised as 'styles of leadership'. This area has probably attracted most attention from practicing managers.

Contingency or Situational Leadership 1. Fiedler's Contingency Model 2. The Hersey-Blanchard Model of Leadership 3. Reddin's Tri-Dimensional Leadership Effectiveness Model 4. Tannenbaum & Schmidt's Leadership Continuum 5. House path goal theory	This approach sees leadership as specific to the situation in which it is being exercised. For example, some situations may even require an autocratic style, others may need a more participative approach. It also proposes that there may be differences in required leadership styles at different levels in the same organisation
Transactional Theory	This approach emphasises the importance of the relationship between leader and followers, focusing on the mutual benefits derived from a form of 'contract' through which the leader delivers such things as rewards or recognition in return for the commitment or loyalty of the followers
Transformational Theory	The central concept here is change and the role of leadership in envisioning and implementing the transformation of organisational performance

L.1. Trait Approach To Leadership

What type of person makes a good leader?

- Early researchers studied the personality characteristics that make a person a leader and concluded that leaders are born and not made (Great Man Theory)

- For example, famous personalities like **Napoleon and Alexander** were natural leaders and would have become leaders even if they had to face situations different from what they actually faced.

- The Trait Approach arose from the **"Great Man"** theory as a way of identifying the key characteristics of successful leaders. It suggests that you can identify a potential leader by examining the personality traits of the person and matching them to the characteristics "real" leaders possess.

- The philosophy of the trait approach is quite simple and would seem, at least initially, quite logical. Successful leaders are assumed to possess more (or less) of certain traits than unsuccessful leaders.

- This is the notion of the ideal leader, or the ideal leader profile which describes which traits a good leader should possess a lot of and which traits he should possess in only minimum amount.

- The emphasis in this approach is on the personal characteristics of good and bad leader.
- Three assumptions of trait theory are:-
  - Leaders are born, not made.
  - Some traits are particularly suited to leadership
  - People who make good leaders have right combination of traits.

L.1.1.Stogdill Traits and Skills

- Stogdill completed two comprehensive reviews by synthesising more than 200 studies of the trait approach. His two surveys identified a group of traits that were positively associated with leadership such as intelligence, self-confidence, initiative, and persistence" (Liu and Liu 8).
- Stogdill's extensive research helped him develop the main key traits and skills that are found in leaders.
- The following table illustrates Stogdill's trait studies from 1949 through 1970:

Main Traits Studied

- Adaptable to situations
- Alert to social environment
- Ambitious and achievement-oriented
- Assertive
- Cooperative
- Decisive
- Dependable
- Dominant (desire to influence others)
- Energetic (high activity level)
- Persistent
- Self-Confident
- Tolerant of stress
- Willing to assume responsibility

Main Skills Studied

- Clever (intelligent)
- Conceptually skilled
- Creative
- Diplomatic and tactful

- Fluent in speaking
- Knowledgeable about group task
- Organised (administrative ability)
- Persuasive
- Socially skilled

L.1.2. Ghiselli Personal Traits

- Edwin Ghiselli conducted probably the most widely publicised trait studies. He studied over 300 managers from 90 different businesses in United States and published his result in 1971.
- He concluded that certain traits are important to effective leadership, though not all of them are necessary for success.
- Ghiselli identified the following six traits, in order of importance, as being significant traits for effective leadership:

    i. **Supervisory ability:** Getting the job done through others.

    ii. **Need for occupational achievement:** Seeking responsibility and having the motivation to work hard to succeed.

    iii. **Intelligence:** The ability to use good judgment and clear reasoning.

    iv. **Decisiveness:** The ability to solve problems and make decisions competently.

    v. **Self-assurance:** Viewing oneself as capable of coping with problems and behaving in a manner that shows others that you have self esteem.

    vi. **Initiative:** Self starting, or being able to get the job done with minimum of supervision from one's boss.

Criticism of Trait Approach

There are a number of important difficulties involved in the trait method of studying leadership.

i. Firstly, there is the problem of defining and agreeing upon traits. The number of descriptive adjectives which can be used to "type" people is tremendously large. For example, helpful, cheerful, courteous, kind, obedient etc. Thus, there are nearly as many traits of people as there are adjectives. Which ones should we measure since we obviously cannot study them all?

ii. A second difficulty exists in trying to measure traits. There are many personality tests available, each of which lists the traits it purports to measure. Unfortunately, all too often, two tests which claim to measure the same trait turn out on close examination to be quite different and two tests which ostensibly are designed to measure traits quite different from each other may turn out to have very similar contents. Thus, there are no reliable measuring tools (tests) to measure traits.

iii. The last objection to the trait approach is probably the most important of all. As a method it does not provide the psychologist with much insight into the basic dynamics of the leadership process.

L.2.Behavioural Theories

What does a good leader do?

- Since the trait theories failed to establish the relationship between traits and effective leadership, researchers turned their attention to the behavioural aspects of successful leaders.

- The behavioural approach is also simple in its philosophy. It states that the best way to study and to define leadership is in terms of **what leaders do** rather than in terms of what leaders are. Thus one is concerned with leader "behaviours" rather than leader traits.

- They attempted to identify the behaviours that were unique to leaders, and which distinguished them from non- leaders.

- Following are the important behavioural theories:

L.2.1. McGregor's Theory X & Theory Y Managers

- Although not strictly speaking a theory of leadership, the leadership strategy of effectively-used participative management proposed in Douglas McGregor's book has had a tremendous impact on managers. McGregor summarised two contrasting sets of assumptions made by managers in industry.

Theory X managers believe that:	Theory Y managers believe that:
<ul><li>The average human being has an inherent dislike of work and will avoid it if possible.</li><li>Because of this human characteristic, most people must be coerced, controlled, directed, or threatened with punishment to get them to put forth adequate effort to achieve organisational objectives.</li><li>The average human being prefers to be directed, wishes to avoid responsibility, has relatively little ambition, and wants security above all else.</li></ul>	<ul><li>The expenditure of physical and mental effort in work is as natural as play or rest, and the average human being, under proper conditions, learns not only to accept but to seek responsibility.</li><li>People will exercise self-direction and self-control to achieve objectives to which they are committed.</li><li>The capacity to exercise a relatively high level of imagination, ingenuity, and creativity in the solution of organisational problems is widely, not narrowly, distributed in the population, and the intellectual potentialities of the average human being are only partially utilised under the conditions of modern industrial life.</li></ul>

L.2.2. Blake and Mouton's Managerial Grid

- Blake and Mouton developed a two-dimensional matrix model of leadership styles based on their own research and the results of the earlier studies.

- The model consists of nine rows and columns. The rows represent the leader's concern for production, while the columns represent the concern for the people.

- According to Blake these two dimensions are independent , a manager can be high on both, low on both, high on one and low on the other, etc.

- Blake and Mouton found five intersection points in his model of 9x9 grid, illustrated below:

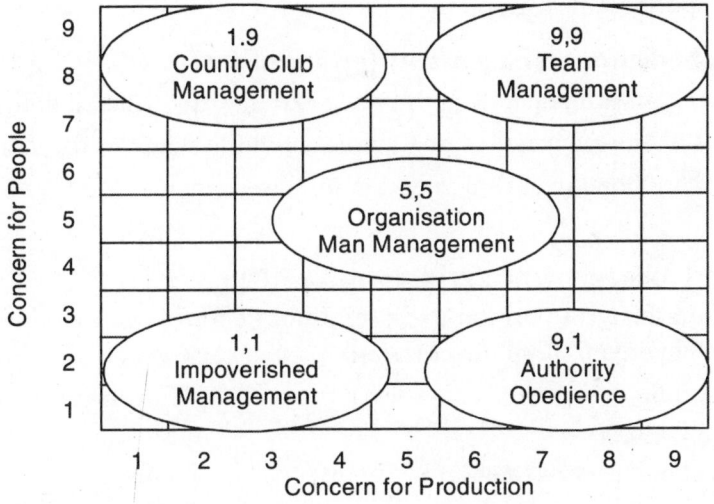

- A 1,1 style shows a low concern for results and alow concern for people – impoverished don't care.

- A 9,1 style shows a high concern for results and a low concern for people – compliance management.

- A 1,9 style shows a low concern for results and a high concern for people – the country club.

- A 9,9 style shows a high concern for results and a high concern for people – team approach.

- A 5,5 style shows a moderate concern for results and a moderate concern for people – middle road.

- Blake and Mouton suggested that managers who practice 9, 9 style of leadership are more effective compared to 9, 1 style or the 1, 9 style. Leaders whose behaviour falls into 5, 5 styles are also considered to be fairly effective.

Country club management: (grid position 1, 9)

- Here we find all the managers with a high concern for people and a low concern for production.
- This kind of manager pays thoughtful attention to the needs of people for satisfying relationships, which leads to a comfortable, friendly organisation and work environment.
- They always have lots of social interaction and put service projects as well as company sports teams high on their list.

Authority- obedience management: (grid position 9, 1)

- All the managers who operate at the other extreme are included in this position.
- They focus on the efficiency in operations with little concerns for individuals.
- They get work done in such a way that human elements interfere to a minimum degree.

Impoverished management: (grid position 1, 1)

- Managers in this grid position exert minimum effort to get required work done and to sustain organisation membership.
- They have little concern for either the human element or the production level of the team.
- This kind of manager has a short life in responsible organisations.

Organisation management: (grid position 5, 5)

- These kinds of managers constantly try to balance the necessity to get work done while maintaining morale of people at a satisfactory level, but not excellent.
- Organisation production will be close to expectations, but without exceeding them.

Team management: (grid position 9, 9)

- This is the ideal manager identified by Blake and Mouton.
- This manager develops a relationship of trust and respect with employees and others. There is also certain interdependence through a common stake, which leads to an enhancement of the productivity.

L.2.3. Michigan and Ohio State Leadership Studies

The most prominent studies were those undertaken by the University of Michigan and by Ohio State University. Interestingly, both studies arrived at similar conclusions. Both studies concluded that leadership behaviours could be classified into two groups.

L.2.3.1. Michigan Leadership Studies

The University of Michigan **(Rensis Likert)** identified two styles of leader behaviour:

i. Production centred behaviour

- When a leader pays close attention to the work of sub-ordinates, explains work procedures, and is keenly interested in performance.
- It emphasises on production and technical aspects of jobs and employees are taken as a tool for accomplishing the jobs.

ii. Employee centred behaviour

- When the leader is interested in developing a cohesive work group and in ensuring that employees are satisfied with their jobs.

L.2.3.2. Ohio State Leadership Studies

The Ohio State studies were begun in 1945 to identify the dimensions of leadership behaviour. The staff of Ohio State created a Leader Behaviour Description Questionnaire (LBDQ) which was designed to discover how leaders carry out their activities. Questions focused on two elements of leadership.

i. Initiating Structure Behaviour

- When the leader clearly defines the leader-subordinate relation, establishes formal lines of communication, and determines how tasks are to be performed.
- Initiating structures are items that indicate the degree of structure that a leader imposes on subordinates (e.g., deadlines, assigning tasks, and following standard procedures).

ii. Consideration Behaviour

- The leader shows concern for sub-ordinates and attempts to establish a warm, friendly, and supportive climate.
- Consideration included those items that indicated a leader's friendliness, supportiveness, and compassion.
- An important finding of the Ohio State studies was that these two dimensions are independent. This means that *consideration for workers* and *initiating structure* exists

simultaneously and in different amounts. A matrix was created that showed the various combinations and quantities of the elements.

	Low Initiating Structure	High Initiating Structure
High Consideration	HIGH CONSIDERATION AND LOW STRUCTURE	HIGH STRUCTURE AND HIGH CONSIDERATION
Low Consideration	LOW STRUCTURE AND LOW CONSIDERATION	HIGH STRUCTURE AND LOW CONSIDERATION

- The Ohio state leadership quadrant shows various combinations of initiating structure and consideration. In each quadrant, there is a relative mixture of initiating structure and consideration and a manager can adopt any one style.

L.3. Situational Approaches To Leadership

- Although the behavioural approaches state that a positive, participative and considerate style of leadership is the most effective, there is evidence that such a style may not be successful in some situations.

- This implies that there is not one style of leadership that is appropriate for all situations. Situational theories of leadership postulate that leaders have to change their style depending on the situation they face.

- The theories also suggest that a leader should carefully analyse the nature of the situation before deciding on the appropriate style of leadership to be adopted.

- Situational theory is also known as **Contingency Theory**.

- This theory was first applied in year 1920 in the armed forces of Germany with the objective to get good Generals under different situations.

- The prime attention in this theory is given to the situation in which leadership is exercised.

- Effectiveness of leadership is affected by the factors associated with the leader (Leader behaviour) and the factors associated with the situation (Situational factors) and so certain leaders are effective in one situation but not in others.

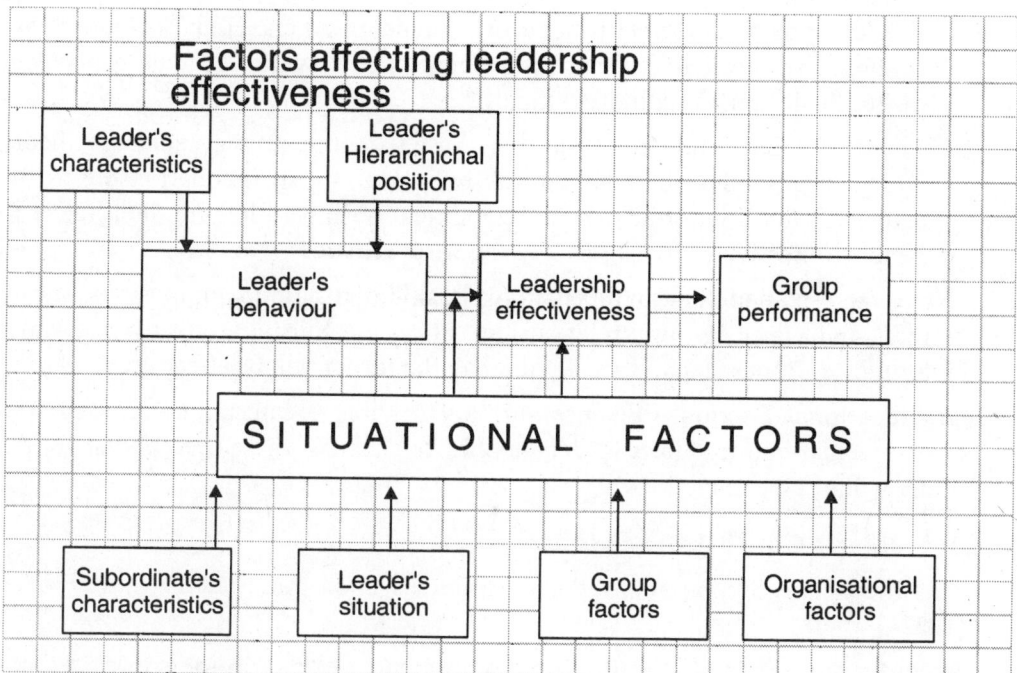

Leader Behaviour

Leader behaviour is further affected by two variables:-

i. **Leader characteristics:** The behaviour of the individuals is influenced by intelligence and ability, his characteristics like his personality characteristics, attitude, interest, motivation, and physical characteristics such as age, sex, and physical features.

ii. **Leader's Hierarchical Position:** Leader's hierarchical position in the organisation is very important because persons at different levels face different kinds of problem which affect the degree of participation between the superiors and his subordinates in arriving at decisions to solve the problems.

Situational Factors

The various situational factors are grouped into four categories:-

i. **Subordinate Characteristics:** It includes personality characteristics, attitude, interest, motivation , physical characteristics such as age, sex and physical features.

ii. **Leader's Situation:** The variables which determine the leader's situation are:

    a. **Leader's position power:** It helps in influencing others. High position power simplifies the leader's task of influencing others, while low position power makes the leader's task more difficult.

    b. **Leader's subordinate relation:** It is based on the classic exchange theory which suggests that there is two-way influence in a social relationship. If the leader has good subordinates, and good relationship with them, he is likely to be more effective.

iii. **Group factors:** Various group factors like task design, group composition, group norms, and peer group relationship affect leadership effectiveness and performance. If these factors are favourable, the leader will be effective.

iv. **Organisational Factors:** Organisational factors like organisational climate and organisational culture affect leadership effectiveness. If these are conducive, the leader will be effective.

L.3.1. Fiedler's Contingency Model

- This theory was proposed by the Austrian psychologist Fred Edward Fiedler (1922-).

- According to this model, leadership requirements depend on the situation faced by the leader; and the choice of the most appropriate style of leadership depends on whether the overall situation is favourable or unfavourable to the leader.

- **Identifying leadership style**: Fiedler believes a key factor in leadership success is the individual's basic style. So he begins by trying to find out what that basic style is. Fiedler created the least preferred co-worker (LPC) scale for this purpose; it purports to measure whether a person is task or relationship oriented.

- **Least Preferred Co-worker (LPC) scale**: Fiedler identified a Least Preferred Co-Worker scoring for leaders by asking them first to think of a person with whom they worked, whom they would like least to work with again, and then to score the person on a range of scales between positive factors (friendly, helpful, cheerful, etc.) and negative factors (unfriendly, unhelpful, gloomy, etc.). A high LPC leader generally scores the other person as positive and a low LPC leader scores them as negative.

- **Situational Favourableness:** According to Fiedler, there is no ideal leader. Both low-LPC (task-oriented) and high-LPC (relationship-oriented) leaders can be effective if their leadership orientation fits the situation. The contingency theory allows for predicting the characteristics of the appropriate situations for effectiveness. Three situational components determine the favourableness or situational control.

i. **Leader member relations**: this indicates the extent to which a leader is accepted by his subordinates. If a leader has friction with majority of his subordinates, then he scores low on this dimension.

ii. **Task structure:** this refers to the degree to which the task on hand can be performed efficiently by following a particular method.

iii. **Position power**: it refers to the power, (or formal authority) that the leader is bestowed within the organisation.

Category	I	II	III	IV	V	VI	VII	VIII
Leader member relations	Good	Good	Good	Good	Poor	Poor	Poor	Poor
Task structures	High	High	Low	Low	High	High	Low	Low
Position power	Strong	Weak	Strong	Weak	Strong	Weak	Strong	Weak

- The next step in the Fiedler model is to evaluate the situation in terms of these three contingency variables. Leader-member relations are either good or poor, task structure is either high or low, and position power is either strong or weak. Fiedler perceived eight possible combinations of these three contingency variables as shown in the box. A situation is considered to be favourable to the leader if the scores on all the three dimensions are high.

- **Leader-Situation Match and Mismatch:** With the knowledge of an individual's LPC score and an assessment of the three contingency dimensions, the Fiedler model proposes matching them up to achieve maximum leadership effectiveness. Based on his research, Fiedler came to the following conclusions.

  i. A task-oriented, tough natured leadership style is most effective in highly favourable or highly unfavourable situations (see below Fielder contingency model).

  ii. A people–oriented, lenient type of leadership is most appropriate in moderately favourable or unfavourable situations (see below Fielder contingency model).

Fiedler Contingency Model

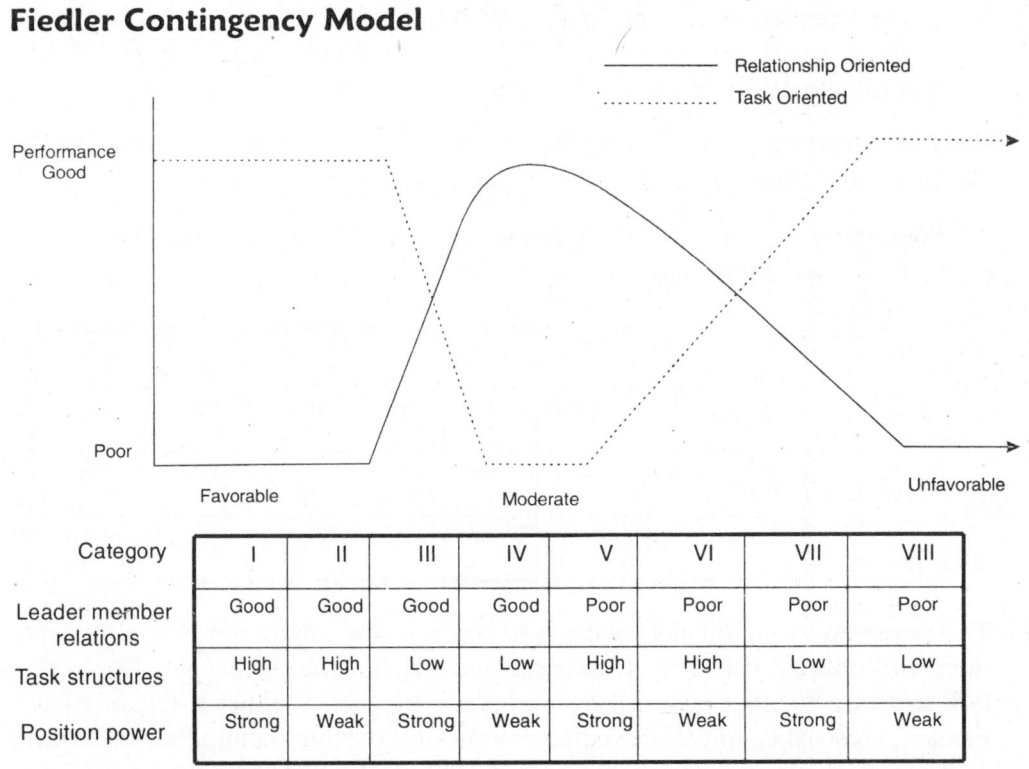

Category	I	II	III	IV	V	VI	VII	VIII
Leader member relations	Good	Good	Good	Good	Poor	Poor	Poor	Poor
Task structures	High	High	Low	Low	High	High	Low	Low
Position power	Strong	Weak	Strong	Weak	Strong	Weak	Strong	Weak

L.3.2. The Hersey-Blanchard Model of Leadership

According to Heresy and Blanchard, leadership styles can be categorised into four types – telling, selling, participating and delegating - which vary in the kind of guidance and support offered by the superior to his subordinate, so the maturity level of the subordinate plays a major role in influencing the leadership style of the superior.

- **Telling (S1)** – Leaders tell their people exactly what to do, and how to do it.

- **Selling (S2)** – Leaders still provide information and direction, but there's more communication with followers. Leaders "sell" their message to get the team on board.

- **Participating (S3)** – Leaders focus more on the relationship and less on direction. The leader works with the team, and shares decision-making responsibilities.

- **Delegating (S4)** – Leaders pass most of the responsibility onto the follower or group. The leaders still monitor progress, but they're less involved in decisions.

As you can see, styles S1 and S2 are focused on getting the task done. Styles S3 and S4 are more concerned with developing team members' abilities to work independently.

- The leadership style selected by an effective manager depends on the development level of employee. If an employee is low in his ability to perform as well as willingness to perform, the manager needs to adopt the telling style i.e. he must constantly give directions to the employee.

- If the employee is low in ability but high in willingness to perform, the manger has to use selling style of leadership. He has to give directions as well as the required support to the employee to perform the task.

- If an employee is capable of performing but not willing to perform the task, the manager has to apply participating style of leadership. He has to give less direction and more responsibilities but extend support to the employee in carrying out his responsibilities.

- If an employee is capable, and is also willing to carry out the task then the manager can simply delegate the tasks and responsibilities to the employee.

Maturity Levels

According to Hersey and Blanchard, knowing when to use each style is largely dependent on the maturity of the person or group you're leading. They break maturity down into four different levels:

- **M1** – People at this level of maturity are at the bottom level of the scale. They lack the knowledge, skills, or confidence to work on their own, and they often need to be pushed to take the task on.

- **M2** – At this level, followers might be willing to work on the task, but they still don't have the skills to do it successfully.

- **M3** – Here, followers are ready and willing to help with the task. They have more skills than the M2 group, but they're still not confident in their abilities.

- **M4** – These followers are able to work on their own. They have high confidence and strong skills, and they're committed to the task

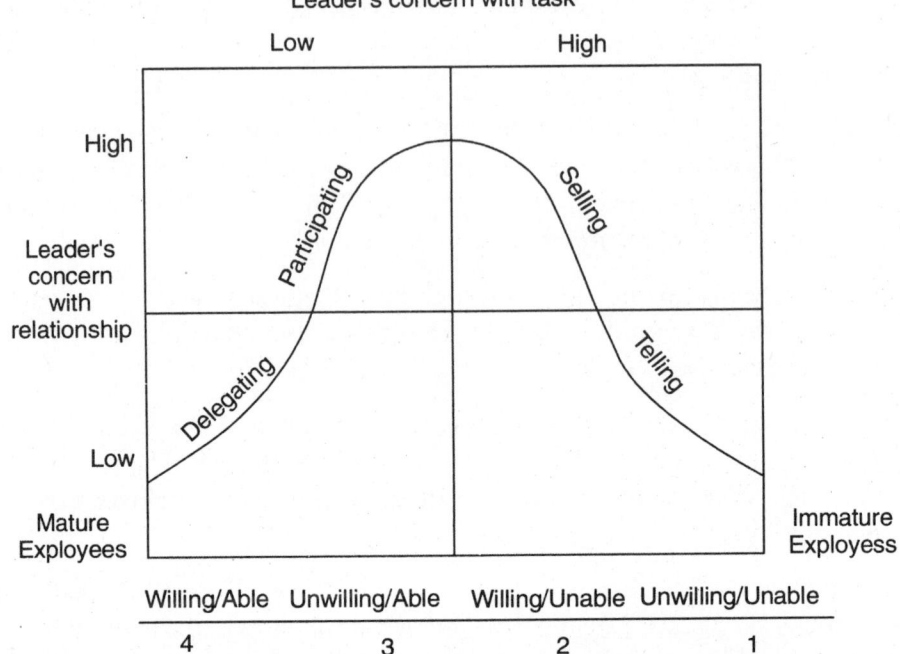

- The Hersey-Blanchard model maps each leadership style to each maturity level, as shown below:

Maturity Level	Most Appropriate Leadership Style
M1: Low maturity	S1: Telling/directing
M2: Medium maturity, limited skills	S2: Selling/coaching
M3: Medium maturity, higher skills but lacking confidence	S3: Participating/supporting
M4: High maturity	S4: Delegating

L.3.3. Reddin's Tri-Dimensional Leadership Effectiveness Model

Reddin combined Blake and Mouton's Managerial Grid with Fiedler Contingency leadership style theory. The outcome was a Three-Dimensional Theory of Management, the dimension being adapted from:

1. Managerial Grid Theory
2. Contingency Leadership Style Theory
3. Effectiveness theory

- Its axis represents **Task-Orientation (To), Relation-Orientation (Ro), And Effectiveness.**

- The below table shows the Less Effective & More Effective Leadership styles in each basic types

Less Effective	Basic types	More Effective
Deserter	SEPARATED	Bureaucratic
Missionary	RELATED	Developer
Autocratic	DEDICATED	Benevolent Autocratic
Compromiser	INTEGRATED	Executive

- These possible combinations result in four basic types (shown in figure)
- i. **Separated,** in which both task orientation and relationship orientation are minimal.
- ii. **Related,** in which task orientation is low and relationship orientation is high. Related leaders relate primarily to their subordinates.
- iii. **Dedicated,** in which task orientation is high and relationship orientation is low. Dedicated leaders are dedicated only to the job.
- iv. **Integrated,** in which both task orientation and relationship orientation are high. Integrated leaders focus on managerial behaviour, combining task orientation and relationship behaviour.

i. Separated Basic Types

Deserter (Less Effective Leadership Style)
- This is essentially a hands-off or laissez-faire approach.
- It involves avoidance of any involvement or intervention which would upset the status; assuming a neutral attitude toward what is going on during the day; looking the other way to avoid enforcing rules; keeping out of the way of both supervisors and subordinates; avoidance of change and planning.
- The activities undertaken (or initiated) by managers who use this approach tend to be defensive in nature.

Bureaucratic (More Effective Leadership Style)
- This is a legalistic and procedural approach.
- It involves adherence to rules and procedures; acceptance of hierarchy of authority; preference of formal channels of communication.
- This function at its best in well structured situations where policies are clear, roles are well defined and criteria of performance are objective and universally applied.
- Because they insist on rational systems, these managers may be seen as autocratic, rigid or particular.
- Because of their dependence on rules and procedures, they are hardly distinguished from autocratic managers.

ii. Related Basic Types

Missionary (Less Effective Leadership Style)

- This is an effective (supportive) approach. It emphasises congeniality and positive climate in the work place.
- In this leaders are sensitive to subordinates' personal needs and concerns. They try to keep people happy by giving the most they can.
- Supportive behaviour represents the positive component of this style.
- However, this type of leaders may avoid conflict, feel uncomfortable enforcing controls and find difficulty in denying requests or making honest appraisals.

Developer (More Effective Leadership Style)

- This is the objective counterpart of the missionary style. Objective in a sense that concern for people is expressed professionally.
- Subordinates are allowed to participate in decision making and are given opportunities to express their views and to develop their potential.
- Their contribution is recognised and attention is given to their development.
- These types of leaders have optimistic beliefs about people wanting to work and produce.
- Their approach to subordinates is friendly: they like to share their knowledge and expertise with their subordinates and take pride in discovering and promoting talent.

iii. Dedicated Basic Types

Autocratic (Less Effective Leadership Style)

- This is a directive and controlling approach. Its concern for production and output outweighs the concern for workers and their relationship.
- This type of leader tends to be formal. They assign tasks to subordinates and watch implementation closely. Errors are not tolerated, and deviation from stated objectives or directives is forbidden.
- They make unilateral decisions and feel no need to explain or justify them. They minimise interaction with people, or limit communication to the essential demand of the task at hand.
- They believe in individual responsibility and consider group meetings a waste of time.
- They tend to be formal, straightforward and critical.
- For that reason, they are likely to be perceived as cold and arbitrary, particularly by subordinates who have strong need for support and reassurance.

Benevolent Autocratic (More Effective Leadership Style)

- This is the communicative counterpart of the autocratic style. It is still directive and interventionist.
- This type of leaders devote themselves comfortably to the accomplishment of production objectives. They enjoy tackling operational problems and may have less patience dealing with problems of human relation.
- They keep in touch with subordinates, instructing them, answering their questions and helping them with operational problems.
- They structure daily work, set objectives, give orders or delegate with firm accountability.
- They would not hesitate to discipline or reprimand, but do that fairly and without antagonising their subordinates.
- They meet group needs but ignore one-to-one personal relationship.

iv. Integrated Basic Types

Compromiser (Less Effective Leadership Style)

- It expresses appreciation of both human relations orientation and task orientation.
- This type of leader however admits to difficulties in integrating both task orientation and human relations orientation. Therefore they may fluctuate between task requirements and demand for human relations.
- In order to lessen immediate pressures, they may resort to compromise solutions.
- They may be sensitive to reality considerations which stand in the way, and willing to delay action for whatever reason, internal or external.
- Their realistic assessment of situations may explain why they do not use freely the approach they actually prefer, that is, the Executive approach.

Executive (More Effective Leadership Style)

- This approach integrates task orientation and human relations orientation in response to realistic demand.
- It is best described as **Consultative, Interactive,** and **Problem Solving** approach.
- This approach is called for while managing operations which require exploration of alternative solutions, pooling different resources, and integrating opposing perspectives.
- It favours a team approach in problem solving, planning and decision making and stimulate communication among subordinates, thus obtaining collective ideas and suggestions.

- Leaders who use this approach are usually perceived as good motivators who tend to deal openly with conflict and who try to obtain collective commitment.

- As in other theories of leadership, the effective behaviour of leader is relative to the situation. Effective leaders apply leadership styles after assessing the situation.

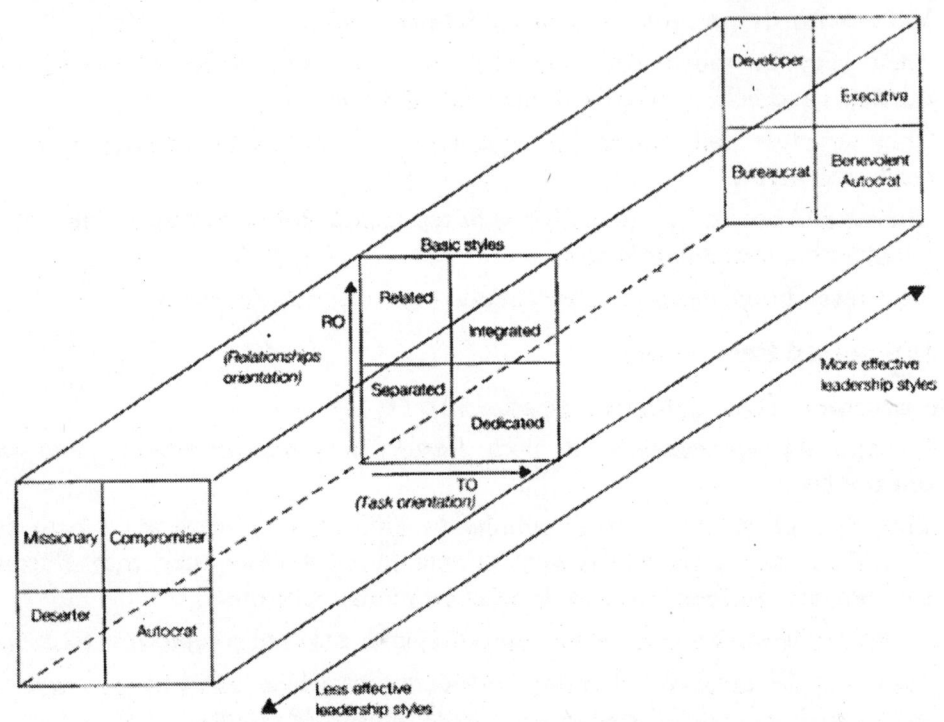

Reddin's Tri-Dimensional Leadership Effectiveness Model

L.3.4. A Continuum of Leader Behaviour by Tannenbaum-Schmidt

- The Leadership Continuum model of Tannenbaum and Schmidt (1973) suggests that autocratic leaders (manager-oriented leadership) are more likely to make their own decisions and not engage their subordinates, whereas a more democratic leader (laissez-faire manager i.e. subordinate-oriented leadership) gives subordinates a greater degree of delegation in decision-making.

- In 1938, Lewin and Lippitt proposed classifications of leaders based on how much involvement leaders placed into task and relationship needs. This range of leadership behaviours was expressed along a continuum by Tannenbaum & Schmidt in 1973, ranging from manager-oriented (task) to subordinate-oriented (relationship).

To choose the most appropriate style and use of authority, the leader must consider:

- **Forces in the manager**: belief in team member participation and confidence in capabilities of members.
- **Forces in the subordinate**: Expectations, need for independence, readiness to assume decision-making responsibility, tolerance for ambiguity in task definition, interest in the problem, ability to understand and identify with the goals of the organisation, and knowledge and experience to deal with the problem.
- **Forces in the situation**: team has requisite knowledge, team holds organisational values and traditions, teams work effectively.
- **Time pressure**: need for immediate decision under pressure mitigates participation.

Although there are a number of different styles indicated in this model, there are four main categories that are frequently described:

Tells

The leader identifies appropriate solutions to problems & the appropriate courses of action & thereafter tells the subordinates what they are supposed to do.

Sells

The leader still decides upon the appropriate course of action in any given situation but attempts to overcome disagreement & resistance among the workforce by selling the decision to them. Often this involves justifying the decision (determined by the boss) as the best course of action in the circumstances.

Consults

The leader allows time for subordinates to discuss the problem & present ideas & solutions to the boss. These are then used by the leader to make decisions which are then announced to, and action is taken by the subordinates.

Joins

The leader defines the nature of the issue to be decided along with any constraints & presents these to the group. The leader then becomes part of the group in finding & implementing acceptable solutions.

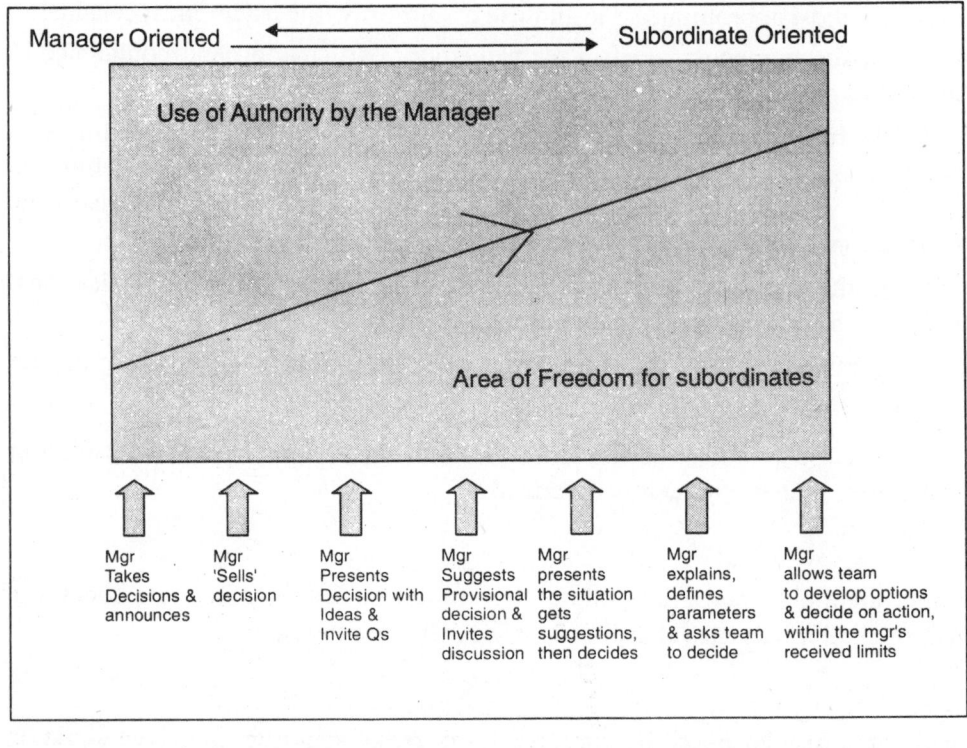

Manager Oriented ⟵———————⟶ Subordinate Oriented

Use of Authority by the Manager

Area of Freedom for subordinates

| Mgr Takes Decisions & announces | Mgr 'Sells' decision | Mgr Presents Decision with Ideas & Invite Qs | Mgr Suggests Provisional decision & Invites discussion | Mgr presents the situation gets suggestions, then decides | Mgr explains, defines parameters & asks team to decide | Mgr allows team to develop options & decide on action, within the mgr's received limits |

⟵————————— Range of Behaviour —————————⟶

Advantages of the Leadership Continuum Model Include

i. Gives managers a range of choices for involvement.

ii. Presents criteria for involvement and delegation.

iii. Focuses decision maker on relevant criteria (e.g. forces & time).

iv. Emphasises employee development and empowerment.

v. Is heuristic—encourages research to see how effective delegation may be under the model.

Some Limitations of The Leadership Continuum Theory

i. Involves only the initial step of assigning a task to someone, not the following processes that may determine the effectiveness of the outcome.

ii. Assumes the manager has sufficient information to determine disposition to self or team.

iii. Assumes "neutral" environment without social bonds or politics.

iv. Simplifies complex decisions to a two-polar dimension; more simple than reality is.

L.3.5. House Path Goal Theory

- According to path goal theory, the leader should provide required support and guidance to his followers and help them achieve organisational goals.

- He should also establish individual (or group) goals for employees that are compatible with the broad organisational goals.

- Thus, the leader defines the path to achieve goals; he also removes any obstructions that come in the way of employees achieving these goals.

Robert House suggested four types of leadership with the help of the path – goal theory:

i. **Directive leader:** lets others know what is expected; gives directions, maintains standards.

ii. **Supportive leader:** makes work more pleasant; treats others as equals, acts friendly, shows concern.

iii. **Achievement-oriented leader:** sets challenging goals; expects high performance, shows confidence.

iv. **Participative leader:** involves others in decision making; asks for and uses suggestions.

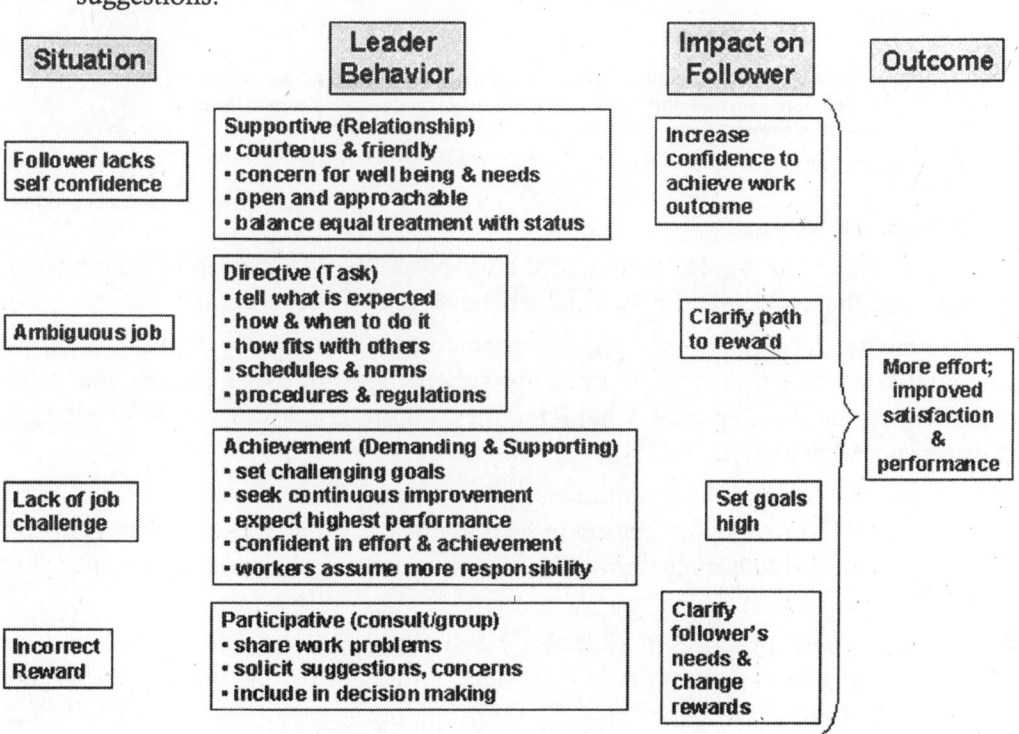

- Supportive behaviour increases satisfaction of the group, especially in stressful situations, while directive behaviour is suited to uncertain and ambiguous situations. It is also proposed that leaders who have influence upon their superiors can increase group satisfaction and performance.

- There is also evidence that more directive leadership is preferred by certain people under some circumstances as shown in the figure below:

Interaction Between Followers' Locus of Control and Leader Behavior in Decision Making

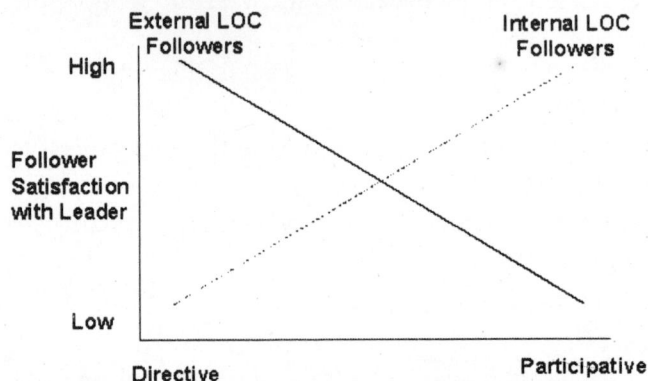

Internal LOC followers who believed outcomes were a result of their own decisions were more satisfied with participative than directive leaders; External locus of control followers were more satisfied with directive leaders)

Mitchell, T. R., Smyser, C. M., & Weed, S. E. (1975). Locus of control: Supervision and work satisfaction, Academy of Management Journal, 18, 623-30.

Path Goal Variables

- As shown in the figure, path-goal theory proposes two classes of contingency variables that moderate the leadership behaviour and effects the outcome-

Environmental factors: those in the environment that are outside the control of the employee (task structure, formal authority system, and the work group) and those that are part of the **Personal Characteristics** of the employee (locus of control, experience, and perceived ability).

Environmental factors determine the type of leader behaviour required as a complement if follower outcomes are to be maximised, while personal characteristics of the employee determine how the environment and leader behaviour are interpreted.

- So, the theory proposes that leader's behaviour will be effective when it is redundant with sources of environment structure or incongruent with the employee characteristics.

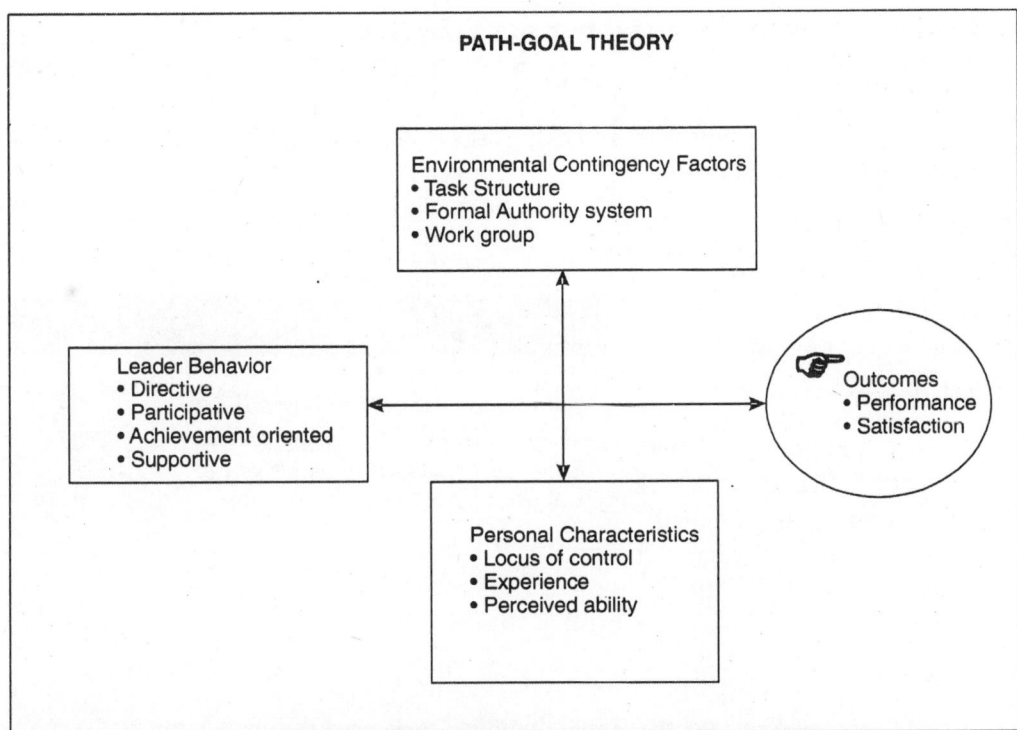

PATH-GOAL THEORY

Environmental Contingency Factors
• Task Structure
• Formal Authority system
• Work group

Leader Behavior
• Directive
• Participative
• Achievement oriented
• Supportive

Outcomes
• Performance
• Satisfaction

Personal Characteristics
• Locus of control
• Experience
• Perceived ability

O. SUCCESSFUL VERSUS EFFECTIVE LEADERSHIP

- Successful leadership has been defined as the ability to get others to behave as the manager intends them to behave. The job may get done, and the leader's needs may be satisfied, but the subordinate's needs are ignored.

- In effective leadership, the subordinates perform in accordance with the leader's intentions and, at the same time, find their own needs satisfied. The positive feelings of the subordinates usually contribute to long term benefits such as team loyalty, support, and enjoyment of participation, an important component of intrinsic motivation.

- Leadership effectiveness refers to the ability to influence others and achieve collective goals, according to **Judge, Bono, Ilies, & Gerhardt** study. Some researchers, however, suggest that leadership success ought to be based on the effectiveness of the team, group, or organisation. But, leadership effectiveness is "often based on the perceptions of subordinates, peers, or supervisors.

- ## Leaders who are Successful but not Effective

Bureaucrat

Product more important than process; Tasks necessary to win are more important than family and personal needs.

Machiavellian

Takes advantage of others' weaknesses; exploits others; must win at any price.

Missionary

Prizes harmony over conflict. Low task orientation, gets emotionally involved, does what is popular, ignores "tough" decisions.

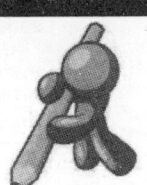

Wisdom Tooth

"Success has to do only with getting the job done, whereas effectiveness adds to the concept of satisfaction on the part of those who do the job."

Climber

Able to manoeuvre into the limelight; high task orientation but for self-serving purposes, not for the team's good.

Exploiter

Exerts constructive control. Hurts anyone who is vulnerable. Uses pressure and fear to get things done.

- ## Leaders who are Effective

Co-operator

Concerned about the good of the team; wins respect; high task orientation; polished and professional; makes people feel needed.

Developer

High people orientation; people considerations may take precedence over achievement, although is very productive.

Integrator

Shares the leadership role, Welcomes the ideas of others. Gives great freedom and authority to others.

Games person

Wants to win from good strategy; enjoys fair competition. Eliminates the weak and non-achievers.

TEST YOUR GREY MATTER

Q 1) What are the different theories of Leadership and what are the factors they consider?

Q2) What are the leadership qualities that a manager should possess? Discuss innate and acquired qualities with examples.

Q3) Discuss Trait theory of Leadership in detail and give the reasons for its criticism.

Q4) What are the different types of management according to Blake and Mouton's Managerial Grid?

Q5) Under what category of leadership theory does Michigan And Ohio State Leadership Studies lie? How are they different from each other?

Q6) "Leadership is situational." Explain this statement by bringing out the situational factors important for effective leadership.

Q7) "Great leaders show concern for both, task and people". Comment on its validity giving a theoretical framework of the theory behind it?

Q8) What is the central theme of the Contingency theory of leadership? Explain Fiedler's model of Leadership.

Q9) Describe Managerial Grid. How can it be used to impart training in leadership.

Q10) What are the implications of House Goal theory of leadership. How is this theory different from other theories?

Q11) Describe The Hersey-Blanchard Model Of Leadership.

Q12) What factor was added by Reddin to the pre-existing theories of leadership? Explain giving brief outline of his Tri Dimensional Theory.

Q13) Write a short note on the Effectiveness of leadership. How are effective leaders different from successful leader?

CHAPTER

10

Group Dynamics

By the end of this chapter, you would be able to :

- Learn about Groups and Group Dynamics.
- Understand how groups form, what is their effect and what it depends on.
- Know about group conflict and learn ways to tackle it.

The chapter contains :

- Group
- Characteristics of a group
- Group dynamics
- Causes for formation of a group
- Effects of groups
- Role of groups
- Types of groups
- Stages of group development
  - Five stage model
  - Punctuated Equilibrium Model
- Theories Of Informal Group Formation
  - Propinquity Theory
  - Humans Interaction Theory
  - Balance Theory
  - Exchange Theory
- Factors Affecting Group Performance
  - Group Roles
  - Group Norms
  - Group Cohesiveness
  - Group Homogeneity
  - Stability of Membership
  - Isolation
  - Group Size
  - Personality of Group Member
- Group Conflict

A. THE INSIGHT

25th June 1983. Not even 20% of India was aware of this event taking place, as Lords in England got jam-packed for the final showdown. A total of 232,081 fans strolled in, nearly equalling the combined total of the past two finals (160,000 for 1975 & 132,000 for 1979).

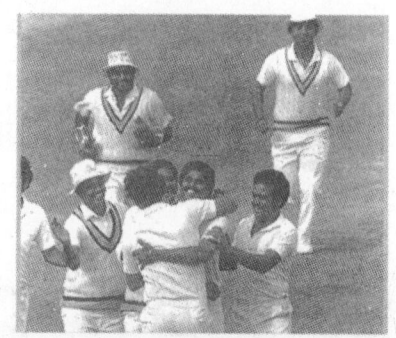

They were underdogs, and they knew it. They were quoted 66:1 before the competition started.

Their mission: To represent their country, India in the World Cup Cricket.

Their task: To defeat teams such as England and Australia.

Their Major Obstacle: West Indies.

West Indies dominated World cricket and had already won the World Cup 2 times consecutively and this was their hatrick chance.

But strange things happen when groups compete with groups and a strange thing did happen when India faced West Indies in the finals.

India was put to bat. The idea was to blow up Indian batting and India scored 183 all out.

But thanks to Indian bowling, fielding and due to sheer group effort, India won by 43 runs.

They showed what a group is all about and what it is capable of doing and gave us the idea about the power of group dynamics.

B. GROUP

Definition: A group is a collection of two or more individuals, interacting and interdependent, who have come together to achieve a particular objective.

Criteria for a collection of people to be called a group:

i. The members of a group must see themselves as a unit.

ii. The group must provide rewards to its members.

> ### You should know
>
> *Group of: 2 people is called Diad. 3 people is called Triad. 4 to 20 is called Small Group.*

iii. Anything that happens to one member of the group affects other members.

iv. The members of the group must share a common goal.

C. CHARACTERISTICS OF A GROUP

As discussed, collection of people is called a group because of the following characteristics:

i. Group Perception

Basic criteria for a being a group is that it should have multiple members and they should consider themselves as a single unit.

ii. Group Rewards

There must be a reward for each member for joining the group. Thus, it forms the reason as to why people join the group and then remain in it.

iii. Interaction and Corresponding Effects

The members of the group must interact with each other and each member influences the behaviour of the others and gets influenced by others. Also, any event that affects a group member should affect all group members.

iv. Common Goals

All group members must have a common goal or purpose. Achievement of the objective is the concern of each member of the group and every member must contribute for its attainment.

D. GROUP DYNAMICS

- Group Dynamics is made up of two words- Group and Dynamics. We have already discussed the definition of Group. Dynamics is defined as follows-

- **Dynamics:** It is the branch of science concerned with forces and their effects on motion.

- **Group Dynamics**: Group dynamics concern the forces operating within groups that affect the way members relate to and work with one another.

Group dynamics is viewed from the nature of groups, their formation, their structure and process and also on how their functionality affects individual members, other groups and the organisation.

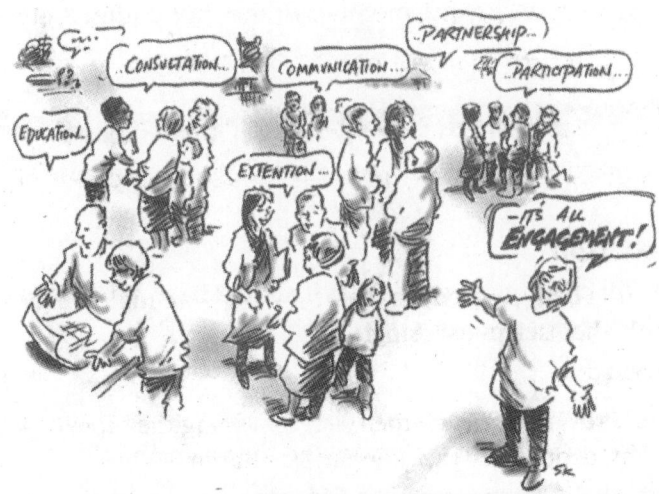

E. CAUSES FOR FORMATION OF A GROUP

i. Affiliation
- It involves the need to be with other people.
- Man is a social animal and he wants to be with other people, talk to them and express his feelings and emotions with others.

ii. Identification
- Many people have the desire to be identified as a member of a social group, thus providing them recognition and status.
- E.g. people join religious cults, sports clubs, Social Service Society etc. to be linked to these groups and be identified socially by them.

iii. Common Interests and Goals
- People who have common interest and goals form groups to share and improve upon their interest and also to attain the goal.
- E.g. musical bands are formed for this reason

iv. Emotional Support
- People who need emotional support also join groups.

v. Personal characteristics
- Skills, attitudes and personality characteristics permit members to be attracted to one another and form groups.

vi. Goal accomplishment

- As different people have different knowledge, skills and resources, it helps in the achievement of goals by careful division of labour among group members.

vii. Security

- People join groups for security, also to reduce the insecurity of "standing alone"; feel stronger and more resistant to threats

- Be it a group of a society or in an organisation, a group gives a sense of security and safety to its members from external forces.

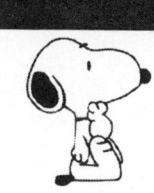

Thinking Time !!

Think about the types of groups you form when you are at college, in the hostel, at home… and what are the reasons due to which you form groups? Do they match with the cause given above or do you have any additions to make?

viii. Monotony

- Informal groups in the organisation are formed to remove monotony and boredom caused by the nature of their job and to refresh themselves.

ix. Assignment

- Groups may be formed with or without the consent of the workers in organisations where work is assigned to a group of people.

- Committees, departments etc. are the result of such group formations.

F. EFFECTS OF GROUPS

i. Effective groups achieve high levels of

- Task performance.
- Member satisfaction.
- Team viability.

ii. Synergy

- Effective groups offer synergy.

- With synergy, groups accomplish more than the total of the members' individual capabilities.

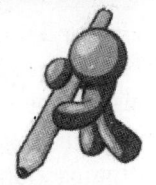

Wisdom Tooth

"The thing I loved the most - and still love the most about teaching - is that you can connect with an individual or a group, and see that individual or group exceed their limits."

Mike Krzyzewski

- Synergy is necessary for organisations to compete effectively and achieve high performance in the long-term.

iii. Social loafing as a performance problem

- Social loafing is the tendency of people to work less hard in a group than they would individually.
- Reasons for social loafing:

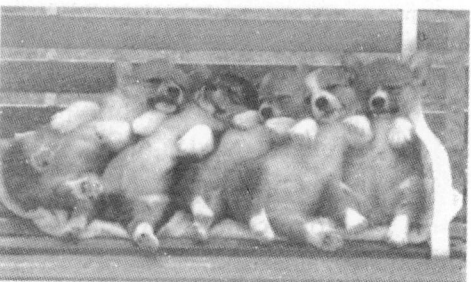

  i. Individual contributions are less noticeable in the group context.

  ii. Some individuals prefer to see others carry the workload.

- Ways of preventing social loafing:

  i. Define member roles and tasks to maximise individual interests.

Example of Social Loafing☺

  ii. Link individual rewards to performance contributions of the group.

  iii. Raise accountability by identifying individuals' performance contributions to the group.

iv. Social Facilitation as a Performance Problem

- It is the tendency of a person's behaviour to be influenced by the presence of others.

- It results in positive effects on the performance when a person is proficient in the task. Also, it has been found that performance of simple, routine tasks tends to increase in the presence of others.

> **Wisdom Tooth**
>
> *"The productivity of a work group seems to depend on how the group members see their own goals in relation to the goals of the organisation."*
>
> **Ken Blanchard**

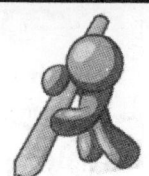

- It results in negative effects on task performance when the task is not well-learned or when the task is more complex and requires more attention.

G. ROLE OF GROUPS

- Group dynamics primarily focuses on the value addition through group efforts. However, sometimes the interpersonal considerations of the group members and also those of the inter-groups results in conflicts (Conflicts are dealt with at the end of chapter). Such conflict situations are detrimental to the person, group, organisation and society at large.

- Thus, it becomes inevitable to eliminate such conflicts and harness the group efforts towards efficiency and value maximisation. Such situations can be created through the development of positive roles and favourable attitudes of the group towards the attainment of the organisational objectives. Such favourable attitudes of a group are classified as below:

i. Task roles

ii. Social roles

iii. Decisional roles

iv. Positive roles

- Each role is briefly explained below:

i. Task Roles

Every group member performs a specific task in the organisation. Such tasks are defined by the formal organisation and are accepted by an employee as a part of the service condition. A group can help the member in performing his task as under:

i. To make member under the group objectives and group problems so that the member can perform his task accordingly.

ii. To invite opinions and suggestions from the group member so that the group activities can be evaluated, improved and adjusted.

iii. To avail new ideals, procedure, and techniques to other groups through experience sharing.

  a. Complex tasks and decisions should be properly structured and presented to the members and should be made available to the group members for their examination and adoption.

  b. To ensure that any conflict area or disputable matter has been settled properly to the satisfaction of the members. Such situation will eliminate any grievance arising in the in the mind of the member.

ii. Social Roles

The groups should play the following social rules:

a. To recognise and appreciate the contribution of any group and to encourage and motivate the group.

b. In case of disagreement among members on any issues, efforts should be made to eliminate or mitigate it.

c. If a group has committed any mistake, then, to accept it and to try to improve it.

d. To facilitate the participation in the discussion.

e. To evaluate the efficiency and effectiveness of the group from time to time.

iii. Decisional Roles

a. To accept the broad, strategic and appropriate decisions of the higher management.

b. To improve the quality of decision through supplying the correct and reliable information as fast as possible.

c. To enhance the decision competence of the members through assigning authorities and responsibilities and giving freedom for decision making.

d. To create the environment that will increase the amenability for developing the consensus in a group decision.

iv. Positive Roles

a. To accelerate the speed of the group work and to try for the economic use of the resources in the group activities.

b. To discourage the tactics of the well-knit small group developing the control on the whole group through polarization.

> ### Wisdom Tooth
>
> *"It'll be all of our efforts together. It won't ever be exactly the way I imagined it. And that is, I think, an important lesson as well, is that in any group enterprise it's going to be the sum total of the group."*
>
> **James Cameron, Director 'Titanic'**

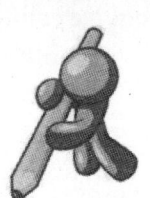

c. To develop and maintain the attitude of divided responsibility. Sometimes it so happens that people tend to develop an attitude that, "every-body responsible means no-body responsible." Divided responsibility develops "a sense of propriety" in the group member who always strive to protect and preserve the resource of the organisation.

H. TYPES OF GROUPS

Groups can classified on many basis, some of which are:

1) Based on the Size Of Group
   i. Small Group.
   ii. Large Group.

2) Based on Closeness of Membership
   i. Primary Group.
   ii. Secondary Group.

3) Based on Permanency of Activities
   i. Temporary Group.

ii. Permanent Group.

4) Based on Formality
    i.   Formal Group.
    ii. Informal Group.

1.i. Small Group

- It is compact and contains few members.
- Members have more interactions and are closely related to each other.
- Dependence on each other is high.

1.ii. Large Group

- It comprise of large number of members or even many smaller groups.
- Members are not so closely related to each other as of a smaller group have less cohesiveness.
- E.g. A Country is an example of large group.

2.i Primary Group

- Primary Group is a very small group which remains in constant contact with each other.
- E.g. A family in a home, a student in a hostel etc.
- They commonly last for years.
- They are similar to small group but its members also have similar interest, values and goals.
- Thus, a primary group is a sub-set of small group.

2.ii. Secondary Groups

- In contrast to primary groups, they are large groups involving formal and institutional relationships.
- The role and position of the members are fixed and they have to act within given set of norms.
- They may last for years or may be disband after a short time.
- Primary groups can be present in secondary settings. For example, attending a university exemplifies membership of a secondary group, while the friendships that are made there would be considered a primary group that you belong to.

3.i Temporary Groups

- Temporary Groups are formed to handle some temporary or ad-hoc activity.

- Such groups are dissolved after the completion of that temporary work.
- E.g. Admission committee is formed to conduct the admission work.

3.ii Permanent Groups

- Permanent group is formed when the activity is repetitive and recurring in nature.
- E.g. Board of Directors of an organisation.

4.i. Formal Group

- These groups are formed by the organisation to carry out specific task. The tasks and responsibilities of the members of formal groups are concerned with achieving organisational goals.
- E.g. The board of editors of a publishing company is a type of a formal group. The organisation forms the group and selects the people who constitute the groups.
- Types of Formal groups include **Command groups** and **Task groups.**

a. Command Group

- Command group is a formal group which is represented in the organisation chart and is relatively permanent in nature.
- The employee who are members of a command group report to a common superior. Thus, they have a functional reporting relationship.
- It handles the routine and regular organisational activities.
- It continues to exist unless a decision is made to change or reconstitute the organisational structure.
- For instance the dean of a Engineering Institute and his faculty members form a command group. Others examples of a command groups in organisation are the quality-control department and the marketing department.
- All the functional departments in an organisational can be considered command groups.

b. Tasks groups

- They are formed to carry out specific task and are generally involved in non routine tasks of organisation.
- Such groups are temporary in nature. They are generally dissolved once the task is over or the problem has been solved.
- Even though people may be made members of a task group, they continue to remain members of their respective command groups or functional departments.

- If a task group member has to spend a lot of time in carrying out the duties of the task group, his command group duties may get affected. Therefore, to reduce his burden, the command group duties are decreased for a short period of time.
- A command group may also be considered a task group, but the reverse is not true since task groups out across boundaries of functional departments and are not characterized by a functional reporting relationship.
- E.g. When shop floor employee, engineers and managers come together to tackle a particular quality problem, a task group is said to have been formed.

Reasons for Formation of Formal Groups

i. To accomplish task that cannot be done by an individual employee.

ii. To bring a number of skills and talents to bear on complex, difficult tasks.

iii. To provide an efficient means for control of employee behaviour.

iv. To satisfy important personal needs as social acceptance and affiliation.

v. To increase organisational stability by transmitting organisational values and believes to employees.

4.ii. Informal Group

- While Formal groups are established by the organisation, informal groups are formed by the employee themselves. Since these groups are not formed by the organisation, they are not structured.
- Common interests and the need for companionship, recreation, growth and support lead to the formation of informal groups.
- A lunch group and a car pool can be considered as informal groups.
- They co-exist along with the formal groups.
- Informal groups are broadly of three types, **Friendship Groups, Interests Groups and Cliques.**

a. Friendship Groups

- They are more permanent in nature. They are formed because of the cordial relationships that the members share with one another.
- The relationship in these groups can be based on similarity in age, ethic heritage, or views.
- The members of the group enjoy each other's company and like to spend time together.

b. Interest Groups

- They are relatively temporary and organised around a common activity or interest.

- E.g. A group of employee coming together to organise a picnic for the department compose an interest group.

c. Cliques

- Cliques consist of colleagues or those employees who associate with each other.

- Number of members is generally smaller and is mostly between five or six.

- They not only provide recognition to each other but also exchange information of mutual interest.

- Cliques are classified into four types.

(1) Vertical Clique

❑ In this case, the superior may be a member in the group consisting mainly of subordinates.

❑ It exists generally when the superior lacks some abilities and is dependent upon the subordinates.

(2) Horizontal Clique

❑ This group consists of people of almost same position and rank and doing more or less same work.

❑ They have some common points and similar objectives.

(3) Random or Mixed Clique

❑ This group contains members from different positions, departments and locations.

❑ The members may form group because they may be members of same club or may be residing in the same locality etc.

(4) Sub-Cliques

❑ In this type, members of a clique inside the organisation forms a group along with persons outside the organisation

Informal Groups are classified on one more factor which is, on the basis of pressure tactics. It was done by **L.R Sayles**, who identified four kinds of groups in the organisations which are discussed below:

a. Apathetic Groups

- This group hardly uses pressure tactics and very less problems occur in it.
- This type of group generally does not contain any clearly defined leader.
- E.g. Low skilled Assembly line workers lack unity and power and hardly ever use pressure tactics.

b. Erratic Groups

- This group lack consistency in their behaviour. Sometimes they oppose the management while on other occasions, they may be cooperative.
- In such a group, any active member could become the leader.
- E.g. Semiskilled workers who work together in performing jobs that require some interaction with each other.

c. Strategic Groups

- The members of such a group are able to prepare a strategy for putting pressure on other groups and the management.
- These people are highly united and participate actively in union activity.
- Members of such groups generally perform technologically independent jobs and are comparatively better placed than members of earlier categories.

d. Conservative Groups

- This group uses controlled pressure and only for highly specific objectives.
- The members of the group are professionals and highly skilled employees.
- They are found at higher levels of the organisation and display considerable self confidence.
- They work independently and are capable of shutting down the plant if they so desire.
- They have moderate unity among its members but the group on whole is very strong and very stable.

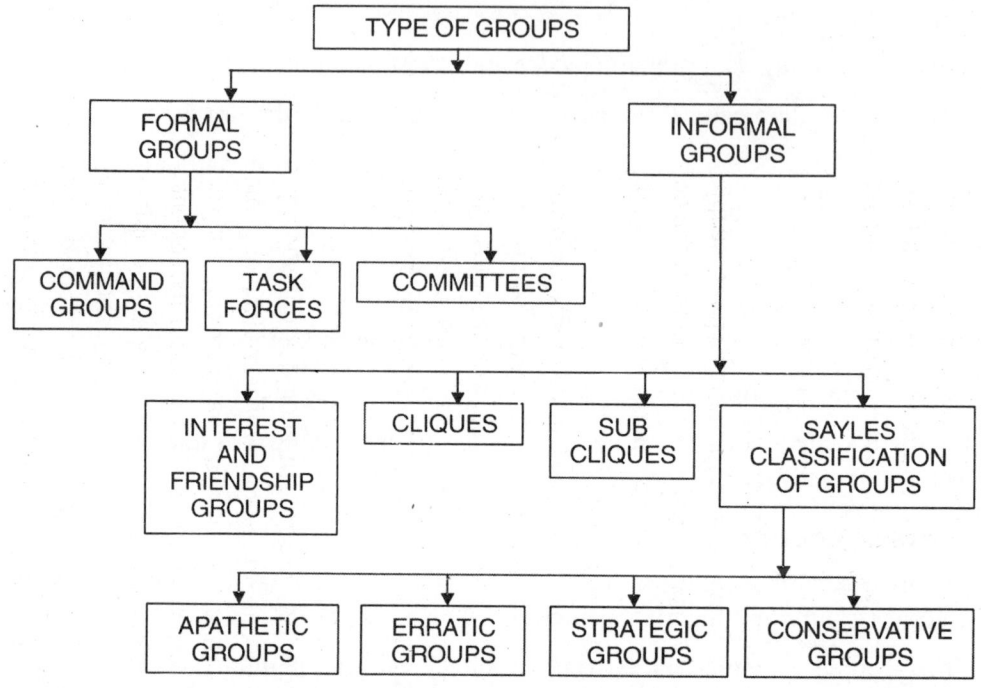

Characteristics of the Informal Groups

i. It is natural outcome and is not planned or designed.

ii. It evolves constantly over time.

iii. It is formed on the basis of some similarity among members as of age, sex, caste, interests, personality etc.

iv. Members are formed voluntarily and may join several informal organisations at the same time.

v. Behaviour of members is controlled by group norms and standards.

vi. Informal Groups are more humane and friendly towards its members and has high degree of Group cohesiveness and cooperation.

Functions of Informal Groups

i. They perpetuate the cultural and social values that the group holds dear. Certain values are usually already held in common among informal group members.

ii. They provide social status and satisfaction that may not be obtained from the formal organisation. In a large organisation (or classroom), a worker (or student) may feel like an anonymous number rather than a unique individual.

iii. They promote communication among members. The informal group develops a communication channel or system (i.e., grapevine) to keep its members informed about what management actions will affect them in various ways.

Benefits/Advantages of Informal Groups

i. Blend with Formal System

- Formal plans, policies, procedures, and standards cannot solve every problem in a dynamic organisation; therefore, informal systems must blend with formal ones to get work done.
- As early as 1951, Robert Dubin recognised that "informal relations in the organisation serve to preserve the organisation from the self-destruction that would result from literal obedience to the formal policies, rules, regulations, and procedures."

ii. Lighten Management Workload

- Managers are less inclined to check up on workers when they know the informal organisation is cooperating with them.
- This encourages delegation, decentralization, and greater worker support of the manager, which suggests a probable improvement in performance and overall productivity.

iii. Fill Gaps In Management Abilities

- If a manager is weak in financial planning and analysis, a subordinate may informally assist in preparing reports through either suggestions or direct involvement.

iv. Encourage Improved Management Practice

- They encourage managers to prepare, plan, organise, and control in a more professional fashion. Managers who comprehend the power of the informal organisation recognise that it is a "check and balance" on their use of authority.
- Changes and projects are introduced with more careful thought and consideration, knowing that the informal organisation can easily kill a poorly planned project.

v. Work Problem Solutions

- Members of informal group share their knowledge and experience and thus helps other members in solving any work related problem

vi. Speedy Communication

- It is a very fast way of communication as it is free from barriers of status and position.
- Thus management can use it when fast communication is required.

vii. Social Function

- Employees experience frustration, tension, and emotional problems with management and other employees. The informal group provides a means for relieving these emotional and psychological pressures by allowing a person to discuss them among friends openly and candidly.

viii. Discipline

- Informal groups have set of norms and code of behaviour.
- Thus they check the behaviour of its members and helps in maintaining discipline and order.

Negative Aspects of Informal Group

i. Resisting Organisational Changes

- Sometimes, informal groups reject the introduction of change within the organisation.
- This may hamper the growth of organisation as new ideas may be difficult to implement.

ii. Role Conflict

- An employee may experience role conflict if the informal group and the organisation place demands on him.
- By integrating the interests, goals, methods, and evaluation procedures of the formal organisation with those of the informal group, the management can ensure higher productivity and employee's satisfaction.

iii. Increased Scope for Rumors

- Rumors often start in informal groups and spread quickly throughout the organisation, causing immense damage if they are not dealt with promptly.
- The best way to handle rumors is to provide people with adequate information.

iv. Pressure To Conform To Group Norms

- Members are often pressurized to comply with the norms of the group.
- Conformity to the norms of the group becomes a problem when the leaders of the group try to manipulate the members of the group to satisfy their own selfish motives.

v. Restriction of Output

- It has been shown in Hawthorne experiments that informal groups may restrict the output by pressurising the members of the group.

vi. Politics for Power

- Informal leaders may undermine organisational values and norms in order to gain dominance over management.

vii. Group Rivalry

- Certain groups could be turned to an unnecessary hatred between themselves due to difference in interest or to gain power over other

- Thus, while useful information is passed within one group, another group may communicate malicious rumor.

Management Response to Informal Groups

Top management is quite suspicious of powerful informal groups, and generally tries to abolish them. However, many studies on group dynamics have revealed that informal groups cannot be abolished. Therefore, in order to ensure the smooth functioning of the organisation, the management should understand the dynamics of the informal groups operating within it. Management should –

i. Accept and understand the informal organisations.

ii. Identify various levels of attitudes and behaviours within it.

iii. Consider possible effects on informal group systems when taking any kind of action.

iv. Integrate as far as possible the interest of informal groups with those of the formal organisations.

v. Keep formal activities from unnecessarily threatening informal organisations.

vi. Should maintain good relations with leader of the informal group by consulting him in certain matters and also seeking his advice to improve the performance of workers.

Difference Between Formal And Informal Groups

Informal Group	Formal Group
i. Evolves spontaneously and naturally.	i. Created deliberately and consciously.
ii. Formed for social and psychological satisfaction.	ii. Formed to achieve objective of organisation.
iii. Members have a common liking, interest etc.	iii. Members may not have anything in common except for the completion of organisational target.
iv. Unstable in nature.	iv. Very stable in nature.
v. Cohered by Trust and Reciprocity	v. Bound together by codified rules and order.
vi. All members are equal. Some may command authority due to their personality.	vi. Authority flows from higher to lower levels.
vii. Members behave according to norms and values.	vii. Members behave as per formal rules and regulations.
viii. Larger in Size	viii. Smaller in size

TEST YOUR GREY MATTER?

Q1) Define Group and Group Dynamics?

Q2) What are the characteristics by which you will identify whether an entity is a Group or not?

Q3) Give the reasons for group formation?

Q4) Define and explain meaning of Synergy?

Q5) What do you understand by social loafing?

Q6) Give briefly the various roles played by a Group?

Q7) Explain with a flowchart, the various types of Group? Also define Formal and Informal Group?

Q8) How many types of Formal Groups are there? Describe each of them?

Q9) How many types of Informal Groups exists? How are they different from each other?

Q10) What is a Clique? Describe different types of Cliques?

Q11) Why do an individual joins a Informal Group?

Q12) List out various characteristics of an Informal Group?

Q13) Do Informal groups have negative effects? Comment.

Q14) Differentiate between Formal and Informal Groups?

Q15) Enumerate various methods which management must use to tackle Informal Groups?

I. STAGES OF GROUP DEVELOPMENT

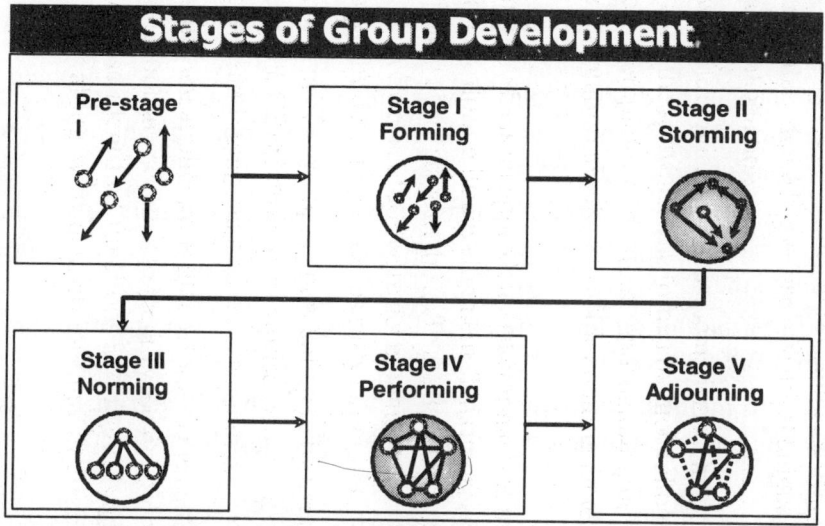

I.1. Five stage model

- American organisational psychologist Bruce Tuckman presented a model in 1965.
- According to this model, all groups pass through five stages – Forming, Storming, Norming, Performing and Adjourning.

i. Forming

- In the Forming stage the group comes together for the first time.
- The members may already know each other or they may be total strangers. In either case, there is a level of formality, some anxiety, and a degree of guardedness
- Members try to identify what behaviour would be acceptable to others in the group and try to mould their own behaviour accordingly.
- At this stage, members are uncertain about the group's purpose, structure, tasks and leadership.
- This stage is often characterized by abstract discussions about issues to be addressed by the group; those who like to get moving can become impatient with this part of the process.
- This phase is usually short in duration, perhaps a meeting or two.

ii. Storming

- Once group members feel sufficiently safe and included, they tend to enter the Storming Phase. This stage is characterized by conflicts and confrontation within the group.
- Members begin to explore their power and influence and they often stake out their territory by differentiating themselves from the other group members rather than seeking common ground.
- They may resist the constraints imposed by the group and may raise conflicting points of view and values, or disagree over how tasks should be done and who is assigned to them.
- It is not unusual for group members to become defensive, competitive, or jealous. They may take sides or begin to form cliques within the group.
- Once group members discover that they can be authentic and that the group is capable of handling differences without dissolving, they to enter the next stage.

iii. Norming

- This stage is characterized by the development of close relationships and cohesiveness within the group.
- Members develop a strong sense of group identity and find it easy to establish their own ground rules (or norms) and define their operating procedures and goals.
- It is hoped at this point the group members are more open and respectful toward each other and willing to ask one another for both help and feedback. They may even begin to form friendships and share more personal information.
- This is completed when a common set of expectation defining appropriate behaviour has been developed.

iv. Performing

- In this stage, the group becomes fully functional and involved in activities aimed at achieving the goals defined in a norming stage.
- Members are not only getting the work done, but they also pay greater attention to how they are doing it.
- Although the members may be involved in independent activities, they are committed to the achievement of the group.

v. Adjourning

- Just as groups form, so do they end. For example, many groups or teams formed in a business context are project-oriented and therefore are temporary

- The feelings of members vary at this stage. While some may be happy about the group's accomplishments, others may be depressed that they would be losing each other after the group is dispended.

1.2. Punctuated Equilibrium Model

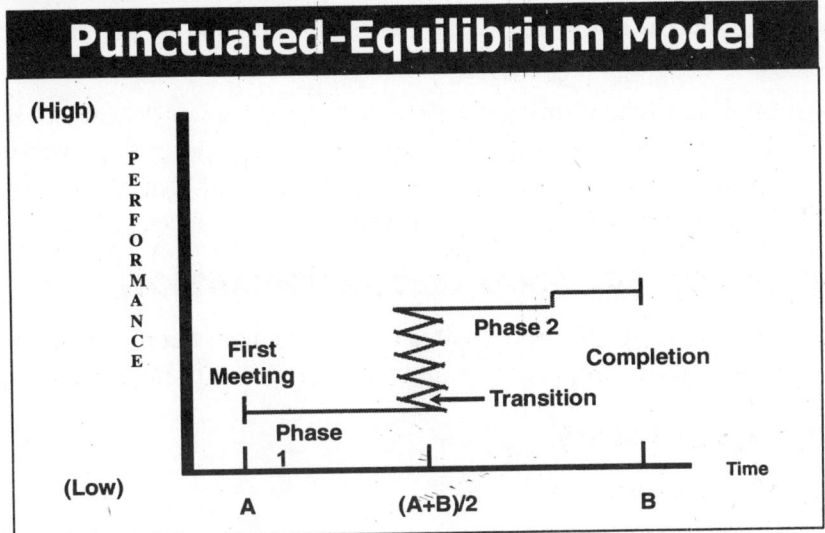

- Joy H. Karriker, found that the life of a group is much more dynamic and cyclical in nature than proposed by Five Stage Model. For example, a group may operate in the Performing stage for several months. Then, because of a disruption, such as a competing emerging technology that changes the rules of the game or the introduction of a new CEO, the group may move back into the Storming phase before returning to Performing.

- The concept of punctuated equilibrium was first proposed in 1972 by paleontologists Niles Eldredge and Stephen Jay Gould, who both believed that evolution occurred in rapid, radical spurts rather than gradually over time.

- According to punctuated equilibrium model, the process of group formation is characterized by long periods of inertia, punctuated or interspersed with brief periods of activity.

- These periods of activity primarily take place when the members become aware of the time and the approaching project deadline

- The first meeting of the group sets the direction of the group. This direction is unlikely to change during the first half of the duration of the project. The first half of the project is characterized by a period of inertia. During this period, no new insights or behavioural patterns develop that challenge the initial patterns of behaviour and assumptions made by the group.

- Halfway through the project duration, the members of the group suddenly experience a heightened sense of awareness of the lapse of time and the lack of progress in the project. This stage marks the transition into the second phase of the project, wherein a new equilibrium is established among the members and a revised direction is set for the group.

- The last meeting of the group just before the completion of the project is marked by a period of intense activity. During this period, the group works toward completing the project on time by finishing all the tasks that remain to be done and resolving all details pertaining to the project.

J. THEORIES OF INFORMAL GROUP FORMATION

Informal groups are not deliberately created by management but they emerge on their own. Various theories are proposed to explain the formation of informal groups.

J.1. Propinquity Theory

- Propinquity means nearness.

- This theory states that people affiliate with each other or forms informal groups because of geographical or spatial closeness.

- Thus it simply states that people working together forms group because they are near to each other.

- Its drawback is that it does not explain the complexities of group formation.

J.2. Humans Interaction Theory

- It is based on three concepts namely Activities, Interactions and Sentiments.

- According to George C. Homans, "The more activities persons share, the more numerous will be their interactions and the stronger will be their shared activities and sentiments, and the more sentiments people have for one another, the more will be their shared activities and interactions. The members of a group share activities and interactions. The members of a group share activities and interact with one another not just because of physical proximity but also to accomplish group goals. The key element is interaction because of which they develop common sentiments for one another."

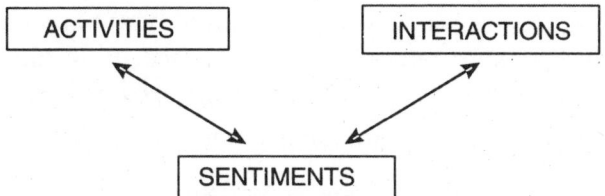

- William G. Scott observes that interactions helped in attaining goals, resolve tension and achieve stability.

J.3.Balance Theory

- It was given by Theodore M. Newcomb.
- He states that "Persons are attracted to one another on the basis of similar attitudes towards commonly relevant objects and goals. Once a relationship is formed, it strives to maintain a symmetrical balance between the attraction and the common attitudes. If an imbalance occurs, attempts are made to restore the balance. If the balance cannot be restored, the relationship dissolves."

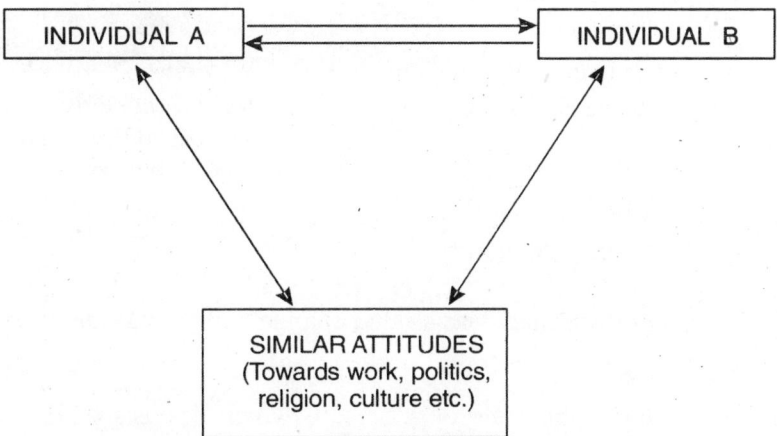

- All the group formation may not be a result of similarity of attitudes. Thus, this theory does not completely explain group formation.

J.4.Exchange Theory

- This theory is propounded by John W.Thaibaut and Harold H.Kelly.
- it is based on Reward-Cost outcomes of interactions which says that to be attracted towards a group, a person thinks in terms of what he will get in exchange for interaction with group members.

- A minimum positive level (rewards greater than costs) of an outcome must exist in order for attraction or affiliation to take place. Rewards from interactions gratify needs while costs incur anxiety, frustrations, embarrassment or fatigue.
- Propinquity, interaction and common attitudes, all have roles in the exchange theory.

K. FACTORS AFFECTING GROUP PERFORMANCE

K.1. Group Roles

Role played by the member affects the performance of the group.

Determinants of Role

Following are the factors which determine the role of its members:

i. Role Identity

- Role identity reflects the attitude and behaviour required for a position from the member of the group.
- Role changes when situation or job demands changes.
- E.g., in a particular work place when some workers were promoted to supervisory jobs, their attitudes changed from pro union to pro management within a few months of their promotions. It means there was a rapid change in their role identities.

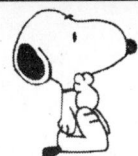

Thinking Time !!

Think about all the friends you had in your life. Which of the above theories justifies your reason for having those friends?

ii. Role Perception

- Role perception is the view of a person, which consists of those activities or behaviours the individual believes are supposed to be fulfilled in the given situation.
- For example, every scientist is certainly influenced by Mr. A.P.J Abdul Kalam.
- Because of role perception, apprenticeship programmes exist in many trade and professions, in which beginners watch an 'expert', so that they can learn to act as they are supposed to.

iii. Role Expectations

- Role expectations are defined as how others believe or expect a member to act in a given situation.

- When role expectations are not met, there are negative repercussions from both the sides.

iv. Role Inaction

- Role inaction is the way the person actually behaves and acts.
- It comes from the perceived and expected role.

v. Role Conflict

- Role conflict occurs when an individual is confronted by divergent role expectation.
- It includes situations in which two or more role expectations are mutually contradictions.

Type of Roles

- There are three types of roles identified
  Task Oriented Roles, Social Roles and Individualistic Roles.
- For a group to be successful, role of its members must either relate to the task aspect of the group or promote social interaction.
- A third set of roles are self-centered and can be destructive for the group.

(i) Task-Oriented Roles	Researchers Benne and Sheats identified several roles which relate to the completion of the group's task: ➤ **Initiator-Contributor:** Generates new ideas. ➤ **Information-Seeker:** Asks for information about the task. ➤ **Opinion-Seeker:** Asks for the input from the group about its values. ➤ **Information-Giver:** Offers facts or generalization to the group. ➤ **Opinion-Giver:** States his or her beliefs about a group issue. ➤ **Elaborator:** Explains ideas within the group, offers examples to clarify ideas. ➤ **Coordinator:** Shows the relationships between ideas. ➤ **Orienter:** Shifts the direction of the group's discussion. ➤ **Evaluator-Critic:** Measures group's actions against some objective standard. ➤ **Energizer:** Stimulates the group to a higher level of activity. ➤ **Procedural-Technician:** Performs logistical functions for the group. ➤ **Recorder:** Keeps a record of group actions.

(ii) Social Roles	Groups also have members who play certain social roles: ➤ **Encourager**: Praises the ideas of others. ➤ **Harmonizer:** Mediates differences between group members. ➤ **Compromiser:** Moves group to another position that is favoured by all group members. ➤ **Gatekeeper/Expediter:** Keeps communication channels open. ➤ **Standard Setter:** Suggests standards or criteria for the group to achieve. ➤ **Group Observer:** Keeps records of group activities and uses this information to offer feedback to the group. ➤ **Follower:** Goes along with the group and accepts the group's ideas.
(iii) Individualistic Roles	These roles place the group member above the group and are destructive to the group. ➤ **Aggressor:** Attacks other group members, deflates the status of others, and other aggressive behaviour. ➤ **Blocker:** Resists movement by the group. ➤ **Recognition Seeker:** Calls attention to himself or herself. ➤ **Self-Confessor:** Seeks to disclose non-group related feelings or opinions. ➤ **Dominator:** Asserts control over the group by manipulating the other group members. ➤ **Help Seeker:** Tries to gain the sympathy of the group. ➤ **Special Interest Pleader:** Uses stereotypes to assert his or her own prejudices.

K.2. Group Norms

Definition: "Group Norms are a set of beliefs, feelings, and attitudes commonly shared by group members. These are also referred to as rules or standards of behaviour that apply to group members".

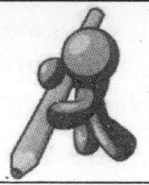

Wisdom Tooth

"The productivity of a work group seems to depend on how the group members see their own goals in relation to the goals of the organization."

Ken Blanchard

Characteristics of Group Norms

i.   Norms are the basis of behaviour of member in the group.

ii. Norms identify the values and ethics of the group members.

iii. The norms are also the basis for predicting and controlling the behaviour of group members.

iv. The norms are applied to all members. For example, if a code of dress for the meetings or for the work place is there, it is to be followed by all the members.

v. Formalised norms are written up in organisational manuals which set out rules and procedures for employees to follow, but by far the majority of norms in organisations are informal.

Types of Norms

i. Performance Norms

- These norms regulate the performance and productivity of the individual members.
- By this work groups provides their members with performing details as how hard they should work, how to get the job done, their level of output etc.

ii. Appearance Norms

- These norms include things like appropriate dress. Some organisation have formal dress codes.
- Appearance norms also involve loyalty or confidentiality on the part of members and organisation.

iii. Arrangement Norms

- These norms are from informal work groups and primarily regulate social informal interactions within the group.

iv. Allocation of Resource Norms

- These norms cover things like pay, assignment of jobs and allocations of new tools and equipment.

v. Behaviour Norms

- These norms include the rules and guidelines defining the day to day behaviour of people at work.
- It includes punctuality, completing any given assignments within the required time framework, not losing temper, showing respect for other members opinions and so on.

Development of Norms

Most norms develop in one of the following four ways:

i. Explicit Statement Made by a Group Member

- Explicit statements made by the supervisors or a powerful member may become norms.
- For example, the supervisor may explicitly say that tea breaks are to be kept to ten minutes and this will become a norm.

ii. Critical Events in the Group's History

- For example, a person who was standing too close to a machine was injured in a work group.
- Thus it became a norm that no person other than the operator gets within five feet of any machine

iii. Primacy

- Primacy refers to the first behaviour pattern that emerges in a group.
- If the first group meeting is marked by very formal interaction between supervisors and subordinates then the group considers it to be a norm and expects future meetings to be conducted in the same way.

iv. Past Experience

- Many norms develop because members may bring their past experiences from other groups and organisations.

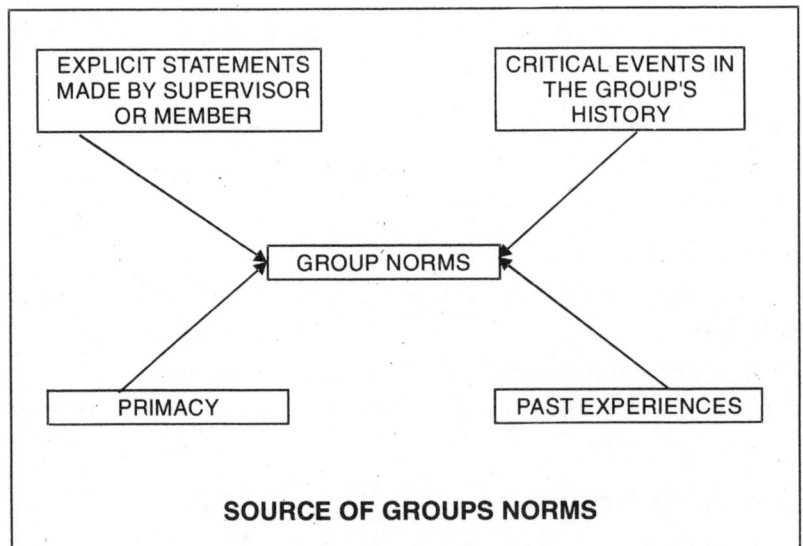

SOURCE OF GROUPS NORMS

Advantages of Norms

Norms are enforced because of the following reasons:

i. It facilitates the group's survival
- Groups strongly enforce those norms that increase their chances of success.
- They also protect them from interference of other groups or individuals.

ii. It increases the predictability of group member's behaviour
- Norms that increase predictability enable group members to anticipate each other's actions and to prepare appropriate responses.

iii. It reduces embarrassing interpersonal problems
- Norms are important if they ensure satisfaction to their members and prevent as much interpersonal discomfort as possible.

iv. It helps in expressing values
- It allows members to express the central value of the group and clarify what is distinctive about the group's identity.

v. It reflects the preferences of the supervisor
- Norms are likely to reflect the preferences of supervisor or other powerful group members.

You should know

Ostracism - Rejection by the group for violation of its norms.

K.3.Group Cohesiveness

- Group cohesiveness is the extent to which group members trust one another, are committed to accomplishing a team goal, and share a feeling of group pride.
- Two dimensions of Group Cohesiveness:

  ### i. Emotional (or personal) Cohesiveness
  - The emotional aspect of cohesiveness is about the

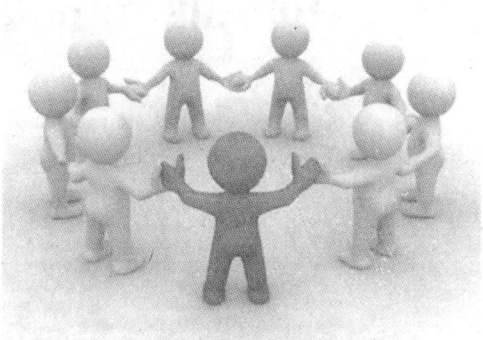

connection that members feel to other group members and to their group as a whole.

- It tells about how much do members like to spend time with other group members? Do they look forward to the next group meeting?

ii. Task-cohesiveness

- It refers to the degree to which group members share group goals and work together to meet these goals.

- That is, is there a feeling that the group works smoothly as one unit or do different people pull in different directions?

Factors Influencing Group Cohesiveness

The forces that push group members together can be positive (group-based rewards) or negative (things lost upon leaving the group). The main factors that influence group cohesiveness are: members' similarity, group size, entry difficulty, group success and external competition and threats.

i. Members' Similarity

- The more group members are similar to each other on various characteristics the easier it would be to reach cohesiveness.

- By Social Identity Theory, people feel closer to those whom they perceive as similar to themselves in terms of external characteristics (age, ethnicity) or internal ones (values, attitudes).

- Similar background also makes it more likely that members share similar views on various issues, including group objectives, how to communicate and the type of desired leadership.

- In general, higher agreement among members on group rules and norms results in greater trust and less conflict. This, in turn, strengthens both emotional and task cohesiveness.

Working with idiots can kill you!

IDIOTS in the office are just as hazardous to your health as cigarettes, caffeine or greasy food, an eye-opening new study reveals.

In fact, those dopes can kill you! Stress is one of the top causes of heart attacks — and working with stupid people on a daily basis is one of the deadliest forms of stress, according to researchers at Sweden's Lindbergh University MedicalCentre.

The author of the study, Dr Dagmar Andersson, says her team studied 500 heart attack patients, and were puzzled to find 62 percent had relatively few of the physical risk factors commonly blamed for heart attacks.

"Then we questioned them about lifestyle habits, and almost all of these low-risk patients told us they worked with people so stupid they can barely find their way from the parking lot to their office. And their heart attack came less than 12 hours after having a major confrontation with one of these oafs.

"One woman had to be rushed to the hospital after her assistant shredded important company tax documents instead of copying them. A man told us he collapsed right at his desk because the woman at the next cubicle kept asking him for correction fluid — for her computer monitor.

"You can cut back on smoking or improve your diet," Dr Andersson says, "but most people have very poor coping skills when it comes to stupidity — they feel there's nothing they can do about it, so they just internalise their frustration until they finally explode."

Stupid co-workers can also double or triple someone's work load, she explains. "Many of our subjects feel sorry for the drooling idiots they work with, so they try to cover for them by fixing their mistakes. One poor woman spent a week rebuilding client records because a clerk put them all in the 'recycle bin' of her computer and then emptied it — she thought it meant the records would be recycled and used again."

ii. Group Size

- Smaller groups are more cohesive than larger groups as it is easier for fewer people to agree on goals and to co-ordinate their work.

- Task cohesiveness may suffer, though, if the group lacks enough members to perform its tasks well enough.

iii. Entry Difficulty

- The more elite the group is perceived to be, the more prestigious it is to be a member in that group and consequently, the more motivated members are to belong and stay in it.

- This is why alumni of prestigious universities tend to keep in touch for many years after they graduate.

iv. Group Success

- Group success, increases the value of group membership to its members and influences members to identify more strongly with the team and to want to be actively associated with it.

v. External Competition and Threats

- When members perceive active competition with another group, they become more aware of members' similarity within their group as well as seeing their group as a means to overcome the external threat or competition they are facing.

- Both these factors increase group cohesiveness.

- E.g., It is observed when a society faces any natural disaster.

Importance of Group Cohesiveness

- Group Cohesiveness is important as it is related to group productivity.

		COHESIVENESS	
		High	Low
PERFORMANCE NORMS	High	High Productivity	Moderate Productivity
	Low	Low Productivity	Moderate To Low Productivity

- Cohesiveness and productivity depends on performance related norms established by the group.
- For high performance related norms such as high output, quality work etc. a cohesive group will be more productive than will a less cohesive group.
- For high Cohesiveness and low performance norms, productivity will be low.
- For low Cohesiveness and high performance norms, productivity increases but increases less than high cohesiveness-high norms situation.
- For low Cohesiveness and low performance norms, productivity falls to low to moderate range.
- But cohesiveness can also lower group performance, especially in a working setting. When employee becomes too cohesive, they often lose sight of organisational goals. For example, police departments tend to be highly cohesive – so that anyone who is not a police officer is considered an outsider which can make community relations difficult.

K.4. Group Homogeneity

- Homogeneity is the extent to which its members are similar.
- A homogeneous group contains members who are similar in some or most ways, whereas a heterogeneous group contains member who are more different than alike.
- Thus Homogeneity or Heterogeneity affects the performance of group.

K.5. Stability of Membership

- The greater the stability of the group, the greater the cohesiveness.
- Thus, groups in which members remain for long periods of time are more cohesive and perform better than groups that have high turnover.
- Also, the groups whose members have worked together perform better than groups whose members are not familiar with one another.

K.6. Isolation

- Physical isolation is another variable that tends to increase a group's cohesiveness.
- Groups that are isolated or located away from other groups tend to be highly cohesive.

K.7. Group Size

- Groups of small sizes perform best as they are more cohesive.
- Large groups have lower productivity, less coordination and low morale.

- Groups with 5 numbers of people are considered to be best.

K.8. Personality of Group Member

- Personality of a group member affects the performance of a group.
- Employees who are emotionally stable, have urge to learn and perform, are open to experience etc are better suited for group performance.

L. GROUP CONFLICT

Definition: Conflict is the psychological and behavioural reaction to a perception that another persons is either keeping you from reaching a goal, taking away your right to behave in a particular way, or violating the expectancies of a relationship.

When the conflict arises in a group it gives rise to Group Conflict.

- The level of conflict that occur is a function of the importance of the goal, behaviour, or relationship. That is, one person's behaviour may force a change in another's, but if the change in behaviour is not important to the individual, conflict will be less than in a situation in which the change is important.

Types of Conflict

i. Interpersonal conflict

- Interpersonal conflict occurs between two individuals.
- In the workplace, interpersonal conflict might occur between two co-workers, a supervisor and a subordinate, an employee and a customer or an employee and a vendor.

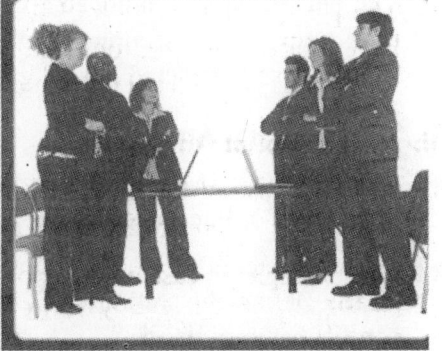

ii. Individual – group conflict

- Individual –group conflict usually occurs when the individual's needs are different from the group needs, goals, or norms.

iii. Group - group conflicts

- The third type of conflict occurs between two or more groups.
- Example, when two departmental groups fight when they want to allocate

Wisdom Tooth

"All men have an instinct for conflict: at least, all healthy men."

Hilaire Belloc

budget to their department.

Causes of Conflict

i. Competition for resources

- In groups, when demand for a resource exceeds its supply, conflict occurs.
- This often true in organisations, especially when there is not enough money, space, personnel, or equipment to satisfy the needs of every group.
- Example, different clubs (e.g. Cultural Club, Sports Club, Hobby Club, Photography Club) of a college try to extract more fund for them and this leads to conflict between them.

ii. Task Interdependence

- Another cause of conflict, task interdependence, comes when the performance of some group members depends on the performance of the other group members.
- For example, a group is assigned to telecast news on television. But if the group which is responsible to write the news does not do the job correctly or in time, it may lead to conflict between the two groups.
- The person who is assigned to type the report cannot do his job unless others have written their sections, and no member of the group is finished until every member has completed the assigned work.

iii. Jurisdictional Ambiguity

- A third cause of conflict, jurisdictional ambiguity, is found when geographical boundaries or lines of authority are unclear.
- For example, in case of Functional Foremen of F.W Taylor, (Refer Chapter 2) to clearly define the authority of 8 foremen may be difficult and thus result in conflict between them.

iv. Communication Barriers

- Communication barriers are the fourth cause of conflict.
- The barriers to interpersonal communication can be physical, such as separate locations on different floors or different buildings; cultural, such as different languages or different customs; or psychological, such as different styles or personalities.

v. Beliefs

A fifth cause of conflict is the belief systems of the individuals or groups. Conflict is most likely to occur when individuals or groups believe that they:

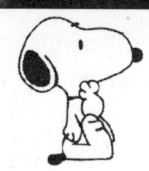

Thinking Time !!
Have you ever been in any conflict with anybody? Why? How did you solve the problem? If the conflict still persists then try to resolve it by reading the methods mentioned below

a. Are superiors to the other people or groups.

b. Have been mistreated by other.

c. Are vulnerable to others .

d. Cannot trust others.

e. Are helpless or powerless.

Resolving Conflicts

Following methods may be used for resolving conflict:

i. Prior to Conflict Occurring

- An organisation should have a formal policy on conflict handling.
- Such policy may state that employee should try to resolve their own conflicts, and if that is not successful, they should utilize a third party intervention.
- Employees should also receive training on the causes of the conflict, ways to prevent conflict, and strategies for resolving conflict.

ii. When Conflict First Occurs

- When conflict fist occurs between co-workers and between a supervisor and a subordinate, the two parties should be encouraged to use the conflict resolution skill they learned in training to resolve the conflict on their own.
- These skills include expressing a desire for cooperation, offering compliments, avoiding negative interaction, emphasizing mutual similarities and pointing out common goals.
- Tension should be reduced and trust should be increased between two parties.
- This helps in resolving minor conflicts easily and in mitigating large conflicts.

iii. Third Party Intervention

- If conflict can not be resolved by the parties involved, then **third-party intervention is preferred.**

This third party usually is provided through mediation, and if that doesn't work, through arbitration.

(a) Mediation

❑ With **mediation,** a neutral third party is asked to help both parties reach a mutual agreeable solution to the conflict.

❑ Mediators do not make decisions rather their role is to facilitate the communication process by providing the parties with a safe and equitable venue so that they are more willing and able to reach a solution.

❑ Mediators can be employees of the organisation (e.g. team leader, supervisor, human resource manager) or professional mediators who work with a variety of organisations.

❑ Mediators are mostly preferred when two parties do not trust on one another and they provide the best results when both sides consider the mediator to be competent and trustworthy.

(b) Arbitration

❑ With arbitration, a neutral third party listens to both sides' arguments and then makes a decision.

❑ Within an organisation, this neutral party is often the manager of the two employees or HR personnel

TEST YOUR GREY MATTER

Q1) Explain (i) Five stage model (ii) Punctuated Equilibrium Model

Q2) Describe various Theories which explains the formation of Informal Groups.

Q3) How does following affects the Group Performance:
   (i) Group Roles
   (ii) Group Norms.
   (iii) Group Cohesiveness

Q4) What are the various types of Roles of an individual in a group?

Q5) Define Group Norms? What are the characteristics of Group Norms?

Q6) Give various advantages of Group Norms? Also describe various types of Norms?

Q7) Explain Group Cohesiveness? What are the factors which affect Group Cohesiveness?

Q8) What is the relation between Group Cohesiveness and Group Performance?

Q9) Define Conflict? What are the various causes of Group Conflict?

Q10) What are various types of Conflicts?

Q11) Personal Beliefs are major reason for conflict in a group? Comment.

Q12) Describe various methods of resolving conflicts?

Q13) What is Third Party Intervention? How is it an important method for conflict resolution?

CHAPTER 11
Work Environment and Engineering Psychology

By the end of this chapter, you would be able to :

- Understand why and how Work Environment affects the performance of workers.

- Know different types of working conditions.

- Understand the effect of different working conditions on the worker and ways to provide adequate environment.

- Learn about Engineering Psychology.

- Appreciate the importance of Ergonomics while working.

The chapter contains :

- Introduction

- Work Environment definition and types

- Different working environmental conditions as noise, illumination, atmospheric condition, cleanliness and music.

- Engineering Psychology definition and fields.

- Definition of Ergonomics

- 5 Aspects/Objectives of Ergonomics

A. THE INSIGHT

Would you like to work here

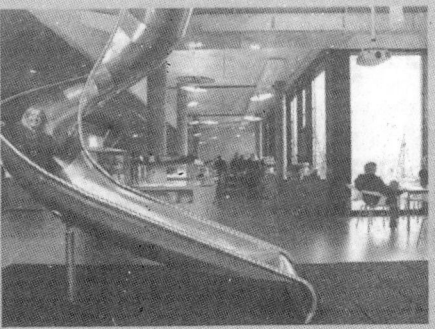

And here?

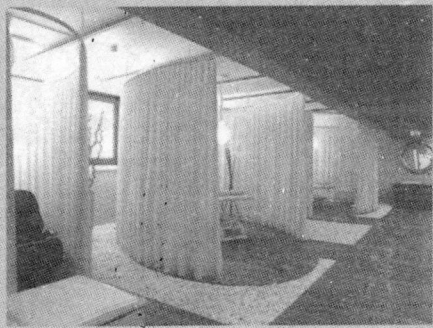

Or here?

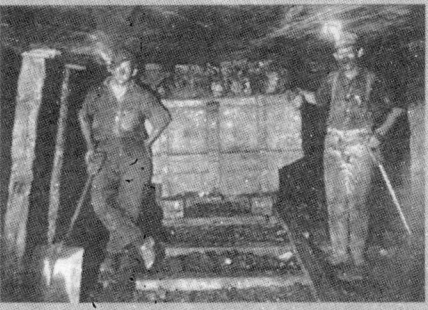

The first two photographs are from the office of Google Inc. while the third is a coal mining work place.

There is only one difference in them, THE WORK ENVIRONMENT...

B. WORK ENVIRONMENT

- As we have seen in the Hawthorne Study Experiment on illumination, change in environment may not be the real cause of decrease or increase in production as there are other factors also which may affect production.
- Improving the working environment may not cause miracles, yet it would always be desirable to have pleasant working conditions.

Also, adverse and bad work environment may have the following effects

i. Health of the worker may be affected which may prevent him from working to his full potential.

ii. Worker may not focus properly on his work and get distracted by poor working facilities.

iii. Bad environment may de-motivate him and he would not give his best efforts.

iv. Absenteeism and attrition may increase.

v. As the worker may not contribute to his optimum efficiency, it would certainly affect the quality and efficiency of the whole organisation.

Definition: Work Environment comprises of the surroundings in which a worker does his work; It can be broadly classified into 3 types –

i. Physical Environment

It includes illumination, noise, colour, vibration, temperature etc. These considerably affect the performance of the worker. We will discuss them in detail later.

ii. Psychological/Mental Environment

It is related to the emotional well-being of the worker. It is the state of his mind, of either stress or happiness which results from the work environment. Mental environment must be created so that worker can contribute more creatively and with motivation.

iii. Social Environment

As we saw in the Hawthorne experiments, social grouping is one of the most important aspects of a worker's performance in an organisation. So, his group of co-workers, his relationship with the management and other people he is associated with at work, constitutes his social environment.

Some working environmental conditions are

1. Noise

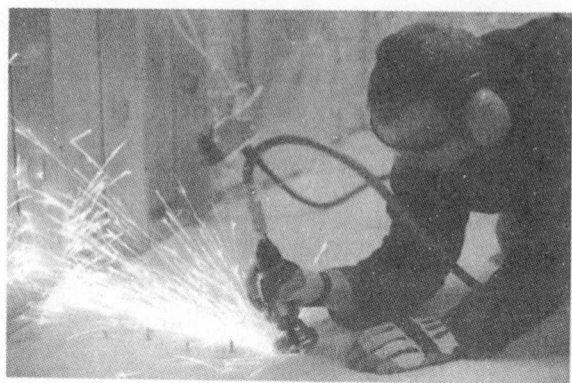

- In simple terms, unwanted sound is called noise.
- Several researches have been conducted to determine the effect of noise at the workplace-

  ❏ Vernor and Warner found that if noise is steady, the person adapts himself to it, but when it is intermittent, it requires greater effort to maintain the efficiency.

  ❏ Park and Payne found that average performance was not affected by intense noise if the task undertaken was of high difficulty.

  ❏ Culbert and Posner found that individuals could adapt to noise in certain time and then no performance change was observed.

  ❏ Morgan found that initially, any irrelevant noise retarded the speed of work but then, speed increased due to the extra effort put in by the worker to overcome the effect of noise.

- Noise at the workplace can be divided into two types –

  a. **Internal:** Caused by machines or people inside the organisation. This noise can be controlled.

  b. **External:** It is caused by factors outside the organisation such as, other

---

You should know

How is noise measured?

Noise is measured in decibels (dB). An 'A-weighting sometimes written as 'dB(A), is used to measure average noise levels, and a 'C-weighting or 'dB(C), to measure peak, impact or explosive noises. You might just notice a 3 dB change in noise level, because of the way our ears work. Yet every 3 dB doubles the noise, so what might seem like small differences in the numbers can be quite significant.

factories, railway lines etc. This noise is not in one's control.

- **Prevention**

High intensity noises should certainly be prevented and there should also be a check on low level noises. Some ways of doing it are –

❑ Ear plugs or ear muffs should be provided

❑ If possible, machinery causing high level noises should be placed in a separate location.

❑ Sound-proof walls, double doors and glass pane windows should be used.

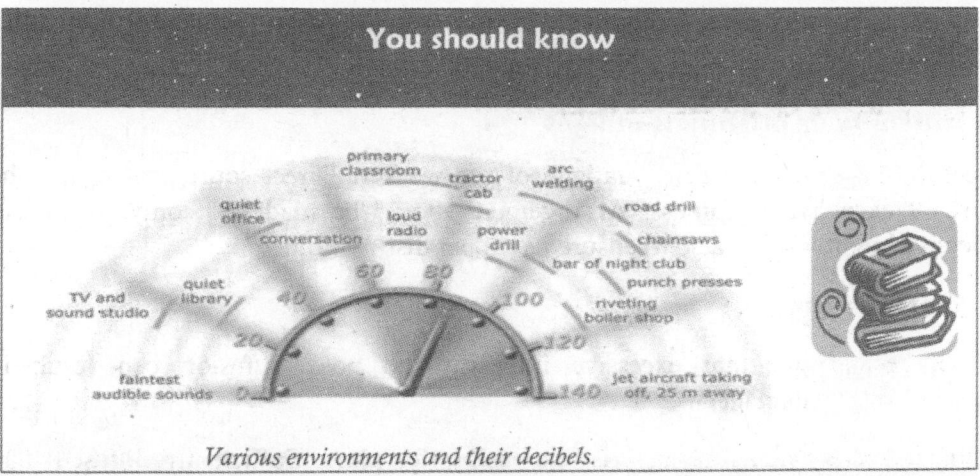

You should know

Various environments and their decibels.

TEST YOUR GREY MATTER

Q 1) What is work environment and how is it broadly classified?

Q 2) How does work environment affect the performance of an employee and the output of an organisation?

Q 3) Write a short note on 'Noise' as an environment factor and ways to overcome its adverse affects?

2. Illumination

The lighting of a workplace affects the

i. Efficiency of the worker

ii. Safety of the worker

iii. Fatigue of the worker

Characteristics of illumination which must be considered are –

a. Type of light

Daylight is found to be the best and then artificial light which closely approximates daylight in colour & composition [yellow light is found to be the best]

b. Distribution and location of lights

Lights are to be placed such that it is evenly distributed in the work area. In uneven lighting (those of us who study under a lamp must have observed this), when we look away from the work area, it requires continual pupillary adjustment and thus causes fatigue.

c. Intensity or brightness of light

Excessive brightness results in fatigue of the worker. Direct source of light is the cause of excessive brightness. Arrangement should be made not only to prevent excessive brightness but also to ensure its proper distribution.

d. Glare of light

It has been found that excessive intensity and poor diffusion can result in considerable eye damage.

Diffusion characteristic of light is responsible for glare. Sufficiently diffused light produces less glare. And that is why daylight is considerably better than artificial light as it produces less glare.

3. Atmospheric Conditions

a. Temperature

- Temperature determines the direction of flow of heat. Heat flows from the body of high temperature to that of low temperature.

- Thus, the temperature of a workplace should be kept at soothing levels, otherwise it may cause discomfort to the worker and affect his performance.

b. Humidity

- Moisture or water vapour content in the air also affects the efficiency of the worker.

- Under high humidity, evaporation of sweat from the skin is decreased and the body cannot maintain acceptable temperature.
- If the atmosphere is warmer than the skin during high humidity, blood brought to the body surface cannot shed heat by conduction to air. Thus, more blood flows to the external surface of the body and less to the muscles, brain and internal organs. This causes fatigue. It also affects the person mentally.

c. Air flow

- Proper air flow ensures circulation of air to prevent the formation of warm or moist air pockets.
- Non-circulation of air may cause fatigue, dizziness and headache to the worker, thus reducing the efficiency.
- It is measured in number of air changes in a room.

Methods to provide adequate atmospheric conditions

- Coolers in summer and heaters in winter.
- Supply and exhaust fans.
- **Air–Conditioning**: It is used to overcome all the 3 atmospheric conditions i.e. it maintains desired temperature, humidity and circulation of air. In addition, it also purifies the air by filtering dust, smoke or fumes.

4. Cleanliness

Various points for a clean workplace are:

i.   Dirt should be removed from the workplace including on machines and tools.

ii. Smoking zones must be provided to prevent non-smokers from passive smoking.

iii. Garbage cans should be provided at various locations.

iv. Diseases caused by pests and insects e.g. rats should be checked and prevented.

Benefits of a clean workplace are:

i.   Reduces injuries

ii. Motivates worker

iii. Reduces attrition

iv. Prevents health hazards

v.   Eliminate waste

Various companies in Japan follow **5S principle** for cleanliness –

i. **Sorting:** Eliminate all files, paper from the desk or cabinets that are not needed.

ii. **Set in order:** Files and other items are categorised and stored at proper place e.g. pencil in pencil box or holders will help the worker to find it easily when needed.

iii. **Shining or sweeping:** To clean up the work area to a new level of cleanliness.

iv. **Standardising:** Create standards for first 3 steps, so that they are easily preserved.

v. **Sustain:** Maintain the process and make the commitment to continue 5S as a way of life.

5. Music

- Several researchers have conducted studies on the effect of music at the workplace but no final conclusion has been derived.

- Some results which have been found are:

    i. Production increases by some percentage, but quality decreases in a musical environment.

    ii. Music is more effective if its rhythm is compatible with the rhythm of work.

    iii. If work is automatic and of repetitive type, music produces effective results, but is distracting when mental work and concentration is required.

    iv. In the long-term, workers adapt to music as they do to noise and no significant efficiency changes were found.

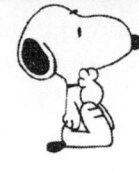

Thinking Time !!

*Find out how music affects you and your friends while studying? Experiment with different forms of music, from **Classical, Instrumental, Old Filmi to A.R. Rehman** and find which form assists you and which breaks your concentration…*

TEST YOUR GREY MATTER

Q1) What are the different characteristics of illumination that have considerable effect on the work environment?

Q2) Write a short note on
   (i)   5S principle of cleanliness
   (ii)   Effects of music on work

Q3) Explain various atmospheric conditions and their effect on workers' performance?

Q4) What is the contribution of good working conditions in maintaining the health of workers? Explain.

C. ENGINEERING PSYCHOLOGY

Definition: Engineering Psychology is a discipline that aims to improve socio-technical systems by considering how human operators interact with

i.   Technologies i.e. machines,

ii. Environment

Its various fields are:

i.   Ergonomics

ii. Human Factors

iii. Applied experimental psychology

iv. Cognitive engineering

We will confine our study to Ergonomics.

Ergonomics or Human Engineering

Definition: It is defined as the scientific study of the relationship between man and his working environment.

- It combines the knowledge of the psychologist, physiologist, anatomist, engineer, anthropologist and a bio-metrician.

- Ergonomics is concerned with "fitting" the job to the worker and to achieve this, it considers-

> **You should know**
>
> - *Ergonomics is derived from two Greek words:*
> - *"Nomoi" meaning natural laws*
> - *"Ergon" meaning work*
> - *Hence, ergonomists study human capabilities in relationship to work demands.*

i.   Job being done and demands of the worker.

ii. Equipment or machine used. Its shape, size and other features with respect to the job and worker.

iii. Information used i.e. how it is presented, accessed and changed.

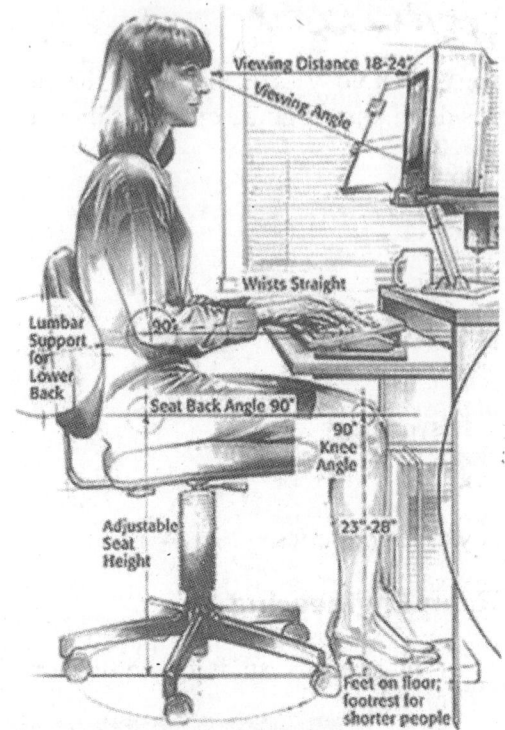

Ergonomic way of working on computers.

- 5 Aspects/Objectives of Ergonomics are–

i. **Safety :** e.g. Machines should be designed such that the worker and those nearby should be protected against dangers of accident.

ii. **Comfort:** e.g. Machine operator should be able to sit and do his job. If it is not possible, rest pauses must be given.

iii. **Ease of use:** e.g. bulky items should be handled mechanically or the machine to be handled should have proper controls at the right place so that the worker needs to make less effort in operating it.

iv. **Productivity/Performance**: e.g. Good working conditions not only motivate the worker to improve his performance but also take care of the mental and physical health of the worker.

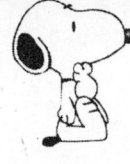

Thinking Time !!

Find out the most ergonomic way of studying.

(Of Course, it is not when you lie on your bed, somehow managing to prevent yourself from falling asleep ☺)

v. Aesthetics: e.g. Signs, posters. charts etc in the work place make the workplace not only aesthetically pleasing but also give useful information.

TEST YOUR GREY MATTER

Q1) Define:

(i) Engineering Psychology

(ii)Ergonomics

Q2) Explain the meaning and need of Human Engineering.

Q3) What are the objectives of ergonomics in an organisation?

12 | Fatigue & Boredom

A. THE INSIGHT

Do you remember that advertisement?

Javed Jaffery is overloaded with work. And just as he thinks the pile on his desk can't get any bigger, the secretary hands him some more papers...

> "Yeh bechaara, kaam ke bojh ka maara!! (he faints)
> Inhein chaahiye Hamdard Ka Tonic Cinkara.

JJ drinks it, and in the next scene, breaks through glass and hands in his reports with a flourish.

> Hamdard ka tonic, Cinkara!"

This is why we should study fatigue and boredom, not to break the glass of our office in front of our bosses (of course you will be fired for that!) but to know the factors which cause us to become *bechaara* and dull and to prevent that from happening.

B. FATIGUE

- **Definition:** Fatigue is a condition characterised by decrease in the output of an activity due to previous activity and is directly proportional to the poorness of output.

- Actually, fatigue is both a psychological as well as a physiological phenomenon. And it results when we spend more energy than we recover.

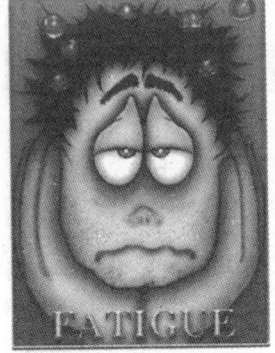

- We can understand this by example- When we run a race, our muscles need energy, which it generates from the aerobic metabolism of fats, but our body re-synthesises it and we continue to run. But after some time, metabolism shifts to anaerobic (absence of oxygen) and slowly the body is not able to re-synthesise it and fatigue occurs. There is lactic acid formation etc. also, but we will not get into the biological aspect of it.

B.1. Types of Fatigue

There are two types of fatigue:

i. Physical Fatigue
- Inability to exert force within one's muscles to the degree that would be expected given the individual's general physical fitness and which results in the decrease in output.

ii. Mental Fatigue
- Mental Fatigue is a psychological phenomenon which results in mental tiredness and decrease of output. It is caused by continual mental effort and attention on a particular task, as well as high level of stress or emotion.

- Mental fatigue is found to be difficult to measure and describe, as many factors are responsible for it. For example, if we take our own case, don't we feel mentally tired very soon when we are studying to complete the course, but when we are reading something of interest, say a novel, we can go on for hours without a trace of tiredness. Thus, it not possible to quantify mental fatigue exactly.

B.2. Symptoms of Fatigue

Following are the symptoms of fatigue –

i. Tiredness

ii. Sleepiness, even falling asleep against one's will (called **micro sleeps**).

[I hope you don't take micro sleeps while studying Industrial Psychology!]

iii. Irritability.

iv. Non-clarity in communication.

v. Slower thinking.

vi. Poor judgment of distance, speed or time.

B.3. Effect of Fatigue at Workplace

If the following effects are seen in an organisation, fatigue may be the culprit for it –

i. Productivity decreases.

ii. Quality of work deteriorates.

iii. Wastage of material or resources increases.

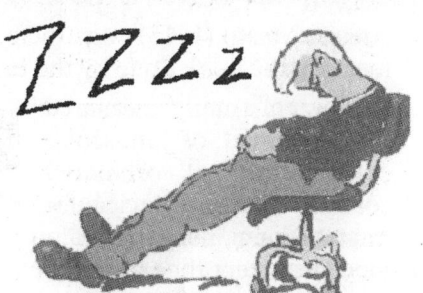

iv. Rework increases.

v. Rate of accidents increases.

vi. Absenteeism increases.

vii. Employee attrition increases.

B.4. Causes of Fatigue

i. Length or duration of work

If working hours are long without proper rest pauses, it causes fatigue.

ii. Speed of work

If some work is carried out at higher speed, it causes fatigue.

iii. Environmental factors

Inadequate illumination, high noise, high temperature etc. result in fatigue.

iv. Type of work

If the work involved causes tension, it may lead to mental fatigue.

v. Shift jobs

As it upsets natural sleep rhythms, it causes fatigue.

vi. Physical and Mental condition of the Person

Age, strength, stamina and health of a person produce stress in different individuals with different intensity.

vii. Training of employee

By proper training, the employee learns to do a job in the most scientific manner which causes least stress.

viii. Workspace layout

If the workspace layout of machine and equipment is not proper or space is not adequate, it results in unnecessary movements by the worker, resulting in fatigue.

ix. Tools, equipment or machinery

Inadequate or inefficient tools, equipment or machinery cause undue expenditure of energy which tires a worker quickly.

B.5. Fatigue Measurement

- Angelo Masso (1915) constructed an instrument called 'Ergograph' to record and measure the work done by the muscles in flexing a finger, to understand fatigue.

- Ergograph usually measured the amount of muscular contraction; it ordinarily consists of some device for immobilising all parts of a member except the part to be measured, and for recording the latter's movements.

You should know

Because of work Fatigue

- *19% of adults report falling asleep at work.*

- *18% of adults indicated that they have called in sick due to a poor night s sleep.*

- *29% of adults indicated that they do not feel well rested when they get up for work.*

- *27% of adults reported dozing off behind the wheel of an automobile.*

Description

- The forearm is laid upon the table, and the strap fixes the wrist in position. The second finger is fixed in the small strap, and the amount of weight on the pulley is graduated from time to time.

- Then, the finger is flexed and extended, the writing point then makes a record on the drum which is moving at a very slow rate.

- By measuring the distance the block travels along the rod, and multiplying it by the weight employed on the pulley and the time taken to do it, you get, as the result, the number of foot-pounds of work performed.

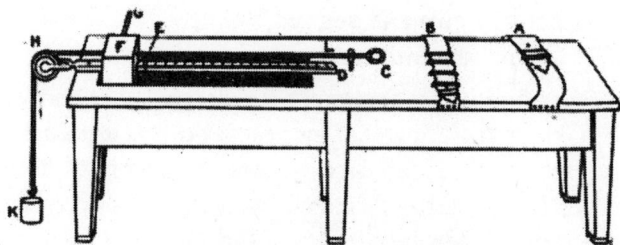

A SIMPLE ERGOGRAPH.

A, strap for fixing forearm; **B,** strap through staples for fixing fingers not in use; **C,** ring for finger to be tested; **D,** brass runner graduated in sixteenths of an inch; **E,** maximum recorder; **F,** pen carrier; **G,** writing pen; **H,** pulley; **K,** weight; **L,** cord. The part shaded in the diagram is cut out of the table.

Work Curve

- A work curve represents a graph between the level of performance and time spent at work.

- As the practices or techniques to minimise fatigue depend to a great extent on the nature of the work curve, its discovery and use are important. No difficulty exists in obtaining such a curve where work is uniform and successive in terms of units produced. However, where work changes are frequent as in ordinary varied office work, work curves are most frequently obtained by the use of laboratory task tests. The results of these tests are then plotted and used as index of fatigue for such jobs. Motivation might be higher in the laboratory tests than on the jobs. The degree of transfer depends on the similarity of task, environment, attitude and neuromuscular process.

Works curves may be divided into 3 types depending upon type of work as, simple muscular, complex muscular and mental work curves.

1. Simple Muscular Work Curve

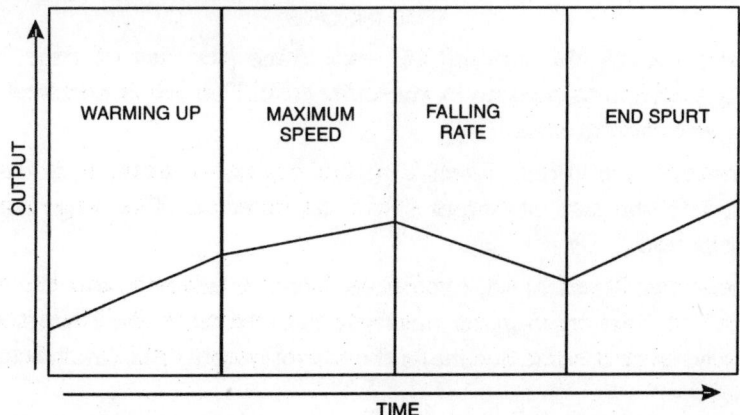

- Simple muscular activity curve is derived by recording the units and output of a group of muscles against the force of some weight or spring. E.g. in Ergograph.
- It can be seen from figure that the curve for simple tasks shows a short warm up period followed by a high level of performance. A gradual tapering off then appears. Subsequently, a sudden drop occurs to appoint of complete exhausting. Such work curves have a general resemblance to motor curves, but they involve simpler coordination of fewer muscles. One can generally conclude from the study of such curves that the more complex and rapid the task, the faster fatigue sets in. Moderate task permits a great total amount of work before complete exhaustion occurs than doing heavier tasks.

2. Complex Muscular Work Curve

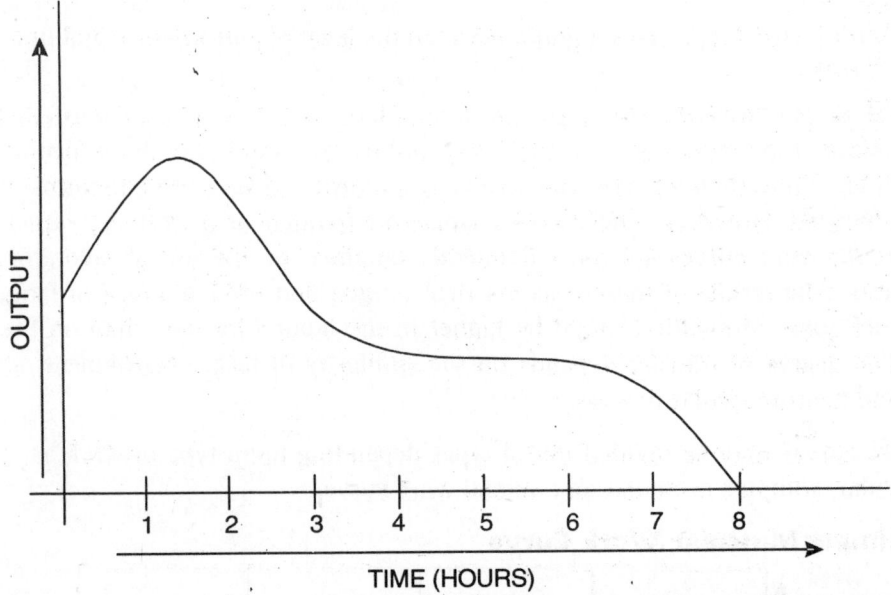

- This curve depicts the amount of work done per unit of time in analytical industrial situation as a complex muscular task. This job is assumed to be motor in nature and monotonous.
- Under normal conditions, when a person begins to work, it is easy and even pleasant, and the rate of output shows an increase. This stage may be called warm up period.
- After about two hours or so, conditions, become uniform, and the output levels off for half an hour or so. After this there is a decline in the interest and pleasure at work and there is some decline in the rate of output until lunch break.

- The productivity immediately after lunch may be lower as compared to the productivity at the time of going to the lunch. But the productivity again increases to the peak and, after some time, it starts declining until the shift ends.
- There are sudden fluctuations in the rate of productivity because of certain factors which are outside the control of the worker.
- It may be noted that post-lunch period output is little higher than when the work began and it soon rises to the peak because of the rest taken by the worker during lunch period.
- If a worker continues his effort even after fatigue sets in, he feels straining of nerves. Sometimes, he may be completely exhausted.
- When there is higher fatigue, the health of the worker deteriorates and his quantity and quality of production will also fall.

3. Mental Work Curve

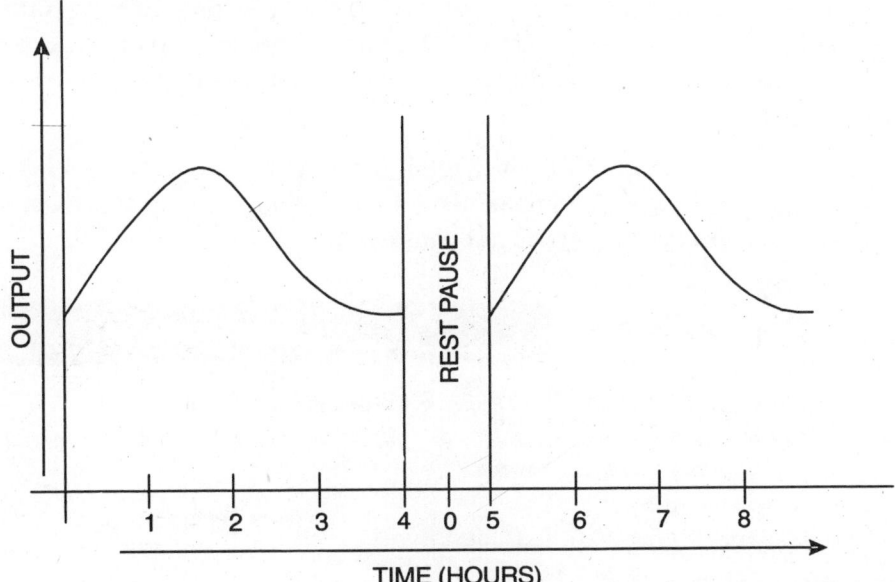

TIME (HOURS)

- As shown in figure, mental work decrement occurs in quantity, speed and accuracy of output as in muscular work. However, the individual differences and the nature of work tend to determine the timing of extent of such declines.
- The work decrement in mental tasks requiring continuous attention has been attributed to interferences known as "blocks".
- Mental fatigue expresses in many different ways the phenomena of monotony and boredom. Monotony is a state of mind caused by performance repetitive tasks. Boredom means lack of interest and is generally characterised by

depression and a desire for change of activity. Boredom is affected by personality, attitude and interest patterns. Boredom can be differentiated from fatigue because it is a desire of change in activity rather than for a rest or relief from the work altogether.

- Prolonged mental work results in an incapacity to evaluate what is being read. Common characteristics of prolonged mental work are increased errors and an increase in the amount of time necessary to assimilate written material or to solve perplexing problems towards the end of the period.

- Consequences of mental overwork in children are - disturbances of vision, headache, bleeding from nose, loss of appetite and indigestion, cerebral disorder and nervousness.

B.6. Remedies for Fatigue

1. Reduced Working Hours

It has been proved that longer work hours do not increase productivity. Rather, it causes fatigue to the worker. So longer work hours should be avoided. For most of the professions, 42 hours per week is considered to be optimum

2. Rest Pauses

Rest pauses help in reducing both mental and physical fatigue to workers and should be given when symptoms of fatigue are visible on workers. Even a tea break, lunch breaks etc. also act as rest pauses.

3. Work Study

Work Study should be done to determine 'A Fair Day's work'. It should determine the optimum speed and method with which a work is to be done so that it causes minimum fatigue.

4. Training

The employee must be given proper training to reduce unnecessary motion which cause fatigue and must be taught the correct way of doing a job.

5. Environmental Factors

Proper Illumination, Noise,

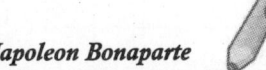

Wisdom Tooth

"The first virtue in a soldier is endurance of fatigue; courage is only the second virtue"

Napoleon Bonaparte

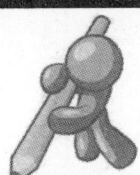

Thinking Time !!

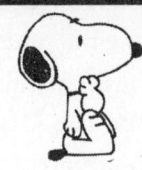

Find out, how giving proper rest pauses between continuous studying, improves your concentration and output. Do different things in the pause such as listening to music, chatting, watching TV, meditating etc. and find out which is more relaxing. But do not increases your rest pause from minutes to hours.

Temperature, Humidity, Cleanliness etc must be maintained to reduce fatigue of workers. (Refer Chapter 11- Work Environment and Engineering Psychology for detail)

6. Workplace layout

Workplace should be properly designed to reduce unnecessary movements which cause fatigue.

7. Ergonomics

Equipment, machinery and tools should be ergonomically designed to reduce the effort and fatigue.

TEST YOUR GREY MATTER

Q1) Discuss what do you understand by fatigue and suggest methods to counter the effects of fatigue.

Q2) What is an Ergograph and how does it work?

Q3) What is mental fatigue and how is it different from physical fatigue?

Q4) What are the effects of fatigue on industry?

Q5) What causes fatigue and what are its counter-measures in the context to industries?

C. BOREDOM & MONOTONY CONCEPTS

Definition: Boredom refers to the dull, uninterested and unfavourable state of mind or attitude of a worker towards his work.

Definition: Monotony refers to a state of mind or attitude of a worker towards his job due to the repetitive nature of work.

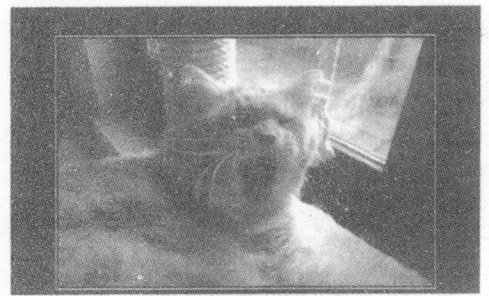

BOREDOM

No really, I love listening to you.

- We sometimes use monotony as a synonym for boredom in our general usage but we should understand that these two are different. Whereas Boredom refers to a particular identified state of mind which is of disliking, Monotony does not refer to a state of disliking or dullness of work, it is just a state of mind caused when we repetitively do the some work.

C.1.Causes of Boredom

1. Personality, Nature and Interest of Person

- Personality and interest of a person affect the way he does a work. Some people find some work interesting while some find it boring.

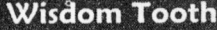
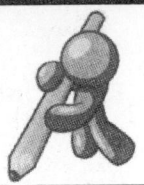

Wisdom Tooth

"The cure for boredom is curiosity. There is no cure for curiosity."

Ellen Parr

E.g. Like Rancho says to Farhan in the movie 3 idiots that you are born to become a photographer but you are studying engineering, then how can you be happy or get success in life.

That means Rancho has studied Industrial Psychology and knew that because of his interest and personality, Farhan felt bored to study engineering☺

2. Intellectual level of person

E.g. Einstein was a clerk, but his intellectual level was so high that his work bored him. So a person should do a work as per his intellectual capacity, to be interested in it.

3. Monotonous Nature of Job

Here, both the nature of Job and the person are important. Some people find repetitive work safe and secure, so they do not get bored of their work. While some people want to learn and face challenges, they get bored by repetitive work.

C.2.Effects of Boredom

i. Decrease in productivity.
ii. Deterioration of quality.
iii. Restlessness in workers.
iv. High attrition.

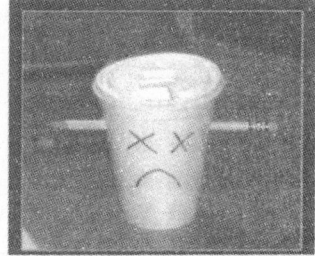

BOREDOM
It Does Terrible Things to the Mind

C.3.Relation between Fatigue and Boredom

Fatigue	Boredom
1. Work capacity decreases.	1. Interest in work decreases.
2. Can be measured to an extent.	2. Cannot be measured and is subjective (varies with each individual).
3. Worker requires rest to overcome fatigue.	3. Generally worker requires change to overcome boredom.
4. Work curve gradually decreases and then there is a spurt.	4. There are irregularities in work curve and intermittent spurts of short durations.

C.4. Remedies for Boredom

1. Rest Pauses

They act as a change for the worker and help in reducing monotony.

2. Importance of Job

It is found that people leave their jobs because they think that the job is of no importance and monotonous. Thus, jobs can be made more interesting if meaning is attached to it and workers are told about the importance of their job.

3. Job Enlargement and Job Rotation

Scope of worker's job should be increased by giving them more duties and responsibilities i.e. Job Enlargement and Job Rotation i.e. to give a worker different jobs. Both these concepts reduce monotony.

4. Social and Recreational Activities

These activities break the monotony of work and give employees a change and an opportunity to recharge themselves.

5. Proper Placement

Tests such as IQ etc., help in placing a person in a job as per his IQ and thus prevent boredom at work.

Thinking Time !!

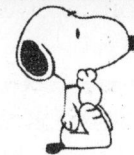

Though all of you are studying Industrial Psychology to become Engineers, yet apart from it, what is the work (painting, music, games, etc.) which really excites your intellect and you naturally have curiosity to learn it? Don t make hypothetical guesses; state only those things in which you actually have done something or have ideas to do. "I wanted to become a musician", but not having any present curiosity or questions or work regarding it, won t be counted!

Wisdom Tooth

"In order to live freely and happily, you must sacrifice boredom. It is not always an easy sacrifice."

Richard Bach

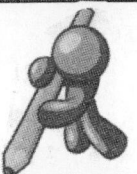

You should know

- *Research indicates that older people are usually less likely to be bored than younger ones.*
- *Males are more likely to be bored than females.*
- *People who are bored are likely to engage in sensation-seeking behavior*
- *If you are bored, you are more likely to be angry and hostile.*

Wisdom Tooth

"Are you bored with life? Then throw yourself into some work you believe in with all your heart, live for it, die for it, and you will find happiness that you had thought could never be yours".

Dale Carnegie

6. Short Term Goals

When goals are set, the worker gets more involved in accomplishing such targets and does not feel bored.

TEST YOUR GREY MATTER

Q1)   What is Boredom and how is it different from

(i) Monotony.   (ii) Fatigue.

Q2)   What are the causes of boredom and how does it affect industry?

Q3)   What are the remedies to prevent boredom?

Q4)   How is the nature of job responsible for causing fatigue?

Q5)   How are rest pauses effective in countering both fatigue and boredom?

CHAPTER
13 | Accidents and Safety

By the end of this chapter, you would be able to :
- Know what an Industrial Accident is.
- Determine the effects of Industrial Accidents.
- Learn to measure Accidents.
- Understand the reasons for causes of accidents and ways to prevent them.
- Appreciate the importance of safety in an organisation and know various ways to ensure safety.
- Know about Safety Management System.

The chapter contains :
- Industrial accidents
- Types of accidents
- Effects of accidents
- Accident proneness principle
- Measuring accidents
- Causes of industrial accidents due to unsafe conditions and unsafe acts
- Safety
- Accident prevention or safety by reducing unsafe conditions and reducing unsafe acts
- Safety Management System

A. THE INSIGHT
- **Location:** Pesticide plant owned by Union Carbide (UCIL), Bhopal, Madhya Pradesh, India.
- **Date:** December 3, 1984
- **Time:** Around 12 am.
- **Deaths:** Agencies estimated 8000 to 10,000 died within 72 hours and 25,000 since then.

- **Cause:** Large amounts of water entered tank 610, containing 42 tonnes of methyl isocyanate. This resulted in an exothermic reaction, which increased the temperature inside the tank to over 200 °C (392 °F), raising the pressure to a level the tank was not designed to withstand. This forced the emergency venting of pressure from the MIC holding tank, releasing a large volume of toxic gases into the atmosphere. The reaction sped up because of the presence of iron in corroding non-stainless steel pipelines. A mixture of poisonous gases flooded the city of Bhopal.

- This was **"Bhopal Gas Tragedy"**, one of the biggest Industrial Accidents in history which raised many questions and changed the way we looked at Industrial Accidents and Safety.

B. INDUSTRIAL ACCIDENTS

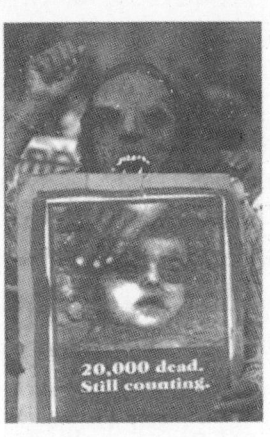

Definition: "An occurrence in an industrial establishment causing bodily injury to a person, which makes him unfit to resume his duties in the next 48 hours"

Indian Factories Act, 1948.

- As the definition states, all the following conditions must be satisfied for it to be called an industrial accident. i.e.

  i. It must be in an industrial establishment or factory.

  ii. It must occur in the course of employment in a factory.

  iii. It makes the person unfit to resume his work in the next 48 hours.

B.1. Types of Accidents

Accidents can be classified as:

i. Major or Minor

- **Major:** Accident resulting in death or prolonged disability.
- **Minor:** Not a severe one but resulting in only a cut or very temporary injury.

ii. External or Internal

- **External -** If the accident results in an injury which can be observed from the outside such as cut etc., it is an external injury.
- **Internal -** An injury such as fracture or cramp etc. which show no signs of injury from outside.

iii. Permanent or Temporary

- **Permanent:** When one cannot recover fully from the disability, it is a permanent accident.
- **Temporary:** When the accident causes an injury which could be cured in a period of time from a day to months, disability is temporary in nature.

iv. Fatal or Non-fatal

- **Fatal:** Accident resulting in loss of life.
- **Non-fatal:** Accident not resulting in loss of life.

B.2. Effects of Accidents/Need for Safety

Accidents can have following consequences:

a. Pain, damage or even death to an individual.

b. Brings down the morale of workers.

c. Even a minor accident leads to a temporary halt of work or wastage of time for worker and organisation.

d. Severe accident may cause stopping of production.

e. Economically expensive to organisation. It involves two components:

- **Direct:** In the form of compensations or medical expenses to the employee or his family member
- **Indirect:** Due to temporary halting of work, slowing down of production, material spoiled, emotional effect on the co-workers, customers lost due to non completion of orders on time etc.

B.3. Accident Proneness Principle

- **Principle:** It says – "Accidents do not distribute themselves by chance but, happen frequently to men and infrequently to others as a logical result of combination of circumstances".
- In simple language, it says that accidents are not a random phenomenon; rather, they can be predicted.

Mathematically, it means –

$$A_T = a_c + a_p$$

A_T = Total Number of Accidents

a_c = Accidents Caused By **Chance** Factors

a_p = Accidents Attributed To **Personal** Characters

Later, other factors were also added to it such as:

$$A_T = a_e + a_p + a_s$$

where, a_s = System Factor

i.e. some systems or machine equipments may be more accident prone than other,

- **Accident Proneness Tendency:** From this principle, it was seen that some employees have more a_p factor than others and were more accident prone as compared to others and this tendency is called Accident Proneness.

  According to T.W. Harrell –

  Definition: "Accident proneness is the continuing tendency of a person to have accidents as a result of his stable and persisting characteristics".

- **'Accident-Prone'** persons are also known as **'Accident Repeaters'** and are more involved in accidents.

B.4. Measuring Accidents

There are two major factors which are used for measuring accidents –

1. Accident Frequency Rate

Wisdom Tooth

"Every twenty seconds of every working minute of every hour throughout the world, someone dies as a result of an industrial accident."

Director General British Council.

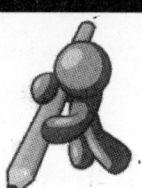

It is defined as the number of injuries which have disabled an employee per 10,00,000 man-hours worked.

$$\text{Accident Frequency Rate} = \frac{\text{Number of injuries}}{\text{Number of human hours worked}} \times 10,00,000$$

2. Accident Severity Rate

It is defined as the total number of days lost because of accidents per 10,00,000 man hours worked.

$$\text{Accident Severity Rate} = \frac{\text{Number of human days lost}}{\text{Number of human hours worked}} \times 10,00,000$$

B.5. Causes of Industrial Accidents

Broadly there are two factors responsible for accidents in industry.

1. Unsafe conditions
2. Unsafe acts

1. Unsafe Conditions

a. Nature of Industry

- Some jobs are rated as highly prone to accident.
- E.g. Coal mining, Chemical industry, Marine transport, Quarry and construction etc.

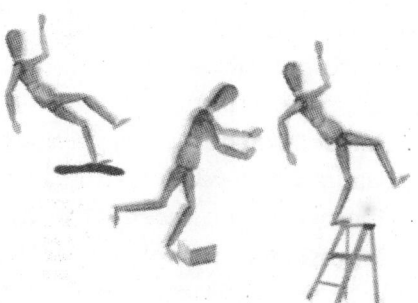

b. Slip or Falls

Falls are of two types -

i.   Fall of a person from heights such as ladder, building or machine etc. into depths such as wells, ditches, holes in the ground.

ii. Fall of person on the same level.

These may happen due to the following reasons –

a.   Surface (floor or staircase etc.), is highly polished & slippery.

b.   Wet or oily surface.

c.   Loose telephone wire or electricity cable.

d.   Improper lighting arrangements or glare.

e.   Parts and tools not stored safely.

f.   No guardrails or handrails.

c. Struck by falling objects

This may be of the following types –

i.   Slides and cave-ins (earth, rock, snow etc).

ii. Collapse of building, walls, ladders, pile of goods etc.

iii. Struck by falling objects during handling.

These may happen due to –

a.   Improper infrastructural design

b.   Improper material used for handling.

d. Striking or Colliding

This may be of following types –

i.   Striking against stationary objects.

ii. Striking against moving objects.

iii. Struck by moving objects (including flying particles and fragments)

This may happen due to –

a.   Layout is not proper and furniture or equipments are placed improperly.

b.   Inadequate lighting arrangements or glare.

c.   Improper work space around machine.

d. Edges of equipment or cutting not covered properly.

e. Exposure or contact with extreme temperatures

It can be of the following types –

a. Exposure to heat.

b. Exposure to cold.

c. Contact with hot substances or objects.

d. Contact with cold substances or objects.

f. Exposure to or contact with electric current

g. Exposure to or contact with harmful substance or radiations

It can be of the following types –

1. Contact by inhalation, ingestion or absorption of harmful substances.

2. Exposure to ionised radiations.

2. Causes Due To Unsafe Acts

- As we have seen in the Accident Prone Principle, there is a factor which is responsible for accidents and is because of personal characteristics.

- It may be further classified into 3 categories –

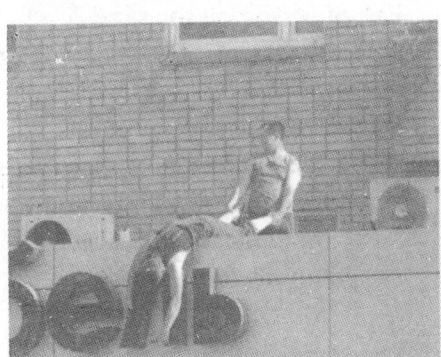

a. Causes due to Medical Reasons

There may be physical difficulties in workers such as, **Defective vision, High Blood Pressure,** etc. which may lead to accidents.

b. Causes due to Personality Problems

Workers may have personality or behaviour problems which may lead to accidents, such as – **Impulsive nature, Irresponsibility, 'Always in a hurry' nature, Aggressiveness** etc.

c. Causes due to Operating Defects

These are due to –

i. Failure of recognizing potential hazard.

ii. Wrong method of operation.

iii. Lack of attention.

iv. Faulty judgment of speed & distance.

v. Fatigue.

vi. Inexperience of operation.

vii. Tension or disturbed state of mind while operating.

You should know

MAJOR ACCIDENTS IN THE LAST DECADE IN INDIA

- Bhopal, December 1984. In the world's worst chemical disaster, methylisocyanate gas leaked from the Union Carbide plant in the city killing over 20,000 people. Thousands suffered irreversible health damage.
- Delhi, December 1985. An oleum leak from a Sriram Foods and Fertilizers plant in Delhi severely affected workers and those living in the neighbourhood.
- Rourkela, December 1985. Blast furnace accident in Rourkela Steel Plant. 18 workers affected.
- Durgapur, June 1987. Chlorine leak in Durgapur Chemicals Factory created panic all round. Long distance trains were halted. Over 100 were affected.
- Bombay, November 1988.Major gas leak at Fertilizers Corporation of India Unit at Ramagundam, killed 7.
- Nagothane, November 1990.Explosion at Indian Petrochemicals, Naghothane Complex, 35 persons killed, over 50 suffered 70 percent burns.
- Bombay,July 1991, Accident in Hindustan Organic Chemicals unit near Bombay killed 7 workers.
- Gwalior, December 1991. Blast at the dyeing department of GRASIM, 14 killed, 22 severely injured.
- Panipat, August 1992. Ammonia leak at the National Fertilizers Plant, 11 killed.
- Khalagaon, October 1992. Boiler explosion in National Thermal Power Corporation. 11 killed and several injured.
- Ahmedabad, August 3, 2003.Over 30 persons killed and several injured in an explosion in an old three storied building that housed an industrial unit to manufacture equipment for diamond cutting and polishing industry.
- Bhadravati (Karnataka), August 1,2003. Eight employees of VISL, including two officers died and 9 others were injured when a powerful explosion occurred in a converter in a steel making section of the plant.
- Mumbai, August 11, 2003. 23 employees of ONGC were killed in a helicopter crash in the offshore Heera Panna Oilfield's Neelam area.
- Jaipur, October 29,2009. The Jaipur oil depot fire broke out at the Indian Oil Corporation (IOC) oil depot's giant tank holding 8,000 kilolitres of oil, in Sitapura Industrial Area on the outskirts of Jaipur, Rajasthan, killing 12 persons and injuring over 200.

Source: Human Resource Management, K Aswathappa, p. 474

TEST YOUR GREY MATTER

Q1) How is industrial accident defined and how does it affect the organisation and worker?

Q2) What is Accident Proneness and how is it responsible for accidents in an organisation?

Q3) Explain Accident Proneness Principle mathematically.

Q4) How are accidents measured? Explain briefly.

Q5) What are the personal factors responsible for accidents in an industry?

Q6) What are unsafe conditions and how are they responsible for accidents?

Q7) State different types of accidents.

Q8) "Accidents do not just happen, they are caused." Comment.

C. SAFETY

Definition: It is the state in which the risk of harm to persons or of property damage is reduced to, and maintained at or below an acceptable level through a continuing process of hazard identification and risk management.

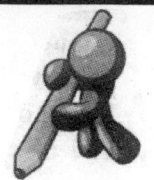

Wisdom Tooth

"Safety doesn t happen by accident."

Meaning of safety at industries can be understood as the fulfilment of the following conditions –

i. Zero accidents.

ii. Freedom from danger or risks i.e. those factors which cause them or are likely to cause them.

iii. Attitude change towards unsafe acts and conditions by employees.

iv. Process of hazard identification and safety management.

C.1. Methods of Accident Prevention or Safety

Safety can be achieved by:

1. Reducing unsafe conditions

2. Reducing unsafe acts

1. Reducing Unsafe Conditions

a. Walking Path

i. Floors or staircases should be properly cleaned and dried. No oil or water should be left on the walking path.

ii. Floors, ramps or staircases should not be defective, which may cause falling or tripping.

iii. Slip reducing floor coatings; floor mats should be used.

iv. Guard rails or handrails on ladders, stairways etc.

b. Lighting Arrangement

i. Proper lighting should be provided at each location to avoid colliding or striking.

ii. There should be no glare.

c. Proper Layout

i. Proper walking spaces must be provided.

ii. There should be adequate space around machinery.

d. Material Handling Equipments

i. Cables, hooks or chains should not be worn out or defective.

ii. Should not be loaded above safe limits.

iii. They should be properly stored.

e. Tools

i. They should not be cracked or worn out or defective.

ii. Power tools must be properly guarded.

iii. Edges of equipment or cutting tools must be covered properly.

iv. Parts or tools must be properly stored.

f. Personnel Protective Equipment

i. Gloves, safety glass, goggles etc. must be worn.

ii. Special attention must be given when dealing with work involving exposure to extreme temperature, current or radiations.

iii. Protective gear must be reliable, durable, easy to put on or off, comfortable, light weight etc.

g. Equipment Redesign

Equipments and tools must be so designed that they become safer to use and cut down chances of accident.

2. Reducing Unsafe Acts

a. Medical Assistance

Those employees suffering from physiological or psychological difficulties must be given medical assistance to overcome them.

b. Personality Readjustment

It can be done in the following two ways:

i. Proper Selection and Placement

By identifying those who have traits which are accident prone and refusing to employ them, accidents can be reduced.

ii. Consultation

Supervisor must talk to the employees who have personality traits which may lead to accidents (irresponsibility, impulsive nature etc.) and give him a clear understanding of his personality difficulties, their probable outcome and ways to correct them.

c. Correcting Operation Defects

i. Through Training

Employees must be trained to follow safe practices and procedures. Correct ways of operation must be taught and they must be warned of the potential hazards.

ii. Through Motivation

Employees must be motivated to develop a safety conscious attitude.

Safety posters, and hoardings, Incentives and positive Reinforcements must be used to motivate employees.

iii. Redesigning of Jobs

Accidents caused by Fatigue or boredom can be prevented by redesigning the jobs. That is, by Job Enlargement or Job Enrichment etc.

You should know

Provisions of Factories Act, 1948

- **Sec 21:** Dangerous part of any machinery shall be securely fenced by safeguards of substantial construction which shall be constantly maintained and kept in position while the parts of machinery they are fencing are in motion or in use.

- **Sec 22:** No woman or young person shall be allowed to clean, lubricate or adjust any part of a prime mover or of any transmission machinery while the prime mover or transmission machinery is in motion.

- **Sec 23:** No young person shall be required or allowed to work at any dangerous machine unless he-

  (a) has received sufficient training in work at the machine.

  (b) is under adequate supervision by a person who has a thorough knowledge and experience of the machine.

- **Sec 24:** (a) Suitable striking gear or other efficient mechanical appliance shall be provided and maintained and used to move driving belts to and from fast and loose pulleys.

  (b) Suitable devices for cutting off power in emergencies from running machinery shall be provided and maintained in every work-room.

- **Sec 25:** No traversing part of a self-acting machine in any factory, be allowed to run on its outward or inward traverse within a distance of forty-five centimetres from any fixed structure which is not part of the machine.

- **Sec 26:** Casing should be done in such a way as to prevent danger.

- **Sec 27:** No woman or child shall be employed in any part of a factory for pressing cotton in which a cotton-opener is at work.

- **Sec 28:** Hoists and lifts should be in good condition and should be examined once in every 6 months.

- **Sec 29:** Similarly, lifting machines, chains, ropes and lifting tackles must be in good construction and should be examined once in every 12 months.

- **Sec 30:** Near each machine, a notice indicating the maximum safe working peripheral speed of every grindstone or abrasive wheel, the speed of the shaft or spindle upon which the wheel is mounted, and the diameter of the pulley upon such shaft or spindle necessary to secure such safe working peripheral speed, is indicated.

- **Sec 31:** If in any factory, any plant or machinery or any part thereof is operated at a pressure above atmospheric pressure, effective measures shall be taken to ensure that the safe working pressure of such plant or machinery or part is not exceeded.

- **Sec 32:** All floors, steps, stairs, passages and gangways shall be of sound construction and properly maintained and shall be kept free from obstructions and substances likely to cause persons to slip.

- **Sec 33:** Fixed vessel, sump, tank, pit or opening in the ground or in a floor, shall be either securely covered or securely fenced.

- **Sec 34:** No person shall be employed in any factory to lift, carry or move any load so heavy as to be likely to cause him injury.

- **Sec 35:** Effective screens or suitable goggles shall be provided for the protection of persons employed on machines that might cause damage to his/her eyes.

- **Sec 36:** No person shall be required or allowed to enter any chamber, tank, vat, pit, pipe, flue or other confined space in any factory in which any gas, fume, vapour or dust is likely to be present.

- **Sec 37:** Effective steps to be taken to prevent explosion on ignition at gas or fume.

- **Sec 38:** All practicable measures shall be taken to prevent outbreak of fire and its spread.

- **Sec 39 :** If it appears to the Inspector that any building or part of a building or any part of the ways, machinery or plant in a factory is in such a condition that it may be dangerous to human life or safety, he may ask for details about them or insist on suitable tests to determine their safety.

- **Sec 40:** If it appears to the Inspector that any building or part of a building or any part of the ways, machinery or plant in a factory is in such a condition that it is dangerous to human life or safety, he may serve a notice to the occupier or manager.

- **Sec 41:** The State Government may make rules requiring the provision in any factory or in any class or description of factories of such further devices and measures for securing the safety of persons employed therein as it may deem necessary.

D. SAFETY MANAGEMENT SYSTEM

Definition: Safety Management System is an organised approach to managing safety, including the necessary organisational structures, accountabilities, policies and procedures. It requires a systems approach to the development of safety policies, procedures and practices to allow the organisation to achieve its safety objectives. It requires planning, organising, communicating and providing direction.

D.1.Steps Involved In Safety Management

Step 1 – Planning

A Safety Manager and a group are selected to conduct the planning phase of Safety Management. Following tasks are performed in the planning stage –

a. Review

- Current capabilities for safety management are identified, such as experience, knowledge, procedure, resources etc.
- Short comings and resources needed are recognised.

b. Safety assessment

It aims at answering the following questions-

- What could go wrong?
- What would be its consequence?
- How often is it likely to occur?

c. Safety Performance indicators and targets

- Various safety performance indicators and targets for the organisation are identified.
- A realistic time line for meeting the targets is also decided.

d. Safety strategy

- Based on the safety targets, a realistic strategy for meeting them is developed.

e. The Plan

- A detailed plan for development and implementation is made.

Step 2: Commitment to Safety

a. Management

- Ultimate responsibility for safety rests with senior management. Success of safety management system depends on the extent of time, resources and attention they give.
- Their commitment to safety is demonstrated to all personnel of the organisation through the stated safety policy and objectives.

b. Safety Policy

Safety Policy outlines the methods and processes that the organisation uses to achieve desired safety outcomes. It reflects the organisation's management and becomes the foundation on which the organisation's Safety Management System is built.

Safety policy issues following statements

i. Overall safety objectives of organisation.
ii. Commitment of senior management to the goal of ensuring that all aspects of the operation meet safety performance targets.

iii. Commitment by the organisation to provide the necessary resources for effective management of safety.

iv. Commitment by organisation to make the maintenance of safety its highest priority.

v. Organisation's policy concerning responsibility and accountability for safety at all levels of organisation.

Roles of Senior Management

i. Gaining safety related information.

ii. Training personnel for safety responsibilities.

iii. Safety related information is given to all affected personnel e.g. through safety posters and film shows.

iv. Potential system features and hazards are promptly inquired and reformed.

v. Regular assessment of safety performance.

vi. New safety ideas are welcomed.

Step 3 – Organisation

Following considerations are important for establishing an effective organisation.

i. Appointing Safety Manager – Safety Manager is appointed to promote safety awareness and level of priority throughout the organisation.

ii. Forming Organisational Structure.

iii. Having a statement of Responsibilities and Accountabilities.

iv. Creating a safety committee.

v. Ensuring training and competency.

Step 4: Hazard Identification

Hazard Identification programs are created for effective Safety Management. It considers identification of all possible sources of failure. It includes the following

i. Equipment.

ii. Operating environment.

iii. Human operators.

iv. Human/machine interface.

v. Operational procedures.

vi. Maintenance procedures.

vii. External services.

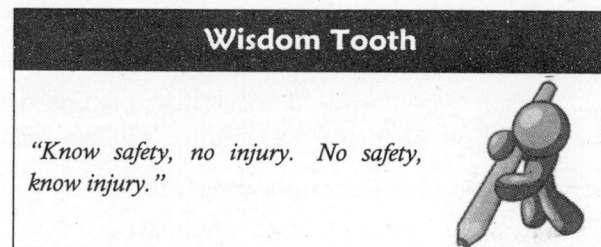

Wisdom Tooth

"Know safety, no injury. No safety, know injury."

Step 5: Risk Management

- All identified hazards are critically assessed and ranked in the order of their risk potential.
- It requires the analysis and elimination (or reduction to acceptable limits) of those hazards that threaten the viability of an organisation

Risk management comprises 3 elements –

a. Hazard identification
b. Risk Assessment
c. Risk Mitigation

Step 6: Investigation Capability

- Investigation is a process conducted for the purpose of accident prevention which includes the gathering and analysis of information, the drawing of conclusions, including determination of causes and when appropriate, making safety recommendations.
- An organisation must have good investigation capability for effective safety management.

Step 7: Safety Analysis Capability

Safety Analysis is the process of organising and evaluating facts objectively. Following the basic rules of logic and drawing upon recognized methodologies and analytical tools, facts are considered in a systematic manner so that valid conclusions can be made.

Step 8: Safety Promotion and Training

Staff is informed about safety issues through relevant training, safety literature, participation in safety courses and seminars etc. It indicates management's commitment towards safety management.

Step 9: Safety Management Documentation and Information Management

To ensure effective safety management, a disciplined

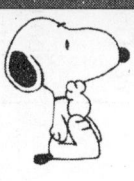

Thinking Time !!

How good is your personal and your family's Safety Management? Are you prepared for any emergency? Do you have contact numbers of Hospitals or Emergency Services? If the answer is 'No', then Go, Think Negatively and list out all possible hazards you, your friends or your family can face and then the safety and prevention methods?

approach to documentation and information management is followed. Generally, information is documented in Safety Management manual, which includes safety policy, individual safety accountabilities, safety procedures etc. Proper tools and skills are used to record, store, secure and retrieve the necessary information.

Step 10: Safety Oversight and Safety Performance Monitoring

For effective working of the 9 steps, feedback is necessary which is achieved through

a. Safety oversight

It is achieved through inspections, surveys and audits. It assures staff and management that organisation's activities are performed safely.

b. Safety Performance Monitoring

It validates the safety management system, confirming that the collective efforts have achieved the organisation's safety objectives. It is achieved through regular review and evaluation.

TEST YOUR GREY MATTER

Q1)   Define Safety. What are the conditions which ensure safety?

Q2)   How will you ensure safety by:
   (i)   Reducing unsafe acts.
   (ii)   Reducing unsafe conditions.

Q3)   What steps should be taken by the management to increase motivation for safety?

Q4)   Briefly describe the steps of Effective Safety Management System?

Q5)   What are the main elements of Risk Management?

14

Job Analysis

A. THE INSIGHT

In 1585, 15 English settlers established a colony on Roanoke Island near what is now the Outer bank of North Carolina coast. When John White arrived at Roanoke Island in 1590, he found no trace of the colony. To this day, it is not known what happened to the settlers of Lost Colony of Roanoke.

Many theories have been put forth to explain the fate of the lost colony - killed by Indians, moved to another location, and so on. One theory is that the members of the colony were not prepared to survive in the new continent: that is the group consisted of politicians, soldiers, and sailors. Although worthy individuals were sent to the New World, few had the necessary training and skills to survive. In fact the colony might have survived if settlers with more appropriate skills, such as farmers, had been sent instead of traditional explorer types. Thus, a better match between job requirements and personnel might have saved the colony.

The story underscores the importance of the process called Job analysis-gathering, analyzing and structuring information about the job's components, characteristics and requirements

(Source: Industrial / Organisational Psychology, Michael G. Aamodt, p. 37)

B. CONCEPTS AND DEFINITIONS

i. Job Analysis

Job Analysis is the process of collecting information about various components of a job. It includes both, duties and conditions of work and individual qualifications of the worker. This information is used in the preparation of job description and job specification.

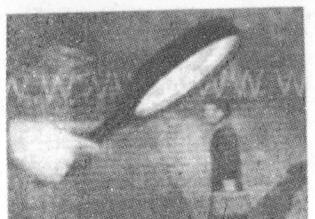

To understand this definition we should understand various terms such as-

ii. Job

Job or work is a physical or mental activity that is carried out at a particular place and time, according to a particular instruction, in return for money.

iii. Job Description

- It is a statement of all tasks and responsibilities attached to a job.
- Job title, work activities, tools and equipment used, job content, work performance, working conditions and compensation information form part of a job.

iv. Job Specification

- It is a statement of capabilities and qualifications required to perform a job.

Job Analysis Matrix

What the Worker Does Duties Tasks Responsibilities	How the Worker Does it Methods Tools Techniques
Why the Worker Does It Products Services	Worker Qualifications Skills Knowledge Abilities Physical Demands

- It includes education, experience, training, judgement, skills, communication, etc.

C. JOB ANALYSIS

C.1. Advantages/Purpose of Job Analysis

A Job Analysis provides information for job description and job specification. It has the following advantages –

i. Human Resource Planning

Job analysis determines the number & kind of jobs and also the qualification required for a job. Thus, it helps in determining as to how many and what type of personnel will be needed in the future.

ii. Recruitment and Selection

- Right person for the right job is a very important activity and this is achieved by Job analysis.
- Job description tells us about the job and the job specification tells us about the type of personnel required.

iii. Training and Development

- Training and Development programs are used to improve employees' skills and knowledge related to a particular task to improve their performance.
- Job description and Job analysis help in determining the content and nature of this training.

iv. Job Evaluation

- Job description and job specification help in determining relative worth of a job. This is important to establish wage and salary grades.

v. Remuneration

- As grades of jobs are decided by Job analysis, so is the remuneration i.e. wages and salaries, fringe benefits, bonus and other facilities.
- This is important to classify jobs as per their worth and thus motivate employees by equitable distribution.

vi. Performance Appraisal

- Performance Appraisal is a method of assessment of an employee i.e. actual performance of employee against what is expected.

- As job analysis facilitates fixing standards of job by job specification, it helps in performance appraisal. This appraisal results in promotions, transfers, increment in salaries, and also assessing training requirements of employee.

vii.Safety and Health

- Job analysis gives an opportunity to know about working conditions and environment.
- Thus, it identifies the hazards and unhealthy factors such as heat, noise, dust etc. and provides an opportunity for a safer environment.

viii. Personnel Information

- Job analysis is vital in building information system of personnel which is useful in two ways-
  a) Increases efficiency of administration by providing the data easily.
  b) This information helps in making lots of decisions regarding human resources such as planning, development, remuneration etc.

ix. Job Design

- Job design is a conscious effort to organise tasks, duties and responsibilities into a unit of work to achieve certain objectives.
- Job analysis sets the basis for Job design.

C.2.Process/ Steps of Job Analysis

There are 8 steps in the job analysis program –

1. Identify Purpose of Job Analysis

Clear purpose of job analysis is to be determined as it will form the basis for other steps.

2. Selecting the Analyst

Company must determine a person who will be in charge of the program.

3. Selecting the Appropriate Method

Before selecting the appropriate method, analyst must carry out the following tasks-

a) He must select representative positions to analyse because there may be too many similar jobs to analyse and it may not be necessary to analyse all of them.

b) He must review background information such as organisational charts, process charts, job descriptions, job specifications, procedure manual of position selected.

After these are done, a job analysis method is identified. The best method must be chosen after considering advantages and disadvantages of each method.

4. Train the Analyst

- If an internal person is employed as an analyst, he must be trained.

5. Preparation of Job Analysis
- Project which is to be done is communicated in the organisation.
- Documentation is prepared e.g. interview, questions, questionnaires etc.

6. Collecting Data
- Data is collected on job activities, employee behaviours, working conditions, human traits and abilities needed to perform the job.
- One or more Job analysis methods are used to collect the data.

7. Review and Verify
- Data which is collected is reviewed and verified to confirm that the information is factually correct and complete.
- Review of data may be done by the person's immediate supervisor, by technical conference etc.

8. Job Description and Job Specification
- Finally, the Job Description and Job specification are prepared.

TEST YOUR GREY MATTER

Q1) Define: (i) Job (ii) Job Analysis.

Q2) Why is Job Analysis important for an organisation. Explain.

Q3) What is Job Analysis and what steps are involved in the preparation of job analysis?

Q4) Explain briefly as to why Job Analysis is an important part of Human Resource Management?

Q5) What role does Job analysis play in the Safety and Health of the employees? Explain.

C.3. Elements of Job Analysis

We need to understand the following things in detail to completely understand the Job Analysis Process.

a. Who should be chosen as an analyst?
b. What is the data which is to be collected?
c. What methods are to be employed to collect the data?
d. Understand Job Description & Job Specification in Detail.

e. Problems which may occur in Job Analysis.

a. Choosing an Analyst

- Three types of persons can be used for collecting the data –
  i. Trained Job Analyst.
  ii. Supervisors.
  iii. Job incumbents. [Incumbent means a person who has any official position or simply, he holds a job in the company]

Comparison of all three is given

Criterion	Trained Analyst	Supervisor	Job incumbent
Cost	Expensive	No extra cost	No extra cost & less expensive than supervisor
Expertise	Expert in Job analysis methods	Needs Training	Needs training
Objectivity & Standardisation	Maximum	Less	Poor
Familiarity of Job	Not completely familiar with job, so may overlook some aspects.	Familiar with job	Greater familiarity with job
Speed of Data Collection	Slow because of non familiarity of job and people	Fast	Fast

b. Types of Job Analysis Data/ Information to Collect

(Source: Leap & Gino, Personal/HRM, p. 127)

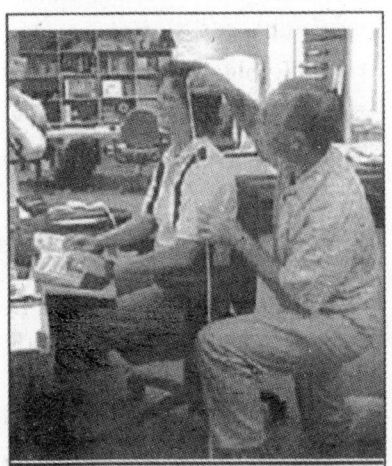

1. Work Activities

i. Description of work activities
   a. How is a task performed.
   b. Why is a task performed.
   c. When is a task performed
ii. Interface with other jobs and equipment.
iii. Procedure used.
iv. Behaviours required on the jobs
v. Physical movements and demands of jobs

2. Machine, Tools, Equipment and Work Aids Used

  i.   List of machines, tools etc. used.

  ii. Materials processed with items listed in II-A

  iii. Products made with items listed in II –A

  iv. Service rendered with items listed in II-A.

3. Job content

  i. Physical Working conditions

     a. Exposure to heat, dust, toxic substances.

     b. Indoor versus outdoor environment.

  ii. Organisational context

  iii. Social context

  iv. Work Schedule

  v. Incentives (financial & non-financial)

4. Personnel Requirement

  i.   Specific skills

  ii. Specific education and training

  iii. Work experience

  iv. Physical characteristics

  v.   Aptitude

c. Methods of Collecting Data

Following methods are used for collecting job-related data-

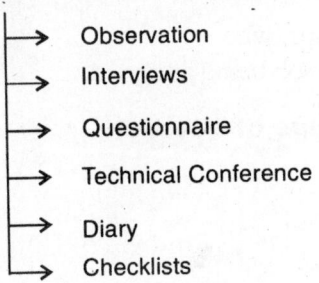

- Observation
- Interviews
- Questionnaire
- Technical Conference
- Diary
- Checklists

i. Observation Method

Here, the job analyst observes the worker performing the job and records the methods or process of doing the job and the time taken to do the job.

Advantages

i. Simple

ii. Accurate method

Disadvantage

i. Time consuming

ii. Not applicable where jobs do not have easily observable job cycles or involves more mental process than physical.

iii. Costly, as training would be involved to teach the analyst, what to observe and how to observe.

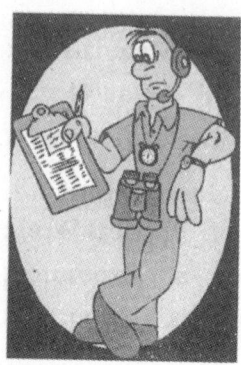

Application

- Analysing repetitive, short cycle, unskilled and semi-skilled jobs.
- Best when used with other methods of job analysis.

ii. Interview Method

- Interview method includes asking questions to both, incumbents and supervisors in either an individual or a group setting.
- Classification of Job Analysis Interview Method.

a. On the basis of People Interviewed

There are 3 types or stages under this category-

i. Individual interviews with each employee.

ii. Group interviews with group of employees having the same job.

iii. Interviewing the supervisor, who is knowledgeable about the job being analysed.

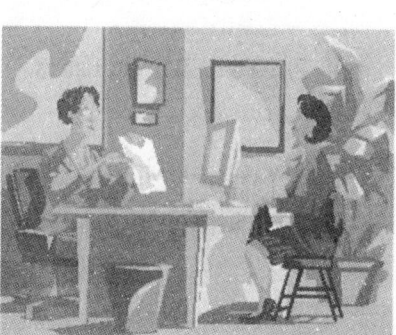

b. On the basis of the type of questions

i. Unstructured

ii. Structured

b.i. Unstructured Interview

- This interview is a conversation with no prepared questions or predetermined line of investigation. However, the interviewer must clarify
  - ❑ Purpose of the study.
  - ❑ Particular focus of interview.

- The role and structure gives some base for the questions to be asked. Listening and taking notes enable the interviewer to follow up the questions to be posed.
- Thus in an unstructured interview, the **interviewer has 3 roles** –
  i. Establish a relationship
  ii. Ask well-structured questions to generate a conversational flow in which the interviewer offers – factual, subjective and objective information about the job.
  iii. To ensure that the information received is heard and understood.

b.ii.Structured Interview

It has a definite format involving -
- Job holder's sequence of activity in performance
- Inventory or Questionnaire.

The Process of Job Analysis Interview has the following steps –

Step 1 –Interview Plan
- Workers who are to be interviewed should be identified
- Interviewee should be notified in advance about the interview.
- Time for the interview must be established.

Step 2 – Role establishment
- Analyst should clearly explain the nature of his role, as often workers being interviewed believe that they are being evaluated and the result may lower their salary, increase their work etc.
- Analyst should build a relationship of mutual confidence with the interviewee.
- Analyst must not dominate the interview and should try to put worker at ease.

Step 3 – Conducting the Interview
- In a structured interview, questions should be followed.
- Worker must be given some open ended questions, not yes/no questions.
- Worker should be helped to think and talk depending on the logical sequence of duties performed.
- Only one question should be asked at a time.
- Analyst must be patient and should encourage the worker.
- Before closing the interview, the information must be summarised.

Step 4 – Closing the interview
- Any questions or comments from workers should be encouraged.

- Worker must be given opportunity to clarify his doubts.

Step 5 – Review and verification of information

- Information collected should be from the best, good, average and poor workers.
- Information collected should be checked from others holding the same or similar jobs.
- Advantages of the Interview Method –
  i. Job holders are most familiar with job and can supplement information obtained through observation.
  ii. Analyst can gather information that never appears on written documents.
  iii. Provides an opportunity to explain the need of analysis.

Disadvantages of the Interview Method

i. Dependent on interviewer's ability.

ii. Workers may not give meaningful responses.

iii. Time consuming and not cost efficient.

iv. Accuracy and objectivity of data depends on non-biased nature of interviewer.

You should know

Job Analysis Interview Questions Include Questions Such As The Following

1. Interview information
- Name of Employee:
- Job Title:
- Job Analyst:
- Department:
- Date:

2. Job introduction
- Describe location of job .

• Job purpose:
- What is the essence of work in your position? What is the job's overall purpose?

4. Job duties
- What are the main duties and responsibilities of your position?
- Describe your duties in the following categories: daily duties, periodic duties, duties performed at irregular intervals
- How long do they take?
- How do you do them?
- Are you performing duties not presently included in your job description? Describe.

- Do you use special tools, equipment, or other sources of aid? If so, list the names of the principal tools, equipment, or sources of aid you use.
- Describe the frequency and degree to which you are engaged in activities such as: pushing, throwing, pulling, carrying, sitting, running, kneeling, crawling, reaching and climbing.

5. Job criteria / results
- How would you define success in your work?
- Have work standards been established (errors allowed, time taken for a particular task, etc.)? If so, what are they?
- Describe the successful completion and/or end results of the job.

6. Records and Reports
- What records or reports do you prepare as part of your job?
- Who do you have to send these reports to?

7. Supervisor
- Who is your supervisor?
- What kinds of questions or problems would you ordinarily refer to your supervisor?
- Are the instructions you receive clear and consistent with your job description?

8. Authority
- What is the level of authority vested in your position?
- What is the level of accountability and to whom are you accountable?
- What kinds of independent action were you allowed to take?

9. Responsibilities
- Are you responsible for any confidential material? If so, describe how you handle it.
- Are you responsible for any money or things of monetary value? If so, describe how you handle it.

10. Compensation
- Consider your level of productivity, and the skill level required to fulfill your responsibilities, do you think that you are underpaid? Overpaid?

11. Knowledge
- What special knowledge of specific work aids is needed for this position?
- Describe the level, degree, and breadth of knowledge required in these areas or subjects.
- Indicate the educational requirements for the job (not the educational background of the incumbent).
- What level of education is required for your position?
- What type of certification and licensing is required for your position?
- Can you specify the training time needed to arrive at a level of competence on the job?
- What sort of on the job training is needed for this position?

12. Skills/ Experience

- What activities must you perform with ease and precision?
- What are the manual skills that are required to operate machines, vehicles, equipment, or to use tools?
- Indicate the amount of experience needed to perform the job.
- What level of experience and skills are required for your position?

13. Abilities required

- What mathematical ability must you have?
- What reasoning or problem solving ability must you have?
- What interpersonal abilities are required? What supervisory or managing abilities are required?
- What physical abilities such as strengths, coordination, visually acuity must you have?

14. Working instruments

- Describe briefly what machines, tools, equipment or work aids the incumbent works with on a regular basis.

15. Health and safety

- What are the safety conditions related to this position?
- Does your work present any type of hazardous or unusual working conditions?

16. Working conditions

- Describe your working conditions.
- Describe the frequency and degree to which you will encounter working conditions such as these: cramped quarters, moving objects, vibration, inadequate ventilation

iii. Questionnaire Method

- It includes a set of questions which are provided to employees and then approved by the supervisors.

- They may be designed specifically for an organisation, or more general to collect information from a large number of people working in many different organisations.

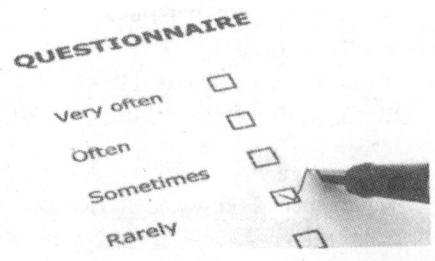

- There are some standard questionnaires which contain the following information:

    i.   The Job title of job holder.

    ii. The Job title of job holder's supervisor.

    iii. Job title and number of staff reporting to job holder.

    iv. Description of purpose of job.

v. Description of tasks and duties to be carried out by job holder.

vi. Tools, Machinery and Equipment used.

vii. Working conditions.

Advantages of the Questionnaire method

i. Short period of time required to collect information on many jobs.

ii. Man-hours saved in carrying out the programme.

iii. All job holders participate, not like the interview method in which only one or two participate.

Disadvantages/Limitations of the Questionnaire method

i. Follow up observations and discussions are necessary to clarify inadequately filled-in-questionnaires and interpretation problems.

ii. It requires specialized knowledge and training.

iii. Employee may not be able to express clearly, the information related to his/her duties.

There are many standard questionnaires. Two of them are:

a. Position Analysis Questionnaire (PAQ)

- Developed by Dr. Ernest J. McCormick and associates at Purdue University.
- PAQ contains 194 job elements on which a job is created depending on the degree to which an element is present.
- These elements are grouped into **six general categories** and are work oriented-
  i. Information Input.
  ii. Mental Processes.
  iii. Work Output (Physical Activities and Tools).
  iv. Relationships with Others.
  v. Job Context (The Physical and Social Environment).
  vi. Other Job Characteristics (Such As Place and Structure).
- Each job element is rated on six scales:
  i. Extent of use.
  ii. Importance.
  iii. Time.
  iv. Possibility of occurrence.
  v. Applicability.
  vi. Special code for certain jobs.

Uses of Position Analysis Questionnaire

The position analysis questionnaire has been used for job evaluation, selection, performance appraisal, compensation planning, assessment-centre development, determination of job similarity, development of job families, vocational counselling, determination of training needs, and job design.

Advantages of PAQ

i. It can be used to analyse almost every job.

ii. It is a highly reliable method.

iii. It provides a comparison of specific job with other job classifications, particularly for selection and remuneration purposes.

Disadvantages of PAQ

It is to be completed by a trained job analyst and not incumbents or supervisor as the language used is difficult.

b. Management Position Description Questionnaire

- It is a highly structured questionnaire containing 208 items relating to managerial responsibilities, restrictions, demands and other miscellaneous position characteristics.

- These 208 items are grouped under 13 categories-

    i. Product marketing and financial strategy planning.

    ii. Co-ordination of other organisational units and personnel.

    iii. Internal business control.

    iv. Product and services responsibility.

    v. Public and customer relations.

    vi. Advanced Consulting.

    vii. Autonomy of actions.

    viii. Approval of financial commitments.

    ix. Staff service.

    x. Supervision.

    xi. Complexity and stress.

    xii. Advanced financial responsibility.

    xiii. Broad personal responsibility.

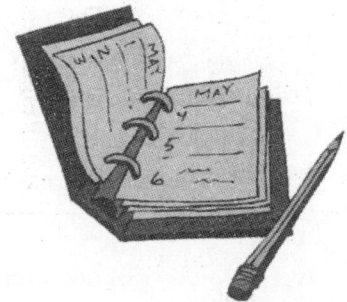

iv. Diary /Log Method

- In Diary method the workers are asked to maintain and keep daily records or list of activities they are doing every day.
- This method is also called **Work / Log Method**

Advantages of diary method

i   May be useful for jobs that are difficult to observe.

ii. Technique is accurate and eliminates the errors caused by job holder in questionnaire and checklist method.

Disadvantages of diary method

i.   Too much variance in writing skills.

ii. Can exaggerate tasks performed.

iii. Remembering what was done earlier is sometimes difficult.

v. Technical Conference

- Technical conference is method of job analysis based on SMEs.
- SMEs are "Subject Matter Experts" that include-
   - Supervisor
   - Incumbents who are familiar with work
   - Human resource staff / supervisor/ manager.
- Technical conference process:

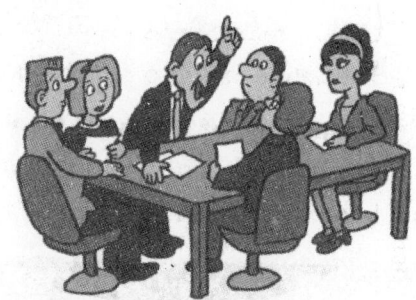

   - The details about the Job are obtained from these SMEs.
   - SMEs conduct brainstorming sessions to identify job elements.
   - SME's assign weights to each of the elements based on the following criteria:
      - Proportion of barely acceptable workers who have the job element.
      - Effectiveness of the element in picking a superior worker.
      - The trouble likely to occur if the element is not considered.
      - The effect of including the job element on the organisation's ability to fill job openings.

Advantages of Technical Conference

i.   Data from experience is superior to observation.

ii. Data is comprehensive.

iii. SMEs chosen have expertise and competence.

Disadvantages of Technical Conference Method

i. SMEs may have trouble breaking work into tasks and describing work.

ii. Time consuming.

iii. Differences in opinion may arise and need to be resolved to consensus.

vi. Checklist

- It is similar to questionnaire, but has lesser subjective judgments and more **'yes' – 'no'** type questions.

- Checklists may cover many activities ranging to 100, but job holder has to tick the one related to his job.

- Checklist preparation is a difficult task and all data related to the job must be collected by consulting supervisors, industrial engineers and others related to the job.

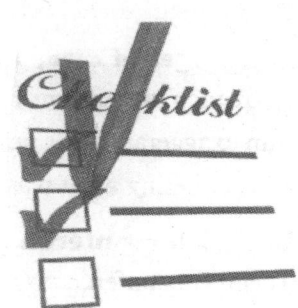

Advantages of Checklist Method

i. Easy to administer.

ii. Useful in large firms which has large number of people assigned to same job.

iii. Tabulation and recording on electronic data processing equipment is possible.

Disadvantages of Checklist Method

i. It may not include important parts of work.

ii. It is expensive for small firms.

TEST YOUR GREY MATTER

Q1) Who all are considered for being a job analyst? Give a comparison between them and analyse their worth as a job analyst?

Q2) What is the information required for Job Analysis purpose?

Q3) Describe briefly the methods used for Job Analysis?

Q4) Describe Interview method of data collection. Also mention its advantages and disadvantages.

Q5) What are Unstructured interviews?

Q6) How is Questionnaire method of Data collection better than other methods? Also describe the method briefly.

Q7) Explain (i) Position Analysis Questionnaire

(ii) Management Position Description Questionnaire

Q8) What is Diary Method? Explain.

D. JOB DESCRIPTION AND JOB SPECIFICATION

D.1.JOB DESCRIPTION

- **Definition:** A Job Description is a clear, concise depiction of a job's duties and requirements in an organised factual statement.

- It is necessary before a vacancy is advertised to tell about the type and requirements of job.

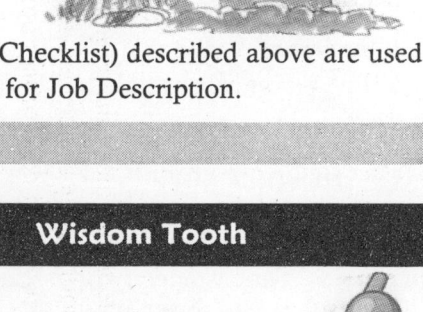

D.1.1. Preparation of Job Description

Various methods (Observation, Interview, Questionnaire, Diary, Technical Conference and Checklist) described above are used to collect the data which provides the information for Job Description.

D.1.2 Importance of Job Description

i. It is important for employment purposes i.e. to attract correct candidates for correct jobs.

ii. For development of realistic standards of performance and increase the effectiveness of training.

> **Wisdom Tooth**
>
> *"The problem is that the job description is constantly changing, almost daily."*
>
> **Bill Horn**

D.1.3. Elements of Job Description

Following are the main elements of Job Description

i. Job Title: It is to describe the nature of the job and should be short and suggestive.

ii. **Job Location:** It is to give the department or place where the job exists.

iii. **Job Summary:** It is a small paragraph giving a summary of the tasks performed by the employee in that job.

iv. **Duties and Responsibilities:** It actually lists down each task to be performed and the responsibilities held by the employee. It is the most important step of job description

v. **Equipment, Machine, Tools, Material used:** It includes the items which are used by the employee to perform his tasks.

vi. **Supervision:** It gives the Nature of Supervision of both, Supervision Received by the employee and Supervision Given by the employee. It enlists the tasks performed in giving and receiving supervision.

vii. **Working Conditions:** It gives the working environment, potential hazards and details of physical surroundings.

D.1.4. Sample Job Description

Job title: Product Developer.

Location: Pune.

Job Summary: Managing a team of engineers for completion of project, maintaining deadlines, communicating to subordinates and seniors about the progress of the project.

Duties and Responsibility: Project Time line, prioritising of bug fixing and features, Client interaction, Support contract, Interacting with Quality assurance, Appraisals of subordinates, Mentoring new recruits, Assisting product manager in internal audits of process, Timely delivery of product

Materials (software) and forms used: Excel, In-house tools-Visible, Bugzilla, Process-specific templates.

Supervision received or given: Supervision received-Time estimates about next release of products, Features to be included in the product, show stopper bugs. **Supervision given-**Assign task based on the expertise, Decide the time estimate, Decide on responsibility of added features.

Working conditions: Flexible working hours, good subordinate and senior relationship.

D.1.5. Accountability for Job Description

- The Personnel Manager and other managers in the organisation, who are heading various departments, are responsible for development and maintenance of job Descriptions.

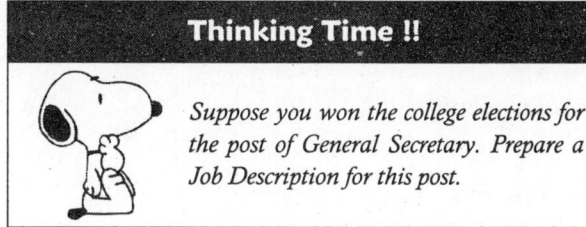

Thinking Time !!

Suppose you won the college elections for the post of General Secretary. Prepare a Job Description for this post.

- Whereas the Personnel Manager is to actually prepare and maintain the Job Description, Other Managers are to supply the required information and should co-operate with the Personnel Manager.

D.2. JOB SPECIFICATION

- Definition: Job Specification is a statement of capabilities and qualifications required to perform a job.
- It tells about the requirements and qualifications of a person who is to be selected to perform a job.

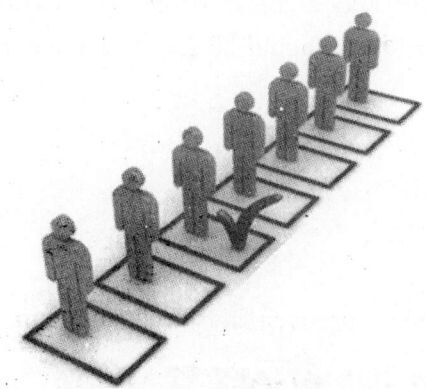

- Preparation and Accountability of Job Analysis:
  - Personnel Manager is responsible for preparation and maintenance of Job Specification but he does it with the co-operation and information received from various other managers and supervisors.
  - The qualities assessed and recorded involve subjective judgement on part of personnel manager, supervisor, job analyst and job holder.

D.2.1.Elements of Job Specification

i.   Education.

ii. Experience.

iii. Training.

iv. Judgement.

v.   Initiative.

vi. Physical Effort.

vii. Physical Skills.

viii. Responsibilities.

ix. Communication Skills.

x.   Emotional Characteristics.

xi. Unusual sensory demands such as sight, smell, hearing.

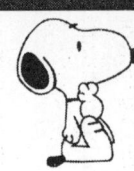

Thinking Time !!

Dream over...you have not won the General Secretary post, but the elections are going to come soon...Make a Job Specification, stating capabilities and qualifications required to perform the job of General Secretary. This will help you realise whether you are fit for the post or not. If you do not contest, it will still tell you whether the person you will be voting for is fit or not.

D.2.2. Sample Job Specifications

- **Education and experience:** B.E - 2 to 5 years of experience in IT domain and MBA - fresher

- **Communication skills:** Very high, since interaction will be with foreign clients

- **Emotional characteristics:** Should be able to handle stress and be considerate towards subordinates.

- **Desired Qualities:**
  - Good Communication
  - Decent background
  - Positive attitude.

- **Special skills:** Aggressive approach and Excellent in communication.

E. PROBLEMS WITH JOB ANALYSIS

i. Lack of Top Management Support

Role of top management is to communicate to incumbents that the purpose of job analysis is to enhance performance in organisation. But this is often not communicated.

ii. Lack of Training of the Analyst and Incumbent

Incumbent should be trained about the purpose of job analysis, otherwise, incumbents may not be able to generate quality data or may distort data of job analysis because employees might think that the process is a threat to them.

iii. Use of only One Method

Each method of Job Analysis has advantages and disadvantages; also job analysis includes both collecting of data and review of data, so using only single method is not a good practice and so combination of 2 methods should be used to provide better data for job analysis.

iv. Other Problems are

- Lack of participation of all stakeholders.
- Job-based rather than person-based.
- Lack of reward for providing quality information.
- Insufficient time allowed for the process.
- Intentional or unintentional distortion by incumbent.
- Absence of a review.
- Time spent on job analysis is too long.

TEST YOUR GREY MATTER

Q1) What is a Job Description? How is it prepared? Explain with the help of an example.

Q2) What is a Job Specification? What are its main elements? Explain with the help of an example.

Q3) How is Job Description different from Job Specification?

Q4) What are the possible problems faced in Job Analysis Process?

15 Recruitment and Selection

A. THE INSIGHT

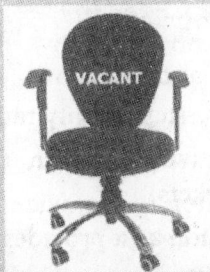

"A picture is worth a thousand words"

B. RECRUITMENT

What is Recruitment?

- **Definition:** Recruitment refers to the process of attracting, screening and selecting qualified people for a job at an organisation or company.
- Recruitment includes the process of receipt of applications from a job seeker and the term is used to describe the entire process of Employee hiring.
- Every organisation has its own recruitment boards to accomplish the process.

B.1.Importance/Purpose of Recruitment

- Recruitment represents the first contact that a company makes with potential employees.
- It is through recruitment that many individuals come to know about a company & eventually decide whether they wish to work for it. A well-planned and well-managed recruiting effort results in high quality applicants, whereas a haphazard effort will result in mediocre ones.

B.2.Main Purposes of Recruitment are

i. Create a talent pool of candidates to enable the selection of best candidates for the organisation.

ii. Determine present & future requirements of the organisation in conjunction with its personnel planning & job analysis activities.

iii. Increase the pool of job candidates at minimum cost.

iv. Help increase the success rate of selection process by decreasing number of under-qualified or over-qualified job applicants.

v. Meet the organisation's legal and social obligations regarding the composition of its work force by creating culturally more diverse workforce.

vi. Help reduce the probability that job applicants once recruited & selected will leave the organisation only after a short period of time.

B.3.Features of Recruitment

The features of recruitment are mentioned below:-

a. Recruitment is a process/ multi-step activity rather than a single act or event.

b. Recruitment is a linking activity between the employer (organisation) and prospective employees (job seekers).

c. Recruitment is a positive function as it provides organisation with the best pool of talented and qualified candidates.

d. Recruitment is an omnipresent (common) function, as all organisations/companies are engaged in recruiting activity.

B.4. Factors Affecting Recruitment

- The recruitment function of the organisation is affected and governed by various internal & external forces.

- The **Internal forces or factors** are factors that can be controlled by the organisation. And **External factors** are all those factors which cannot be controlled by the organisation.

> ### Wisdom Tooth
>
> *"You need massive recruitment to tell the poorest of the poor what is possible".*
>
> *Jonathan Kozol*

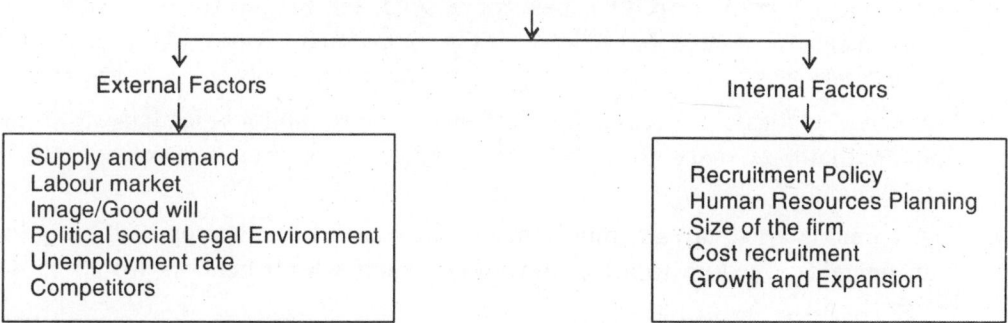

Factors Affecting Recruitment

External Factors	Internal Factors
Supply and demand Labour market Image/Good will Political social Legal Environment Unemployment rate Competitors	Recruitment Policy Human Resources Planning Size of the firm Cost recruitment Growth and Expansion

1. External Factors

a. Supply And Demand

The supply and demand of specific skills in the labour market is of great importance. If the demand of a particular skill is high relative to the supply, an extraordinary recruiting effort may be needed. E.g. The need or demand for programmers and financial analysts is likely to be higher than their supply, as opposed to demand – supply relationship for non-technical employees.

b. Unemployment Rate

When the unemployment rate in a given area is high, the company's recruitment process becomes simpler. The number of unsolicited applications is usually greater, and the increased size of the labour pool provides better opportunities for attracting qualified applicants. On the other hand, as the unemployment rate drops, recruiting effort must be increased and new sources explored.

c. Image/Goodwill

The company's/organisation's image also matters in attracting large number of job seekers. An organisation with positive image and goodwill as an employer finds it easier to attract and retain an employee than an organisation with a negative image.

E.g. Larsen & Toubro Ltd. is the leading, reliable & well-established organisation in the field of manufacturing, construction and many more fields with a positive image, it is able to attract the cream (qualified & skilled) of engineers from reputed institutions.

d. Political – Social – Legal Environment

Various government regulations prohibiting discrimination in hiring and employment have direct impact on recruitment process/practices.

- Government of India (GOI) has introduced legislation for reservation in employment for Scheduled Castes (SC), Scheduled Tribes (ST), physically handicapped etc.
- Preference to locals is another political factor. Some political leaders are of the opinion that preference must be given to people of their respective state in employment.
- Trade unions also play an important role in recruitment thereby restricting the management's freedom to select those individuals who it believes would be the best performers.

e. Labour Market

Employment conditions in the community where the organisation is located will influence the recruitment efforts of the organisation. If there is surplus of manpower at the time of recruitment, even informal attempts at the recruiting time, like notice board display of requisition or announcement in the meeting etc. will attract more than enough applicants.

f. Competitors

The recruitment policies of the competitors also affect the recruitment function of the organisation. To face competition, many times organisations have to change their recruitment policies according to the policies followed by competitors.

2. Internal factors

a. Recruitment Policy

- Creating a suitable recruitment policy is the first step in the efficient hiring process. A clear and concise recruitment policy helps to ensure a sound recruitment process.

- **Definition:** The recruitment policy of an organisation specifies the objectives of recruitment & provides a frame work for the implementation of a recruitment programme.

Factors affecting Recruitment Policy

i. Organisational objectives.

ii. Personnel policies of the organisation & its competitors.

iii. Government policies on reservations.

iv. Preferred sources of recruitment.

v. Needs of the organisation.

vi. Recruitment costs & financial implications.

Components of the Recruitment Policy

i. The general recruitment policies & terms of the organisation.

ii. Recruitment services of consultants.

iii. Recruitment of temporary employees.

iv. Unique recruitment situations.

v. The Selection process.

vi. Job descriptions.

Features of Recruitment Policy of an Organisation

i. It should focus on recruiting the best potential people.

ii. Ensure that every applicant and employee is treated equally with dignity and respect.

iii. Unbiased policy.

iv. Aid and encourage employees in realising their full potential.

v. Transparent, task-oriented & merit-based selection.

vi. Weightage during selection should be given to factors that suit organisational needs.

vii. Optimisation of manpower at the time of selection process.

viii. Abides by relevant public policy and legislation on hiring & employment relationship.

ix. Integrates employee needs with organisation needs.

b. Human Resource Planning

Effective human resource planning helps in determining the gaps present in the existing manpower of an organisation. It also helps in determining the number of employees to be recruited & qualifications they must possess.

c. Size of the firm

The size of the firm is an important factor in the recruiting process.

E.g. Large firms such as Coco Cola has more recruitment needs than any small company.

d. Cost

Recruitment cost to the employee is yet another internal factor that has to be considered. Organisations try to employ that source of recruitment which will bear a lower cost of recruitment to the organisation for each candidate. Thus recruiters must operate within budgets and so cost affects the recruitment process.

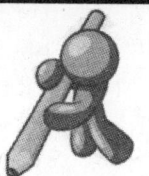

Wisdom Tooth

"Continuing economic growth requires both recruitment of new companies and expansion of existing business."

Phil Bredesen

e. Growth and Expansion

Organisation will employ or think of employing more personnel if it is expanding its operations. Organisation's expansion depends upon its growth & profit.

TEST YOUR GREY MATTER

Q1) Define Recruitment and explain why it is important for an organisation to do an effective job of recruiting?

Q2) How can a company determine if its recruitment processes are working effectively?

Q3) Enlist and briefly elaborate about various internal and external factors which affect the recruitment process?

Q4) What are the advantages and disadvantages of various external recruitment sources and compare them with internal sources?

Q5) Define Recruitment Policy and mention its important features?

Q6) Outline the legal, economic, social and political considerations in recruitment.

B.5.Recruitment Process

- Recruitment process involves a systematic procedure, from sourcing the candidates to arranging & conducting the interviews.
- The ideal recruitment programme is one that attracts a relatively larger number of qualified applicants who would survive the screening process and accept positions with the organisation, when referred.

B.5.1.Loopholes in the process may cause

i.   Failure to attract an adequate applicant pool.

ii. Under-selling/over-selling the firm.

iii. Inadequately screening applicants, before they enter the selection process.

B.5.2.Points to consider

To approach ideal individuals, the following points must be known:

i.   How many & what types of employees are needed,

ii. Where and how to look for individuals with appropriate qualifications and interests.

iii. What inducements to use (or avoid) for various types of applicant groups.

iv. How to distinguish applicants who are unqualified from those who have a reasonable chance of success.

v.   How to evaluate their work.

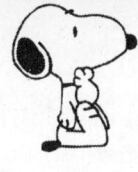

Thinking Time !!

Consider yourself to be the Head of the Human Resource Department of a huge organisation (choose your favourite) and now answer the, 'points to be considered given above. Assume you have all the authority and resources available.

B.5.3.Stages in Recruitment Process

1. Planning.
2. Strategy development.
3. Searching.
4. Screening and
5. Evaluation

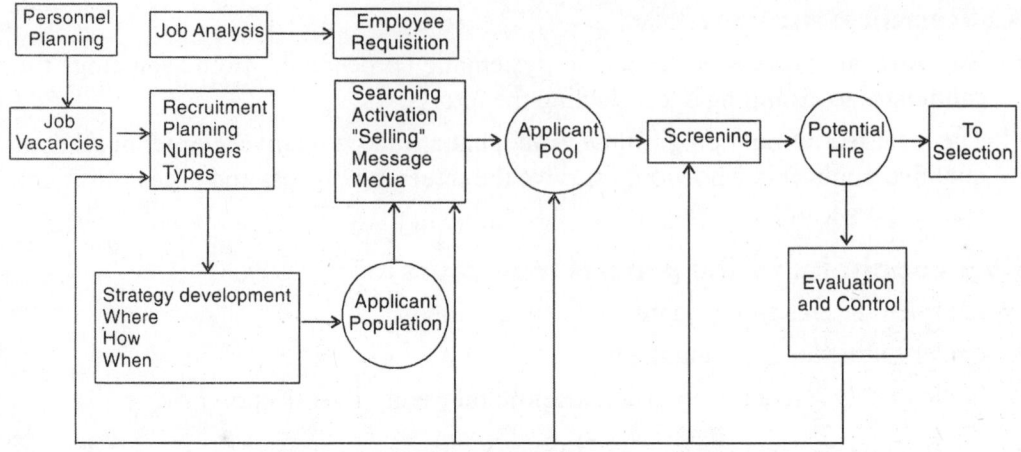

Recruitment Process

Source : Herbert G.Heneman III,et al,Personne/Human Resource Management,p226

1. Recruitment Planning

The first stage in the recruitment process is planning. Planning involves the translation of likely job vacancies and information about the nature of their jobs into a set of objectives or targets and specify the following :

a. **Number of Contacts:** Organisations nearly always plan to attract more applicants than they would hire. Some of these contacted will be uninterested, under-qualified or both.

b. **Type of Contacts:** This refers to the type of people to be informed about job openings. The type of people depends on the tasks and responsibilities involved and the qualifications and experiences expected. These details are available through job description & job specifications.

2. Strategy Development

Once it is known how many and what type of recruits are required, consideration needs to be given to –

a. 'Make' or 'Buy' employees.

b. Technological sophistication of recruitment & selection devices.

c. Geographical distribution of labour markets comprising job seekers.

d. Sources of recruitment.

e. Sequencing the activities in the recruitment process.

a. 'Make' or 'Buy'

Organisations must decide whether to hire less skilled employees and invest on training and education programmes, or to hire skilled labour and professionals. Essentially, this is the 'make' (hire less skilled labour) or 'buy' (here skilled workers & professionals) decision.

b. Technological Sophistication

- The second decision in strategy development relates to the methods used in recruitment & selection. This decision is mainly influenced by available technology.
- The advent of computers has made it possible for employers to check national and international applicant qualifications.

c. Where to Look

- In order to reduce costs, firms look into the labour market most likely to offer the required job seekers.
- Generally, companies look into the national market for managerial & professional employees, regional and local market for technical employees, and local markets for clerical and blue-collar employees.

d. How to Look

How to look refers to the methods of sources of recruitment. There are various sources and they may broadly categorized into (1) Internal sources, and (2) External sources.

d.1. Internal sources

Internal recruitment seeks applicants for positions from those who are currently employed:

i. Present Employees

Those already working in the organisation can be a source of internal recruitment by:

    a. Transfers: The Employees are transferred from one department to another according to their efficiency and experience.

    b. Promotions: The employees are promoted from one position/level to another (higher position) with more benefits and greater responsibility based on their experience and ability to perform.

    Advantages of Promotion
- It builds morale.
- It encourages competent individuals who are ambitious.
- It improves the probability of a good selection, since information on the individual's performance is easily available.
- It is cheaper than going outside to recruit.
- Those chosen internally are familiar with the organisation.

ii. Employee Referrals

- Employee referral is a method in which current employees recommend their friends and family members for specific job openings.

- With this method, employees can develop good prospects for their relatives, by acquainting them with the advantage of a job with the organisation and encouraging them to apply.
- Sometimes, organisation also offers, **"Finder's Fee"** in the form of a monetary incentive for a successful referral.

iii. Retired/Former Employees

- Retired employees can also be recruited once again in case of shortage of qualified personnel or increase in work load.
- It saves time and cost of the organisation as people are already aware of the organisational culture, policies and procedures.

iv. Previous Applicants

- All applicants who have previously applied for the job can be contacted by e-mails etc.
- This is quick and inexpensive way to fill an unexpected opening but is not truly an internal source of recruitment.

d.2. External Sources

i. Advertisements

- Advertisements of vacancy in periodicals such as local newspapers or professional journals are a widely used source.
- Its main advantage is that it reaches a wide number of people.
- There are 4 ways in which newspaper advertisement asks applicants to respond:

  a. Calling: Applicants are asked to respond by calling when a company wants to either quickly screen applicants or hear an applicant's phone voice. E.g. For telemarketing or receptionist positions.

  b. Apply-In-Person Ads: Organisations use this method when they want to get a physical look at the applicants.

  c. Send Resume Ads: Organisations use 'send a resume directly to the company ads' when the organisation expects a large response and does not have

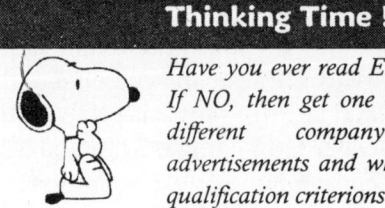

Thinking Time !!

Have you ever read Employment News? If NO, then get one and find out how different company give their advertisements and what are their basic qualification criterions?

(After few years of your college you may need it anyway!!!)

the resources to speak to thousands of applicants.

d. Blind Box: This type of ad directs applicants to send their resume to a blind box, one in which there is no identification of the company. Respondents are asked to reply to a post box number or to a consulting firm that is retained by the organisation.

ii. Employment Exchanges

● Government establishes public employment exchanges throughout the country.

● These exchanges provide job information to job seekers and help employers in identifying suitable applicants.

● Thus, employment exchange acts as a link between the employers and prospective employees.

iii. Campus Recruitment

● Various Management Institutes, Engineering Colleges, Medical Colleges, Research Laboratories etc. are a good source for recruiting well qualified fresh graduates from their institutions.

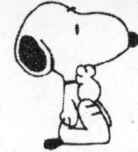

Thinking Time !!

Find out from your seniors what are the various companies which came to your college for recruitment and what are the packages they offered.

● This kind of recruitment done through such educational institutions is called as **campus recruitment.**

iv. Direct Application: Walk-ins, Write-ins and Talk-ins

● Direct application method of recruitment is very common and least expensive for candidates. In this method, job seekers submit unsolicited application letters or resumes.

● Direct applications can also provide a pool of talented and potential employees to meet future needs.

● **Walk-ins** are those in which aspirant directly goes to the place where the interview is to take place without any prior notice or examination. Walk-ins are preferable as they are free from the hassles associated with other methods of recruitment.

● **Write ins** – are those which require written enquiries to be sent. These job seekers are asked to complete applications forms for further processing.

● **Talk-ins**- Under this, job aspirants are required to meet the recruiter for detailed talks. No application is required to be submitted to the recruiter.

Walk-in for TCS for multiple skills at Gurgaon on 13-Mar-10

Tags: C/C++/ Systems, DBA/System Administrator, Experienced, Gurgaon, TCS, Unix/Linuxs

Date	13-March-2010 (Saturday)
Venue	Tata Consultancy Services,249 D & E Udyog Vihar Phase IV, Gurgaon
Registration Time	9.30 am to 12.30 pm

Skills	Experience Band	Requirement (JD)
C++	3+ years	3 + yrs exp in C++, NMS, Networking Management Systems
Unix Admn	3-8 years	3-8 yrs experience on Unix/HP Unix/Solaris Admin/AIX Administrator, different hardware environment, standard operation procedures. Any flavour of Unix is desirable. Administration & Troubleshooting of different Unix Servers
Oracle DBA	3-7 years	3+ yrs experience in Oracle 9i/10g database administration, Oracle software installation, database creation and configuration, RMAN backup and recovery, performance tuning.
Windows Admn	3-7 years	3-7 years experience and at least 3+ years on Windows system administration, Strong working knowledge of the Microsoft Windows Server, Enterprise Level knowledge of Active Directory, WINS, DNS/DDNS and DHCP. Operating systems (WinNT/2k/2k3).

Documents to be carried for the walk-in

- A copy of the resume
- Passport size photo
- Last 3 months pay-slip copies

v. Consultants/Outsourcing

Several private consultancy firms perform recruitment functions on behalf of client companies by charging a fee. These agencies are particularly suitable for recruitment of executives and specialists. It is also known as RPO (Recruitment Process Outsourcing)

E.g. ABC consultants, Aims Management Consultants etc.

vi. Labour contractors

- These (contractors) are the specialist people who supply manpower to factories or manufacturing plants. Through these contractors, workers are appointed or contract basis, i.e. for a particular time period.

- They are under the condition that when these contractors leave the organisation, such people who are appointed also have to leave the concern.

vii. Poaching/Raiding/Competitors

- "Buying talent" (rather than developing it) is the latest mantra being followed by organisations today.

- Poaching means employing a competent and experienced person already working with another reputed company in the same or different industry; the organisation may be a competitor in the market/industry.

- A company attracts talent from another firm by offering attractive pay packages & other terms and conditions, better than the current employer of the candidate. But it is seen as an unethical practice & not openly talked about.

- Indian software & retail sectors are the sectors which are facing the most severe effects of poaching today.

viii. E-Recruitment

- Many big organisations use internet as a source of recruitment. E-recruitment is the use of technology to assist the recruitment process.

- They advertise job vacancies through the world wide web. Jjob seekers send their applications/Curriculum Vitae i.e. CVs through E-mail using internet. Alternatively, job seekers place their CVs in the world wide web, which can be drawn by prospective employers depending upon their requirements.

Advantage of E-Recruitment

i.   Low cost

ii. No intermediaries.

iii. Reduction in time for recruitment.

iv. Efficiency of recruitment process

Disadvantages of E-recruitment

i.   Broader exposure might result in many unqualified applicants applying for job.

ii. More resumes need to be reviewed.

iii. Recruiters are likely to miss out many competent applicants who lack access to internet.

Advantages & Disadvantages of Internal and External Recruitment

i. Internal Recruitment

Advantages	Disadvantages
(i) It is less expensive	(i) The size of prospective applicants is considerably reduced
(ii) Good performance is rewarded	(ii) External candidates might be better suited/qualified for the job.
(iii) Candidates are already oriented towards the company	(iii) Another vacancy will be created that has to be filled
(iv) Organisations have better knowledge about internal candidates	(iv) Politics play greater role.
(v) It offers wonderful opportunities for the current staff to further their career.	(v) It abets raiding.
(vi) May help to retain staff who might otherwise leave.	(vi) Morale problem for those who are not promoted.

ii. External Recruitment

Advantages	Disadvantages
(i) Benefits of new talent, new skills with new ideas	(i) Longer process
(ii) Larger pool of workers from which to find the best candidate	(ii) More expensive process due to advertisement & interviews required.
(iii) Scope of abet raiding can be avoided	(iii) Adjustments of new employees to the organisational culture takes longer time.

e. When to Look

- An effective recruiting strategy must determine when to look i.e. decide on the timings of events – besides knowing where & how to look for job applicants.

3. Searching

Once a recruiting plan & strategy are worked out, the search process can begin. Search involves two steps:

i. Source activation

- If the firm/organisation has planned well & developed its sources & search methods, source activation results in a flood of applications and/or resumes.
- The applications/ resumes must be screened. Those who pass have to be contacted & invited for interview.

ii. Selling

- Selling issue in the searching process concerns communications.
- It involves two extremes, doing anything to attract desirable applicants and also resisting the temptation of over-selling their virtues.
- In selling the company, both the message & media deserve attention.
- **Message** means employment advertisement.
- Effectiveness of any recruiting message depends on the credibility of the media. As there are many forms of media – with low credibility (e.g. Employment Exchange) or high creditability (e.g. Advertisement in business magazines), therefore selection of media needs to be done with a lot of care.

4. Screening

- The main purpose of screening is to eliminate from the recruiting process, at an early stage, all those applicants who visibly do not qualify for the job. Effective screening can save a great deal of time and money.
- The selection process begins after the applications have been scrutinized & short listed.
- With this process, applicant's can be judged on their skills, knowledge, abilities and interests required to do the job.
- The screening techniques used in the organisations vary, depending on the candidate sources and recruiting methods used. E.g.. (i) Campus recruiters use interviews & resumes. (ii) Psychometric testing, Technical skill testing.

5. Evaluation & Control

- Evaluation and control is necessary as considerable costs are incurred in the recruiting process.

The costs generally incurred are –
i. Salaries for recruiters.
ii. The cost of advertisements or other recruitment methods, that is, agency fees.
iii. Management & professional time spent on preparing job description, job specifications, advertisements, agency liaison & so forth.
iv. Recruitment overheads & administrative expenses.
v. Cost of overtime & outsourcing while the vacancies remain unfilled.
vi. Cost of recruiting unsuitable candidates for the selection process.

B.5.4.Evaluation of Recruitment Process

Recruitment has the objective of searching for and obtaining applications from job seekers in sufficient numbers and quantity. Keeping this objective in mind, the evaluation might include:

i. Return rate of applications sent out.

ii. Number of suitable candidates for selection.

iii. Retention and performance of the candidates selected.

iv. Cost of the recruitment process.

v. Time lapsed data.

vi. Comments on image projected.

TEST YOUR GREY MATTER

Q1) What are the consequences of loopholes in the recruitment process and what are the steps which should be taken to avoid them?

Q2) What are stages involved in the Recruitment Process? Explain briefly.

Q3) What are the sources for internal recruitment and external recruitment?

Q4) Differentiate between Internal Recruitment and External Recruitment, stating their advantages and disadvantages?

Q5) What is Screening and how is it done?

Q6) What are the various forms of costs incurred in the Recruitment Process?

Q7) Discuss the methods of making contact with prospective candidates from whom you will be selecting?

Q8) How will you evaluate and control a recruitment programme?

C. SELECTION

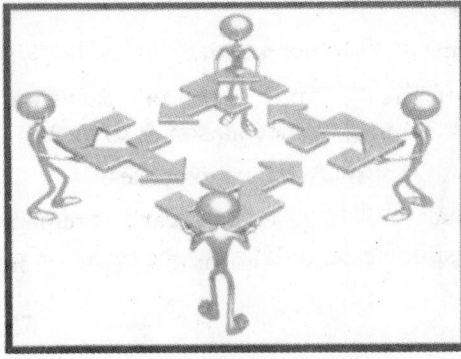

C.1. What Is Selection/Nature of Selection

Next to Recruitment, the logical step in the HR Process is SELECTION, of qualified and competent candidates.

Definition: Selection is defined as the process of differentiating between applicants in order to identify (and hire) those with a greater likelihood of success in a job.

Or

Selection is basically picking applicants from a pool of job applicants, who have the appropriate qualification and competency to do the job in the organisation.

C.2. Difference between Recruitment and Selection

- Recruitment and selection are the two crucial steps in the HR process and are often used interchangeably. There is, however, a fine distinction between the two steps.

- While **Recruitment** is identifying and encouraging prospective employees to apply for a job, **Selection** is selecting the right candidate from the pool of applicants.

- Recruitment is said to be **positive in its approach** as it seeks to attract as many applicants as possible to apply to the jobs in the organisation. In this way, it increases the selection ratio and provides a great opportunity to the management to select suitable applicants. Selection, on the other hand **is negative in its approach** as it seeks to eliminate as many unqualified applicants as possible in order to identify the right candidates.

- Difference between Recruitment & Selection

Basis	Recruitment	Selection
1. Meaning	It is an activity of establishing contact between employers and applicants	It is a process of picking the more competent and suitable employee
2. Objective	It encourages large number of candidates for a job.	It attempts at rejecting unsuitable candidates.
3. Process	It is a simple process	It is a complicated process
4. Hurdles	The candidates need not cross many hurdles	Many hurdles have to be crossed by candidates.
5. Approach	It is a positive approach	It is a negative approach
6. Sequence	It preceeds selection	It follows recruitment
7. Economy	It is an economical method	It is an expensive method
8. Time consuming	Less time is required	More time is required

C.3. Importance of Selection

- Selecting the right person for the job is an extremely important component of a successful organisation. Effective selection is important for at least two reasons-

i. **Work performance** depends on individuals. How employees perform their jobs is a major factor in determining how successful an organisation will be. Job performance is essentially determined by the ability of an individual to do a particular job and the effort the individual is willing to put in to perform the job. Through effective selection, organisation can maximise the profitability, knowledge, skills & abilities to do the jobs they were hired to do.

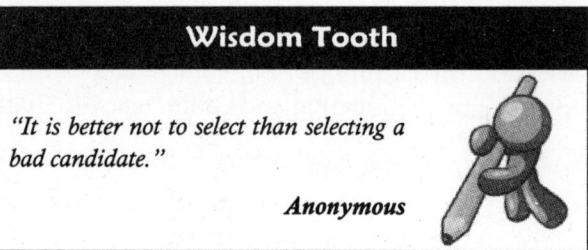

Wisdom Tooth

"It is better not to select than selecting a bad candidate."

Anonymous

ii. **Cost incurred** in recruiting and hiring personnel is a clear indication of the importance of selection. Mistakes done in hiring are costly, in terms of expenditure incurred on selection, induction, training & poor performance of the employee.

- Employee selection also provides the base for other HR practices - such as
  i. Effective job design
  ii. Goal setting and
  iii. Compensation, that motivates workers to exert the effort needed to do their job effectively.

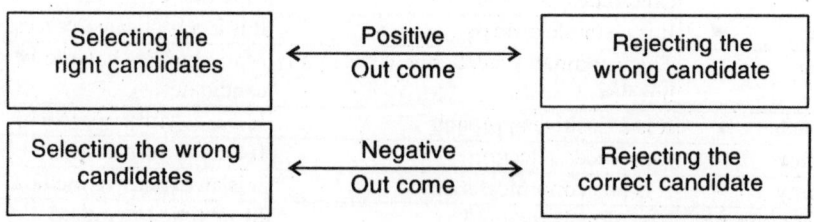

C.4.Selection Process

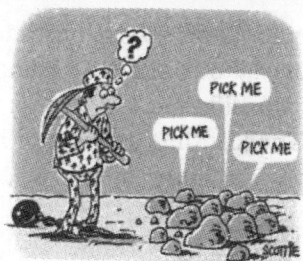

- Selection is a long process, commencing from the preliminary interview of applicants & ending with the contract of employment.

The following chart gives an idea about the selection process:

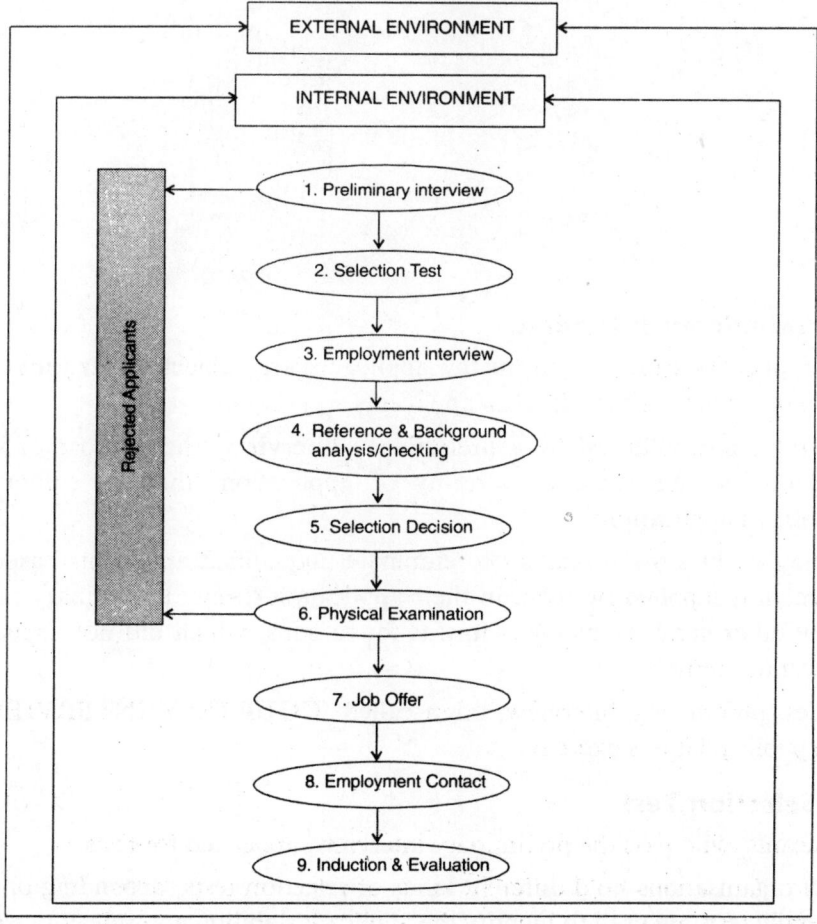

Environmental Factors Affecting Selection

Selection is influenced by several factors. More prominent among them are supply & demand of specific skills in the labour market, unemployment rate, labour market conditions, legal & political considerations, Company policy, Human Resource Planning and Cost of Hiring. The last three constitute the internal environment & the remaining constitutes the external environment of selection process.

Steps in the Selection Process

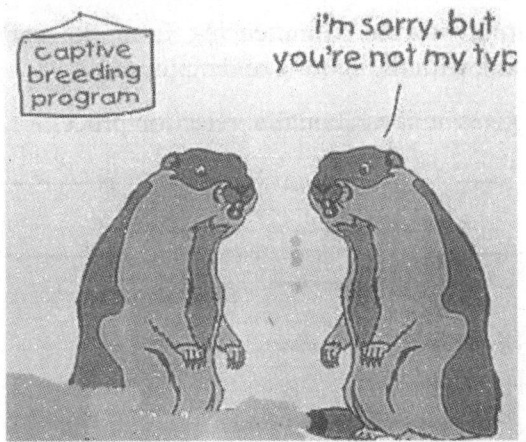

Step 1: Preliminary Interview

- The applications received from the applicants are subject to **scrutiny** so as to eliminate unqualified candidates/applicants.
- This is usually followed by a **preliminary interview**, the purpose of which is more or less the same as scrutiny of application, that is, elimination of unqualified applications.
- Scrutiny enables the specialists to eliminate unqualified applicants based on the information supplied by them in their application forms. Preliminary interview, on the other hand, helps reject misfits for reasons, which did not appear in the application forms.
- Besides, preliminary interview, often called **'COURTESY INTERVIEW'**, is a good public relations exercise.

Step 2: Selection Test

- Applicants, who pass the preliminary interview, are called for tests.
- Many organisations hold different kinds of selection tests, depending on the job. Generally tests are used to identify the applicant's ability, aptitude & personality.

- The following types of tests have gained popularity in organisations these days.
  - i. Intelligence test
  - ii. Ability/Achievement tests
  - iii. Aptitude tests
  - iv. Personality tests
  - v. Interest tests

The details of these tests have been given in 'Chapter 16- Psychological Tests'

Step 3: Employment Interview

Definition: Interview is an essential element of the selection procedure,

- i. Where the information collected through application letter or application forms and tests can be cross-checked.
- ii. Where candidates demonstrate their capabilities & strength in relevance to their academic credentials.

Purpose of Interview

- i. Obtaining information about the background, education, training, work history and interests of candidates.
- ii. Giving information to candidates about the company, the specific job & human resources policies.
- iii. Establishing a friendly relationship between the employer (company) and the candidate so as to motivate the successful applicant to work for the organisation.

> **Thinking Time !!**
>
> *Have you ever faced any interview? Share your experiences with your friends. Aren t interviews fun?*

Step 4: Reference Checks

- The applicant is asked to mention in his application form, the names, addresses and telephone numbers of two or more persons who know him for the purpose of verifying information and perhaps, gaining additional background information on an applicant.
- The reference persons may be his previous employers, heads of education institutions, public figures, neighbours or friends. These people are requested to provide their frank opinion about the candidate without incurring any liability.
- Previous employers are preferable because they are already aware of the applicant's performance. In Government and public sector organisations, candidates are generally required to route their applications through their present

employers, if any. The opinion of references can be useful in judging the future behaviour & performance of candidate, but it is not advisable to rely exclusively on the referees because they are generally biased in favour of the candidate.

Step 5: Selection Decision

- After obtaining information through the preceding steps, the selection decision-the most critical of all the steps-must be made.
- Other stages in the selection process have been used to narrow the number of candidates. The final decision has to be made from the pool of individuals who pass the tests, interview & reference checks.
- Finally, the candidates shortlisted by the department (HRD) are approved by the executives of concerned departments.

Step 6: Physical Examination / Medical Examination

- Applicant who has crossed the above stages is sent for a physical examination either to the company's physician or to a medical officer approved for the purpose.
- A job offer is, often, dependent upon the candidate being declared fit after the medical examination.

Purpose of Physical/Medical Examination

a. It determines whether the candidate is physically fit to perform the job, where those who are physically unfit are rejected.

b. It reveals existing disabilities & provides a record of the employee's health at the time of selection. This record will help in setting company's liability under the **Workmen Compensation Act** for claim for any injury.

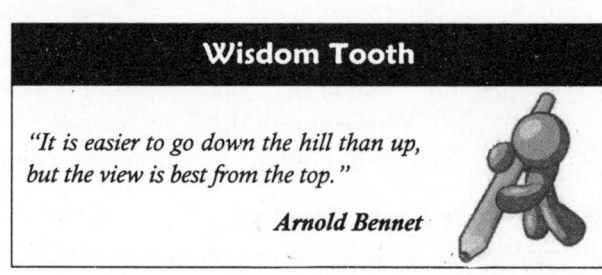

Wisdom Tooth

"It is easier to go down the hill than up, but the view is best from the top."

Arnold Bennet

c. It prevents the employment of people suffering from contagious diseases.

d. It identifies candidates who are otherwise suitable but require specific jobs due to physical handicaps & allergies.

Step 7: Job offer / Employment

- Employment is offered in the form of an appointment letter mentioning the post, the rank, the salary grade, the date by which the candidate should join & other terms and conditions in brief.

Step 8: Contracts of Employment

- After the job offer has been made & candidates accept the offer, certain documents need to be executed by the employer and the candidate.
- One such document is the **Attestation Form**. This form contains vital details about the candidate, which are authenticated and attested by him/her. Attestation form is a valid record for future reference.
- There is also a need for preparing a contract of employment. The basic information that should be included in a written contract of employment will vary according to the level of the job.

Checklist for Employee contract

1. Contract Details

    i. Full name of Employer and Employee.

    ii. Address of Employer.

    iii. Place of work of employee.

    iv. Title of job or nature of the work or a brief job description.

    v. Date of commencement of employment.

2. Pay & Benefits

    i. Wages/salary details

    ii. Rate of overtime work (if eligible for overtime pay)

    iii. Method of payment & method of calculating wages.

    iv. Additional benefits e.g. Achievement of targets.

    v. Pension scheme – whether one exists, and if so, conditions.

    vi. Approvals for any deduction from pay, other than those required by law.

3. Nature of contract

    i. Type of contract – permanent, temporary or fixed term.

    ii. Duration of temporary contract or termination dates for fixed term contract.

4. Hours of work, schedules and overtime

    i. Number of hours in work week & work day.

    ii. Meal and rest periods

    iii. Shift arrangement

5. Leave

    i. Annual leave entitlement

    ii. Sick leave arrangements & conditions of any benefits.

    iii. Details of any other paid leave entitlement.

    iv. Termination due to continued illness.

    v. Notification of illness (medical certificate)

6. Disciplinary Procedures

    i. Details of the disciplinary procedure.

    ii. Conditions under which the employer can terminate the contract. E.g. Gross misconduct.

7. Grievance Procedure

    i. Definition of Grievance

    ii. Employee's right to union representation.

    iii. Explanation of each step in Grievance & time limit at each step.

8. Protection of Business Information

    i. Details of confidential requirements.

    ii. Use/misuse of electronic communications & internet.

9. About Probation Period

    i. Purpose & duration of probation period.

    ii. Benefits that will come into effect after the period of probation.

10. Performance Evaluation

Criteria & frequency of evaluations.

11. Retirement policy

Benefits that will be provided after retirement.

12. Any Other Conditions

13. Acceptance

Acceptance clause whereby employees sign that they accept the contract of employment & conditions therein.

Step 9: Final Step

1. Induction

- The process of receiving employees when they begin work, introducing them to the company and to their colleagues, and informing them of the activities, customs and traditions of the company is called induction.

- Various induction courses are given to new recruits in order to familiarise them with the new working environment.

2. Follow-Up (Evaluation)

- All selections should be validated by follow-up. It is a stage where the employee is asked how he or she feels about the progress till date. The worker's immediate supervisor is asked for comments, which are compared with the notes taken at the selection interview.

- If a follow-up is unfavourable, it is probable that the selection has been a fault; the whole procedure from job specification to interview is then reviewed to see if a better choice can be made next time. Therefore, it is essential to follow-up newly engaged employees, to ensure that they have settled in and to check, how well they are doing.

TEST YOUR GREY MATTER

Q1) Define Selection Process and state why it is important for the organisation?

Q2) Differentiate between Selection and Recruitment Process?

Q3) What are the various steps involved in a selection process. Explain them briefly?

Q4) What is meant by selection tests? What are the different types of tests used in selection process?

Q5) What is a selection interview and what are its purposes?

Q6) What are the factors considered while arriving at a selection decision?

Q7) What is a reference check? Do you agree with the view that reference check has become a mere formality in the selection process in Indian organisations?

Q8) Is physical examination necessary for selection process? Express your views.

Q9) What are the main constituents of a Contract of Employment?

CHAPTER 16

Psychological Tests

By the end of this chapter, you would be able to :

- Know what is psychological testing and assessment and how it is important for the organisation.
- Understand the concept of intelligence and its different classifications.
- Learn about different methods of testing and their purposes.
- Design a test and also check its reliability and validity.
- Learn about all the aspects of Employment Interview Process.

The chapter contains :

- Psychological testing
- Psychological assessment
- Employment tests
- Intelligence
- Types of tests
- Other Classifications of Test
- Reliability of Tests
- Validity of Tests
- Designing of tests
- Guidelines/Principles of testing
- Meaning & Purpose of Employment Interview

A. THE INSIGHT

A little intelligence test for you. There are 10 questions. Do not look at the answers found at the end of this chapter- no cheating. Write each of your answers down, it makes a difference. Good Luck!

1. Some months have 30 days, some months have 31 days. How many months have 28 days?

2. If a doctor gives you 3 pills and tells you to take one pill every half hour, how long would it be before all the pills have been taken?

3. I went to bed at eight 8 'clock in the evening and wound up my clock and set the alarm to sound at nine 9 'clock in the morning. How many hours sleep would I get before being awoken by the alarm?

4. Divide 30 by half and add ten. What do you get?

5. A farmer had 17 sheep. All but 9 died. How many live sheep were left?

6. If you had only one match and entered a COLD and DARK room, where there was an oil heater, an oil lamp and a candle, which would you light first?

7. A man builds a house with four sides of rectangular construction, each side having a southern exposure. A big polar bear comes along. What colour is the bear?

8. Take 2 apples from 3 apples. What do you have?

9. How many animals of each species did Moses take with him in the Ark?

10. If you drove a bus with 43 people on board from Kanpur and stopped at Unnao to pick up 7 more people and drop off 5 passengers and at Amausi to drop off 8 passengers and pick up 4 more and eventually arrive at Lucknow 2 hours later. What's the name of the driver?

B. PSYCHOLOGICAL TESTING

Definition : Psychological testing is a field characterised by the use of samples of behaviour in order to assess psychological constructs, such as cognitive and emotional functioning, about a given individual.

- The technical term for the science behind psychological testing is **Psychometrics.**

- Samples of behaviour, here means, observations over time of an individual performing tasks that have usually been prescribed beforehand, which often means scores on a test.

- These responses are often complied into statistical tables that allow the evaluator to compare the behaviour of the individual being tested to the responses of a norm group.

C. PSYCHOLOGICAL ASSESSMENT

- Psychological Assessment is similar to psychological testing but usually involves a more comprehensive assessment of the individual.

- **Definition:** Psychological Assessment is a process that involves the integration of information from multiple sources such as tests of normal and abnormal personality, tests of ability or intelligence, tests of interests or attitudes, as well as information from personal interviews.

- A useful psychological measure must be both valid (i.e. there is evidence to support the specified interpretation of the test results) and reliable (i.e., internally consistent over time, across raters etc.)

D. EMPLOYMENT TESTS

Definition : A test can be defined in two different ways.

From an 'Assessment View Point': A test is a standardised series of problems or questions that assess a person's knowledge, skills, abilities or other characteristics.

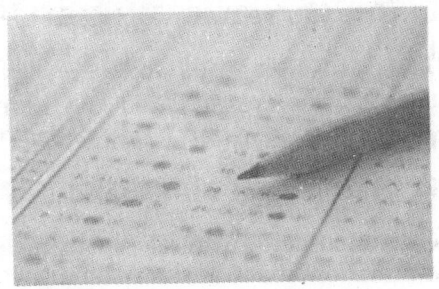

From a 'Legal View Point': A test can be any method which can be used to make an employment decision.

- While using these tests it must be ensured that the tests are both valid and reliable.
- The basis is that if scores on a test correlate with job performance, then it is economically useful for the employer to select employees based on scores from that test.

D.1. Kinds of Tests

There are different kinds of tests-
i. According to their mode of administration (e.g. paper & pencil vs. web-based)
ii. Their content (e.g. interpersonal skills, mathematical ability).
iii. Their level of standardisation or structure.
iv. Their costs.
v. Their administrative case etc.

D.2. Reasons for Testing /Advantages of Testing

i. Testing leads to savings in the decision-making process

Employment tests can be a cost-effective way to cut down the applicant pool. Tests can make the decision process more efficient because less time is spent with individuals whose characteristics, skills, and abilities do not match with what is needed.

ii. The costs of making a wrong decision are high

- For certain employment decisions, a wrong decision can be very costly in terms of training costs, errors due to poor performance, costs of replacement, etc.
- For these types of decisions, investing in testing may be seen as a particularly worthwhile endeavour if testing reduces the number of wrong decisions.

iii. The job requires attributes that are hard to develop/change

Tests are often used to assess characteristics that cannot be developed through training but are acquired over long periods of time or even a lifetime (e.g. a personally trait, in-depth knowledge of a profession).

iv. Hard-to-get information can be obtained more easily & efficiently

One important advantage of using employment tests is that they can often provide information about an individual that is not easily obtained using other methods or that would be much more costly to obtain by other means.

v. Individuals are treated consistently

- Using standardised tools in employment decision making ensures that the same information is gathered about each individual & used in a similar way in decisions.
- Employer often turns to testing because of the unfairness of less standardised processes, in which, all individuals are not treated in a similar way & similar information is not gathered on all individuals. Thus, subjective biases can creep into decisions if the process of making a decision is un-standardised.

vi. Large number of applicants

Sometimes the sheer number of individuals to consider for an employment decision leads an employer to choose testing as the most efficient & fair means of making a decision in a timely manner.

D.3. Reasons for Not Testing/Disadvantages of Testing

i Cost

- Tests are sometimes not preferred because of the cost factor attached to them. Costs of the test vary according to the type of test and are not uniform.
- But the cost of testing may not be considered a huge disadvantage, considering costs of low productivity, errors, retaining and attrition.
- For example, conservative estimates of the cost of attrition range from 1/3 to ½ of the annual salary of the employee that is being replaced. The cost of replacing a management executive and highly skilled talent can easily be 1-2 times the

annual incumbent salary. Further, the costs associated with hiring a wrong employee can be quite high.

ii. Fear of legal action

- Sometimes concerns are raised at the legality of using tests in hiring. As with any other method of making employment decisions, tests can be scrutinized if there is a belief that discrimination in employment decisions has occurred.
- There is an adverse impact when the selection rate of a given demographic group (ex. Females vs. Males, White vs. Black etc) is substantially lower than the selection rate of the majority.
- Employers should have clear documentation regarding any tools used in employment decision-making.

iii. Practical constraints

Tests may not be the best choice if not many individuals are being considered in a particulate employment decision, if

a. the resources to properly administer the test are not available or

b. the timing & logistics of the decision-making process prevents the use of an appropriate test.

D.4. Limitations of Testing

A number of factors can limit the use of selection tests in selection programs. Some of the factors are mentioned below:

i.   Legality of test.

ii. Possibility of rejection of qualified candidates.

iii. Privacy issues i.e. what can & should be asked?

iv. Tests cannot make 100 percent prediction of an individual's on the job success.

v.   Ethical issues:

    a. Test users

    b. Test security

    c. Test interpretation

    d. Test publication

E. INTELLIGENCE

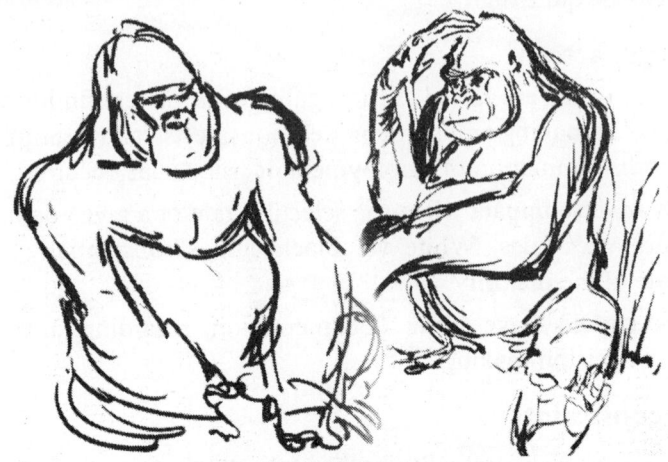

**"...you know, out of all the animal species,
I reckon the human must be about
the nearest to us in intelligence."**

Definition : According to **Thornidke**: Intelligence is the amount of transfer capacity.

- Thornidke developed psychological connectionism. He believed that through experience, neural bonds or connections were formed between **perceived stimuli** and **emitted responses**. Therefore, intellect facilitated the formation of neural bonds. People of higher intellect could form more bonds & form them more easily than people of lower ability.

- He identified three types of intelligence-
  - i. Abstract intelligence
  - ii. Social intelligence
  - iii. Mechanical intelligence

Wisdom Tooth

[Man] survives by means of man-made products, and. . . The source of man-made products is man s intelligence. Intelligence is the ability to grasp the facts of reality and to deal with them long-range (i.e., conceptually). On the axiom of the primacy of existence, intelligence is man s most precious attribute. But it has no place in a society ruled by the primacy of consciousness: it is such a society s deadliest enemy.

Today, intelligence is neither recognised nor rewarded, but is being systematically extinguished in a growing flood of brazenly flaunted irrationality.

AYN RAND

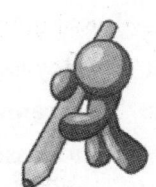

i. Abstract Intelligence

- Abstract intelligence is shown by the manipulation of words, concepts and symbols.

- Abstract intelligence consists of numerical, spatial, and verbal abilities, deductive and inductive reasoning, mental agility and attention span.

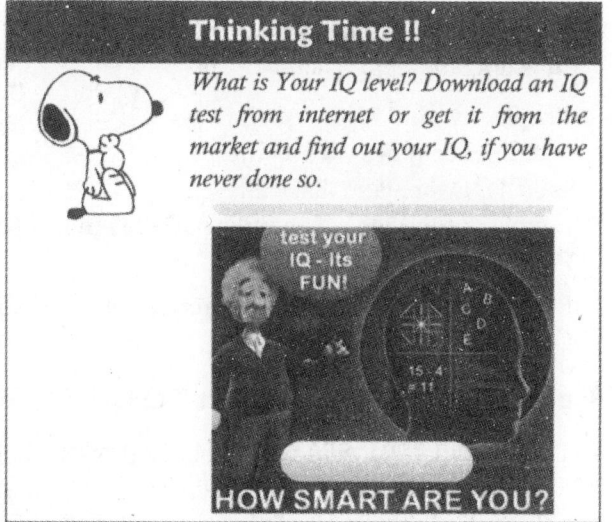

- This is the type of intelligence which is measured by **IQ tests**.

- According to Thorndike, there are four general dimensions of abstract intelligence:

  a. **Altitude:** The complexity or difficulty of tasks one can perform.

  b. **Width:** Variety of tasks of a given difficulty.

  c. **Area:** It is a function of both width & altitude.

  d. **Speed:** The number of tasks one can complete in a given time.

ii. Mechanical Intelligence (Concept object)

- Mechanical Intelligence is the ability to visualise relationships among objects & understand how the physical world works.

- It is shown in the ability to use and understand tools and machines.

- **'Mechanical Aptitude'** is a common term used to refer to this ability.

iii. Social Intelligence (People)

- Social intelligence is the ability to understand, to manage and to act wisely in human relations. It is the ability to function successfully in interpersonal situations.

- Extremes of SI (social intelligence) - very low and very high -in metaphorical terms are, "toxic" or "nourishing" respectively.

- **Toxic behaviours:** Those that cause others to feel devalued, inadequate, intimidated, angry, frustrated, or guilty.

- **Nourishing behaviours:** Those that cause others to feel valued, capable, loved, respected, and appreciated.

- People with **high social intelligence**-those who are socially aware and basically nourishing in their behaviour-are magnetic to others and have a **"Magnetic Personality"**.

- People with **low social intelligence** - those who are primarily toxic to others- are anti magnetic.

Intelligence Factors Used in Tests

For constructing and using psychological tests, the grouping of human abilities into three kinds of intelligence has been very useful. After a long period of study and research on the nature of intelligence, abilities, and personality as they are revealed by tests, psychologists found that mental ability can be expressed in terms of a number of "factors".

i. Mental Ability Factors are mentioned below
- Verbal ability.
- Spatial Visualisation.
- Deductive Reasoning.
- Inductive Reasoning.
- Spatial Orientation.
- Number Ability.
- Memory.
- Perpetual Speed.
- Word Fluency.

ii. Mechanical-Aptitude Factors are believed to be
- Mechanical Information.
- Tapping Speed.
- Eye-hand Coordination.

- Finger Dexterity.
- Space-relation Factors.

iii. Personality Factors

Some of the generally accepted personality factors are
- Reasoning.
- Emotional stability (mature, adaptive).
- Dominance (Dominant).
- Social Boldness (Socially Bold).
- Rule-consciousness (dutiful) etc.

TEST YOUR GREY MATTER

Q1) Define Psychological Tests and Psychological Assessment.

Q2) Discuss the significance of employment tests in the selection of new employees.

Q3) What are the factors which can limit the use of selection tests in selection programs?

Q4) What do you understand by the term 'Intelligence'?

Q5) Briefly define the types of Intelligence which have been identified?

Q6) How has the identification of types of intelligence helped in constructing psychological tests? Enlist the mental factors which help in designing the tests.

F. TYPES OF TESTS

1. Ability Tests/Achievement Tests

- Ability Test helps in determining how well an individual can perform tasks related to the job.
- An excellent example of this is **The Typing Test** given to a prospective employee for a secretarial job.
- Also called as 'Achievement Test', it is concerned with what one has achieved.
- When an applicant claims to know something, an achievement test is taken to measure how well they know it.
- **Trade tests** are the most common type of achievement test. It is also called as **Performance Test**.

- Questions have been prepared & tested for such trades as asbestos worker, punch-press operator, electricians & mechanics.

2. Aptitude Test

- This test helps in determining whether an individual has the capacity or ability to learn a given job if given adequate training.

- The use of aptitude test is advisable when an applicant has had little or no experience along the lines of the job opening.

- Aptitude test indicates the ability or fitness of an individual to engage successfully in any number of specialised activities.

- They cover such areas as - clerical aptitude, numerical aptitude, mechanical aptitude, motor-coordination, finger dexterity and manual dexterity. These tests help to detect positive and negative points in a person's sensory or intellectual ability.

- An example of such a test is the Graduate Management Aptitude Test (GMAT) which many business students take prior to gaining admission to a graduate business school programme.

Forms of Aptitude Test

a. Mental or Intelligence Tests

- They measure the overall intellectual ability of a person and enable him to know whether the person has the mental ability to deal with a certain problem.

- Mental alertness tests are used to measure the speed and accuracy with which an individual understands and reacts to ideas, their symbols and their relationships.

- The mental ability test generally includes-

  i.   Verbal comprehensions.

  ii. Information like word fluency, vocabulary.

  iii. Reasoning (non-verbal reasoning).

  iv. Arithmetic problems

  v.   Spatial visualisation (like cube counting, paper fold etc).

- The scores on the test are usually expressed numerically as intelligent quotient (IQ), where,

$$IQ = \frac{\text{Mental Age}}{\text{Actual Age}} \times 100$$

b. Mechanical Aptitude Tests

- They measure the ability of a person to learn a particular type of mechanical work.

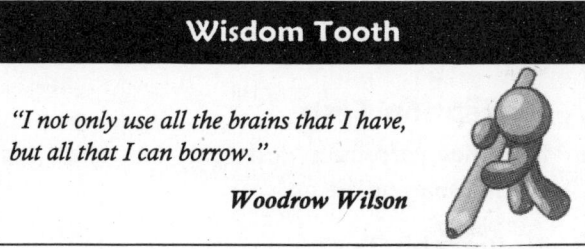

- These tests help to measure specialised technical knowledge & problem solving ability of the candidate.

- **Use:** They are useful in the selection of mechanics, maintenance workers etc.

c. Psychomotor/Skills Test

- They measure a person's ability to do a specific job.
- Such tests are conducted for semi-skilled and repetitive jobs such as packing, testing and inspection etc.

3. Intelligence Test

This test helps to evaluate traits of intelligence, mental ability, presence of mind (alertness), numerical ability, memory & other aspects.

4. Interest Test

- This test is conducted to find out likes and dislikes of candidates towards occupations, hobbies, etc.
- Such a test measures an individual's activity preferences. Such tests also enable the company to provide vocational guidance to the selected candidates & even to existing employees.

5. Personality Test

- It is conducted to judge maturity, social or interpersonal skills, behaviour under stress and strain etc.
- This test is very essential in case of selection of sales force, public relation staff, etc. where personality plays an important role.
- Personality tests are similar to interest tests, as, they also involve a serious problem of obtaining an honest answer.

6. Graphology Test

- It is designed to analyse the hand writing of an individual. It has been said that an individual's hand-writing can suggest the degree of energy, inhibition and spontaneity, as well as disclose the idiosyncrasies and elements of balance and control.

- E.g. Big Letters and emphasis on capital letters indicate a tendency toward domination & competitiveness.

7. Perception Tests

- At times perception tests can be conducted to find out beliefs, attitudes and mental sharpness etc.

8. Polygraph Test

- Polygraph is a lie detector, which is designed to ensure accuracy of the information given in the applications.

9. General Aptitude Test Battery (GATB)

- The General Aptitude Test Battery, also known as the GATB, is a professional career aptitude test which measures **nine** different aptitudes and can be used to help assess the likelihood of success of a person in specific careers or training programmes.
- An aptitude refers to the innate ability of a person to do well at tasks that require a specific type of skill. Aptitude is not dependent on previous learning.

The aptitudes that are measured by the General Aptitude Test Battery are as follows

i. G-General Learning Ability

- The ability to "catch on" or understand instruction and underlying principles, the ability to reason, and make judgments.
- It is closely related to doing well in school.

ii. V-Verbal Aptitude

- The ability to understand the meaning of words and to use them effectively.
- The ability to understand relationships between words & to understand the meaning of whole sentences and paragraphs.

iii. N-Numerical Aptitude

The ability to perform arithmetic operations quickly and accurately.

iv. S-Spatial Aptitude

- The ability to think visually of geometric forms and to comprehend the 2-D representation of 3-D objects.

- The ability to recognise the relationships resulting from the movement of objects in space.

v. P-Form Perception

The ability to perceive pertinent detail in objects or in pictorial or graphic material.

vi. Q-Clerical Perception

- The ability to perceive details in verbal or tabular material.
- Ability to observe difference in copy, to proofread words and numbers, and to avoid perceptual errors in arithmetic computation.

vii. K-Motor co-ordination

- The ability to co-ordinate eyes and hands or fingers rapidly and accurately in making precise movements with speed.
- Ability to make movement response accurately & swiftly.

viii. F-Finger Dexterity

The ability to move fingers, and manipulate small objects with fingers, rapidly or accurately.

ix. M-Manual Dexterity

- The ability to move hands easily & skilfully.
- Ability to work with hands in placing & turning motions.

10. In-Basket Test

- The In-Basket Test is a simulation exercise requiring the performance of a managerial position by dealing with mail and related items which have presumably accumulated in the "In-Basket" of the manager. Each subject is confronted with a standard set of problems in the form of letters, memos, reports, and related materials.
- The exercise provides an excellent training tool for prospective managers, and is widely used for this purpose in industry.
- In addition, several methods of scoring performance on these methods have been worked out, so In-basket is frequently used as a selection aid.
- **Advantage of the In-Basket test:** As a selection aid it has **high face validity.** Since it requires performance of an important aspect of a managerial work, the use of this test as a screening device makes sense to candidates for managerial jobs. It is probably the high face validity of the test that accounts for the fact that there have been few attempts to validate that test as a measure of actual on-the-job managerial performance.

Factors used for Assessing Managerial Behaviour are mentioned below

i. Comprehension ability.

ii. Written communication ability.

iii. Planning and organisation.

iv. Problem analysis.

v. Ability to take risks.

vi. Judgment.

vii. Decisiveness.

viii. Delegation.

ix. Initiative.

11. Career maturity inventory (CMI)

Definition: According to Development Theory of Vocational Behaviour:

Career maturity has been defined as the maturity of attitudes and competencies pertaining to career decision making.

- It has been found to be influenced differentially in different cultures, races & gender groups by certain psychological, educational & demographic factors.

- **Crites** developed a model, according to which Career Maturity Inventory (CMI) consists of six independent dimensions. One dimension is related to the attitude variable and rest of the five dimensions denote competencies pertaining to Career Decision Making:

1. The attitude variable includes

(a) Decisiveness

(b) Involvement

(c) Independence

(d) Orientation and

(e) Compromise in career decision making

2. Competencies are

(a) Self appraisal (SA) or knowing yourself.

(b) Occupational information (OI) or knowing about jobs.

(c) Goal selection (GS) or choosing a job.

(d) Planning (PL) or looking ahead.

(e) Problem solving (PS) or what should they do?

12. Thematic Apperception Test (TAT)

- The Thematic Apperception Test (TAT) is a projective measure intended to evaluate a person's pattern of thought, attitudes, observational capacity, and emotional responses to ambiguous test materials.

- In the case of TAT, the ambiguous materials consist of a set of cards that portray human figures in a variety of setting & situations. The subject is asked to tell the examiner a story about each card that includes the following elements: the event shown in the picture, what has led up to it, what the characters in the picture are feeling and thinking, and the outcome of the event.

- **Purpose : Individual Assessments**

  The TAT is often

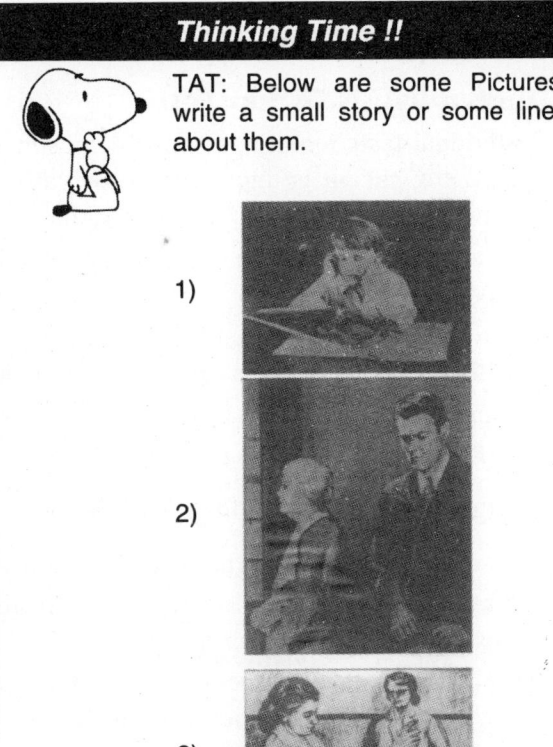

Thinking Time !!

TAT: Below are some Pictures, write a small story or some lines about them.

1)

2)

3)

administered to individuals as part of a battery, or group, of tests intended to **Evaluate Personality**. It is considered to be effective in eliciting information about a person's view of the world & his or her attitudes toward the self and others.

- **Application:** The TAT is often used in individual assessments of candidates for employment in fields requiring a high degree of skill in dealing with other people and/or ability to cope with high levels of psychological stress, such as law enforcement, military leadership position, religious ministry etc. TAT is sometimes also used for forensic purposes in evaluating the motivations and general attitudes of persons accused of violent crimes.

For e.g. TAT was recently administered to a 24yr-old man in prison for a series of murders. The results indicated that his attitudes towards other people are not only outside normal limits but are similar to those of other persons found guilty of the same type of crime.

G. OTHER CLASSIFICATIONS OF TEST

1. Individual Vs Group Test

i. **Individual tests** require one-on-one consultation with the applicants. During the test, the applicant is under keen observation of the examiner who observes his behaviour carefully throughout the testing period and then awards the scores.

The tests involve variable verbal and non-verbal sub tests which can be combined to give on overall IQ.

ii. **Group tests**, on the other hand, are usually used is mass testing situation. In this test, there is no need of observing their behaviour.

Group tests are more objective, because their administration, scoring & interpretation is done in a routine manner.

2. Language Vs Non-Language tests

This test is also known as **Verbal and Non-Verbal** test.

i. **Verbal test** is used to identify the ability to understand, analyse and interpret written information of an applicant.

This test includes a number of short passages of text followed by statements based on the information given in the passage.

ii. **Non-verbal tests** involve the ability to understand and analyse visual information & solve problems using visual reasoning.

- Most of such tests have items in the form of pictures, designs, figures or some other symbols.
- This test can be used for deaf, illiterate and foreign language speaking people.
- It enables people to analyse and solve complex problems without relying upon or being limited by language skills.

3. Performance Tests Vs Paper Pencil tests

i. **Paper & Pencil Test :** The testee simply receives a test paper or printed booklet containing the test questions, and he records his responses in some written manner on the answer sheet that is usually provided.

ii. **Performance Test :** They involve some sort of manipulation activity such as handling pegs or blocks, or assembling mechanical objects.

4. Speed & Power Tests

i. **Speed Test** is based primarily upon the speed with which one works.

These tests are constructed so that every item is very easy, the task is to complete as many items as possible in a short time.

ii. **Power Test** is a test where the items are difficult and the person is given as much time as necessary to complete the items.

In such tests a person's score is based exclusively upon his ability to answer the questions correctly, no matter how long (within reason, of course) it takes.

5. Achievement and Aptitude Test

i. **Achievement Test** is supposedly a measure of a person's potential in a given area.

ii. **Aptitude Test** is a measure of a person's current skill or ability at the moment of testing.

Since the same test can often be considered both an achievement test & an aptitude test depending upon use, this classification system is often a fuzzy one. Thus, with many tests one can

a. Measure the amount of present skill, and

b. Use the present score to predict future performance

H. ESSENTIALS OF GOOD PSYCHOLOGICAL TESTS

H.1. Reliability of Tests

- **Definition:** Reliability refers to the consistency of a measure. A test is considered reliable if we get the same result repeatedly. Thus, it refers to standardisation of the procedure of administering and scoring the test results.

- An individual's intelligence, for example, is generally a stable characteristic so if we administer an intelligence test, a person who scores 110 in March would score 110 if tested in April. Tests which produce wide variation in results, do not serve good purpose in selection.

Reliability can be improved by

i. Getting repeated measurements using same test.

ii. Getting many different measurements using slightly different techniques & methods.

Types of Reliability

There are several types of reliability. Few of them are mentioned below:

i. Test-Retest Reliability

- The test-retest method of estimating a test's reliability involved administering the test to the same group of people at least twice.
- Then the first set of scores is correlated with the second set of scores.
- Correlation ranges between 0 (low reliability) and 1 (high reliability).

ii. Inter-Rater Reliability

- This type of reliability is assessed by having two or more independent judges score the test. The scores are then compared to determine the consistency of the rater estimates.

iii. Parallel-forms Reliability

- Parallel-forms reliability is gauged by comparing two different tests that were created using the same content.
- This is accomplished by creating a large pool of test items that measure the same **Quality** and randomly divide the items into two separate tests.
- The two tests should then be administered to the same subject at the same time.

iv. Internal-Consistency Reliability

- This form of reliability is used to judge the consistency of results across items on the same test. Essentially, test items that measure the same construct are compared to determine the test's internal consistency.

H.2. Validity of Tests

- Validity asks "Is the test measuring what you think it's measuring?"
- It is a test, which helps predict whether a person will be successful in a given job. A test that has been validated can be helpful in differentiating between prospective employees who will be able to perform job well & those who will not.
- Though no test will be 100% accurate in predicting job success, a validated test increases possibility of success.
- Validity of a test is expressed in terms of a **Co-Efficient of Correlation** in which the test score is correlated with some performance criterion.

  For e.g.: the validity of an intelligence test can be determined by correlating the test score with the student's marks in the examinations.

Classifications of Validity

a. Logical Validity

- The term validity in logic is largely synonymous with logical truth; however the term is used in different contexts.

- Validity is a property of formulas, statements and arguments.
- A **logical valid argument** is one where the conclusions follow from the premises. An invalid argument is where the conclusion does not follow from the premises.
- A test consists of many items to measure capacities like intelligence and aptitude.

b. Empirical Validity

- Empirical validity (also called statistical or predictive validity) describes how closely scores on a test correspond (correlate) with behaviour as measured in other contexts.
- E.g. A student's scores on a test of academic aptitude, for example, may be compared with his school grades (a commonly used criterion).
- In empirical validity, therefore, the subject's performance in certain test situation is correlated with certain criteria.
- For instance, intelligence tests scores and scholastic achievements are co-related.
- **Limitation:** One limitation of empirical validity is that unless the choice of external criterion has been widely tested, one cannot conclude whether the test is valid or not. Various other psychological variables and internal conditions of the subject may influence the performance.

c. Factorial Validity

- **Factorial validity** is a form of construct validity that is established through factor analyses.
- **Factor analyses:** A set of mathematical procedures for analysing the interrelationship among a set of variables.
- **Factor:** A hypothetical variable that influences scores on one or more observed variables; Factor = An Unobservable or Latent Variable.

Types of Validity

Validity may be of the following types:-

1. Preductive validity, ⎫
2. Concurrent validity ⎭ criterion-related validity
3. Synthetic validity
4. Content validity
5. Construct validity
6. Face validity

1. Predictive Validity

- It is the most important type of validity for personnel selection. This measures the extent to which a future level of a variable can be predicted from a current measurement.
- It involves using a selection test during the selection process and then identifying the successful candidates.
- The characteristics of both successful & less successful candidates are then identified.

2. Concurrent Validity

- This involves determining the factors that are characteristics of successful employees and then using these factors as the yardsticks.
- According to Burn and Naylor (1968), high concurrent validity of a test does not result in high predictive validity.

3. Synthetic Validity

- **Definition:** Synthetic validity is "the inferring of validity in a specific situation from a logical analysis of jobs into their elements, and a combination of those elemental validities into whole".
- It involves taking parts of several similar jobs rather than one complete job to validate the selection test.
- A basic assumption of synthetic validation is that different jobs involving the same kinds of behaviour should also require the same knowledge, skills, abilities, and other characteristics.
- Synthetic validity subsequently assumes that if a test is valid for a particular job element, then it will be valid for use with any job involving that same element.

4. Content Validity

- A test has content validity if it measures knowledge of the content domain of which it was designed to measure knowledge.
- Another way of saying this is that content validity concerns, primarily, the adequacy with which the test items adequately and representatively sample the content area to be measured.
- For e.g., a comprehensive math achievement test would lack content validity if good scores depended primarily on the knowledge of English, or if it only had questions about one aspect of math (e.g. algebra).

5. Construct Validity

- A test has construct validity if it demonstrates an association between the test scores and prediction of theoretical traits.
- Intelligence tests are one example of measurement instruments that should have construct validity.

6. Face Validity

- Face validity occurs where something appears to be valid.
- This depends mostly on the judgment of the observer.
- In any case, it is never sufficient and requires more solid validity to enable acceptable conclusions to be drawn.
- Unlike content validity, face validity does not depend on established theories for support.

Relationship between Reliability and Validity

If a test is unreliable, it cannot be valid.

For a test to be valid, it must reliable.

However, just because a test is reliable does not mean it will be valid.

Reliability is a necessary but not sufficient condition for validity!

I. DESIGNING OF TESTS

Tests for employment purpose are designed by the personnel department with the help of other department heads, foremen, superintendents and psychologists. Steps involved in good tests are:

1. Job Analysis

- The basic requirement to design a test for a job is to know the job first.
- What does the worker do and what are the working conditions? What are the mental requirements of the job? What are the physical and social demands of the job?
- Answers to these lead to the preparation of job description and job specification which are essential to develop any type of tests.

2. Test Procedure

- Depending upon the job analysis done, a test may be selected either from the battery of existing tests or a test may be devised for checking qualities required for the job.

3. Preliminary Trials and Refinement

- A new test should be tried out and then revisions and refinements may be made accordingly.
- Trials can be done on officers and personnel groups similar to those sought to be tested.
- These trials are used to select items that are not up to the mark and are either too difficult or too easy or items that fail to discriminate between people of different capabilities.

4. Validation of Test Procedure

- Empirical validity should be established during trials of the test.
- Experimental evidence is called for to show that test is discriminating between those who are not successful in a particular job.

5. Combination of Tests into a Battery

- Testing all the required traits by a single test is always not possible so different types of testing techniques are required to assess them.
- When different tests are combined, the validity of these tests and correlation between them should be always considered.

6. Application of Tests

- To maintain the objectivity of tests and to get correct results it should be applied by experts and persons who understand them.

7. Standardisation of Tests

- The tests must be standardized before they are applied to measure an individual's traits or qualities.
- While standardising the tests, the psychologist must see that these fulfil the statistical requirements of validity, reliability and objectivity.

TEST YOUR GREY MATTER

Q1)   Briefly define the types of tests used for employment in organisations.

Q2)   What is General Aptitude Test Battery (GATB)? Mention the aptitudes that are measured by the General Aptitude Test Battery?

Q3)   Define:
   i.   In-Basket Test
   ii.   Career Maturity Inventory (CMI)
   iii.   Thematic Apperception Test (TAT)

Q4) What is the difference between reliability and validity of test?

Q5) What is meant by reliability of psychological tests?

Q6) What is test validity? Explain.

Q7) What are the types of test validity?

Q8) How will you design a test? Mention the points which you will consider while designing a test.

J. MEANING & PURPOSE OF EMPLOYMENT INTERVIEW

Definition: Interview is a formal, in-depth conversation, conducted to evaluate the applicant's acceptability. It is a face to face exchange of views, ideas & opinions between the candidate and interviewer.

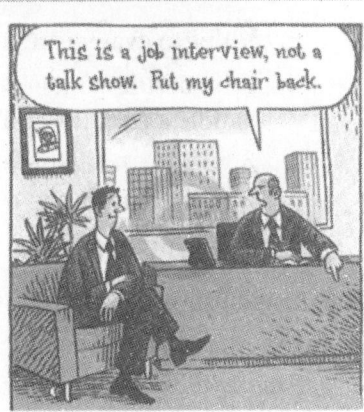

This is a job interview, not a talk show. Put my chair back.

- Basically, an interview is nothing but an oral examination of candidates. Interview can be adapted to unskilled, skilled, managerial & professional employees.

- It is considered to be an excellent selection device.

J.1. Objectives of Interview

i. It helps to obtain additional information from the applicants concerning his attitude about his job, the company, etc. These interviews are referred to as **Attitude Interviews**.

ii. Facilitates giving general information to the applicants such as company policies, job, product manufactured and the like.

iii. To find the suitability of the candidate.

iv. It helps to build the company's image in the eye of the applicants.

> **Wisdom Tooth**
>
> *"I had a job interview at an insurance company once and the lady said "Where do you see yourself in five years?" and I said "Celebrating the fifth year anniversary of you asking me this question".*
>
> ***Mitch Hedberg***

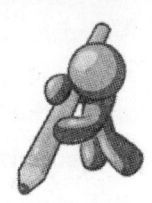

J.2. Significance/Importance of Interview

Interviews are one of the most important hiring tools available to employers, used extensively to judge how appropriate a prospective candidate would fill a role with an organisation.

a. Importance from the Employee point of view

i. The interview provides an opportunity to meet several candidates and screen them to find the ones most suitable for the organisation.

ii. Helps to evaluate a person's skills, capabilities & personality traits.

iii. Provides tremendous insight into the candidate's confidence level & ability to handle a pressure situation.

iv. A chance to communicate the company's policies, beliefs, work culture & expectations to the prospective employee.

v. Finally, narrow down, select & hire the best talent to fill the job vacancy.

b. Importance from the job seeker's point of view

i. The interview presents an ideal situation to make the first impression on the Employer. (And you know, first impression is the last impression!!)

ii. Chance to convince the employer/interviewer that he/she is the best suited candidate for the job.

iii. Time to understand the work culture of the company, its policies & the people.

J.3. Limitations of an Interview

i. Reliability:

No two interviewers offer similar scoring after interviewing an applicant.

ii. Validity:

There is lack of validity because few departments use standardised questions upon which validation studies can be conducted.

iii. Objectivity:

Biases of interviewers may cloud the objectivity of interviews.

iv. Information Gathering:

Interviewers could not extract complete/maximum information from the applicant.

J.4. Types of Interviews

Interviews can be of different types, following are the various types of interview:-

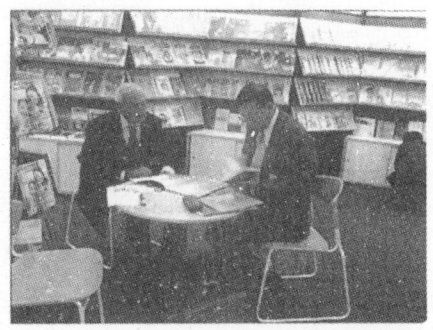

i. Informal Interview

- An informal interview is an oral interview & may take place anywhere. The manager or the personnel manager may ask a few almost inconsequential questions like name, place of birth, name of relatives etc. either in the respective offices or any where outside the company. It is not planned & nobody prepares for it.

ii. Formal Interview

- Formal interviews may be held in the employment office in a more formal atmosphere with the help of well-structured questions, the time & place of the interview will be stipulated by the employment office.

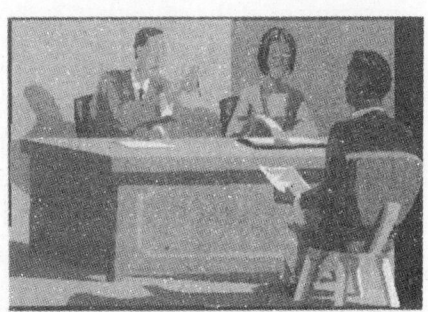

iii. Non-directive Interview

- Non-directive interview is designed to let the interviewee speak his mind freely. The interviewer has no formal or directive questions, but his all attention is on the candidate. He encourages the candidate to talk, whenever he is silent.

- E.g. "Mr. Anuj Veer, please tell us about yourself after you graduated from high school".

- The idea is to give the candidate complete freedom to "sell" himself, without the encumbrances of the interviewer's questions.

- The interviewer must be of higher calibre & must guide & relate the information given by the applicant to the objective of the interview.

iv. In-Depth Interview

It is designed to intensely examine the candidate's background & thinking and to go into considerable detail on particular subjects of an important nature & of special interest to the candidate.

v. Stress interview

- It is designed to test the candidate & his conduct and behaviour by keeping him under conditions of stress & strain.

- The interviewer may start with "Mr. Arun, we do not think your qualifications & experiences are adequate for this position", and watch the reaction of the candidate. A good candidate will not yield, on the contrary he may substantiate why he is qualified to handle the job.

vi. Group Interview

- It is designed to save a busy executive's time and to see how candidates may be brought together in the employment office where they may be interviewed.

vii. Panel Interview

- A panel or interviewing board or selection committee may interview the candidate, usually in the case of supervisory and managerial positions.
- This interview pools the collective judgment & wisdom of the panel in the assessment of the candidate & also in questioning the faculties of the candidate.

viii. Sequential Interview

- The sequential interview takes the interviewee one step further and involves a series of interviews, usually utilising the strength and knowledge base of the interviewer, so that each interviewer can ask questions in relation to his/her subject area to each candidate, as the candidate moves from room to room.

ix. Structured interview

- In a structured interview, the interviewer uses preset standardised questions, which are put to all the candidates.
- This interview is also called as "Guided' or "Patterned' interview.
- It is useful for valid results, especially when dealing with a large number of applicants.

x. Unstructured Interview

- It is also known as **'Unpatterned'** interview, the interview is largely unplanned and the candidate does most of the talking.
- Unguided interview is advantageous in as much as it leads to a friendly conversation between the interviewer and the candidate and in the process, the latter reveals more of his or her desires and problems.
- The unplanned interview lacks uniformity. This approach may overlook key areas of the applicant's skill or background.

xi. Telephone Interview

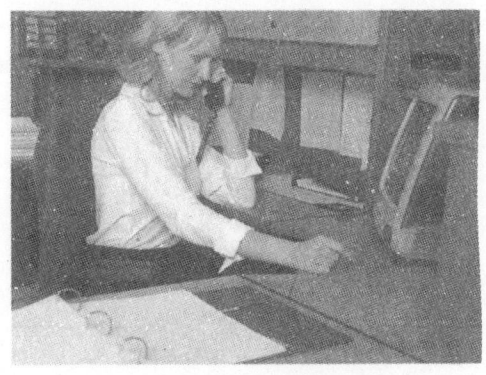

- Employers use telephone interviews as a way of identifying and recruiting candidates for employment.
- Phone interviews are often used to screen candidates in order to narrow the pool of applicants who will be invited for in-person interviews.
- They are also used as way to minimise the expenses involved in interviewing out-of-town candidates.

xii. Written Interview

- Written Interview involves the applicant answering a series of written questions & then sending the answers back through regular mail or e-mail.

J.5. Guidelines for Effective Interview

- In order to make the interview successful, certain established principles are followed in matching the qualification to job requirements. With the help of effective interviewing, more qualities of an applicant can be revealed which could not be obtained during psychological tests and other selection processes.
- Following measures may contribute to making an interview more effective:
  i. Prepare carefully for the interview (no interruption during the interview is to be planned, adequate time is scheduled, job description is studied, person to conduct the interview is decided, format of interview is decided etc.)
  ii. Ask the applicant only job-related questions and these interview questions should be prepared in advance.
  iii. Ask the same questions to each applicant so that each interviewed applicant receives equal treatment.
  iv. Interviewers must be frank and straight forward instead of being shrewd.
  v. Ask questions that require the applicant to describe his/her knowledge experience, and training as related to the job opening (avoid questions that produce "Yes" or "No" answers).
  vi. Document the applicant's answer during or immediately after the interview.
  vii. Check for inconsistencies in interview answers and application information.
  viii. Allow time during the interview for applicants to ask questions about the job, the work unit, etc.
  ix. The feelings of the applicants should not be hurt.
  x. Evaluate the applicant immediately after (not during) an interview & evaluate based on objective, job-related reasons.

J.6. Steps in the Interview Process

- Organising a successful interview requires considerable planning which involves the following main steps

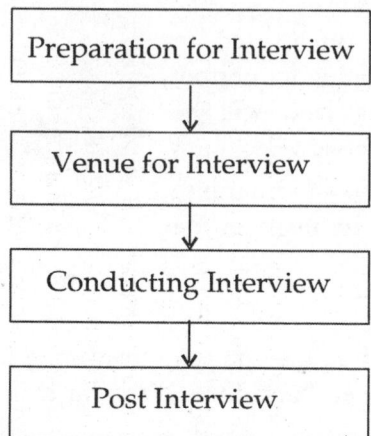

```
┌─────────────────────────────┐
│   Preparation for Interview │
└─────────────────────────────┘
              │
              ▼
┌─────────────────────────────┐
│      Venue for Interview    │
└─────────────────────────────┘
              │
              ▼
┌─────────────────────────────┐
│     Conducting Interview    │
└─────────────────────────────┘
              │
              ▼
┌─────────────────────────────┐
│        Post Interview       │
└─────────────────────────────┘
```

a. Preparation for Interview

- Pre-interview preparation should be such that interview is conducted properly. To achieve this task, the areas mentioned below should be focused on before starting the interview.

i. What the job requires

- Define the job & what qualifications are required.
- Prepare to discuss the job briefly, in terms that the candidate can readily understand.

ii. Outline the interview process

- Include the basic elements in conducting the interview session. This will provide the frame work for interviewing all the candidates on a consistent basis & ensure that all important areas have been covered.
- It will also make it easier for you to observe & assess each candidate & keep the discussion to the point.

iii. Record & summarise observations about the candidates

- Develop a form or standardised format to use in the interview, see the evaluation work sheet.

Evaluation Worksheet

The following are suggested areas to consider in your interview. Keep in mind that questions and decisions must be based on job-related factors. This evaluation worksheet will become a part of the reviewable records file.

Candidate's Name	
Item # Being Filled	Division
Salary Grade	Supervisor
Section	Title

Skills	Very Good	Good	Fair	Poor	Comments

Factors	Very Good	Good	Fair	Poor	Comments
Rapport or confidence established during the interview					
Replies to questions completely and accurately					
Appearance					
Work experience					
Ability to make sound judgments					
Sense of responsibility shown					
Ability to deal with people					
Adaptable and flexible to interruptions/changes in work routine					
Adaptable to highly predetermined and repetitive activities					

Interested in hiring _____   Possible interest in hiring _____

No interest in hiring _____   Candidate has no interest _____

Reasons:_____

_____

iv. Schedule Interview

- Enough time should be scheduled with each candidate to allow for a relaxed, unhurried interview.
- Do not schedule too many interviews for one day.
- Develop a schedule that does not adversely affect your other office responsibilities.

v. Notify the candidate

Typically, the office of human resources telephones the candidate or sends an interview letter to invite him/her to an interview.

vi. Review the candidates Application, Resume or other related material:

Each interviewer should know specific details about the candidates so that questions are directed to that. Hence, a brief resume of all candidates to be interviewed should be prepared.

b. Venue for Interview

Consider the location or venue of the interview such that it is easily accessible to candidates with disabilities & must be at a reasonable distance from the room in which candidates remain seated during their waiting period. The interview venue must be free from noise, phone call interruption & other disturbance.

c. Conducting Interview

This is the most crucial phase of the interview process. Conducting an interview is a six step approach that can be modified to fit your own particular needs & circumstances:-

i. Introduction

- Introduce yourself & greet the candidate with a hand shake and a friendly smile.

ii. Review the Application

- Go over the information supplied on the application and/or resume & ask the candidate to elaborate on his/her previous job responsibilities or special projects.
- The nature, direction and enthusiasm of the candidate's response can provide you with valuable insight into the candidate's communication skills.
- These responses may also give you an indication about what the candidate finds interesting or challenging.

iii. Describe the Job

- Provide a written job description to the candidate, and summarise or review the major job responsibilities.
- The key consideration is that all candidates are left with basically the same impression of what the job is & requires.

iv. Candidate Self Assessment

- Encourage the candidate to assess himself/herself against the job in order to obtain as much information as possible regarding the candidate in relation to job.
- Encourage responses with open ended questions such as "How do you see yourself in relation to the job?" or "What contributions do you think you can make to the work or the company?"

v. Candidate Classification

- Ask the candidate if he/she has any questions about the job requirements, working conditions, prospective co-workers or other considerations.
- Let the candidate know that you & the personnel office will be available to answer any questions that might arise after the interview.

vi. Closing of Interview

- Finally, close the interview by explaining what happens next in the hiring process and thank the candidate for his/her time.

d. Post Interview Final Evaluation

The post-interview process should consist, at a minimum, of the five following elements:

1. Record Your Observations

Immediately after each interview, take time to summarise the observations made during the course of the interview.

2. Narrow the Field

After you have interviewed all the scheduled candidates and before you make your final hiring decision, narrow the field to those you would consider hiring for the position.

3. Check References

Begin with your first choice and check the references the candidate provided. References from former employers may be helpful in finding out about the candidate's work habits and personal characteristics. Inform the candidate beforehand that you will be checking references.

4. Make the Hiring Decision

Review all the information you have obtained on the candidates. Consider the following factors to arrive at your final decision:

- Ability to do the work.
- Interest in doing the job.
- Potential for growth.
- Ability to adjust to the job environment.

After careful thought, make the decision to hire or not to hire. A valid selection occurs when the "merit and fitness" of the candidate are the primary determining factors in the decision. Inform the Personnel Officer of your choice.

5. Notify Selected Candidate

Follow your organisation procedures with respect to notifying selected candidates. Typically, the Personnel Office notifies the selected candidate by telephone to ensure that he or she is willing and able to accept appointment, and follows up with a written confirmation.

If a candidate declines the job offer, the Personnel Officer or the interviewer should secure a written declination from a candidate who refuses an offer of employment. See the next section for guidance in preparing this document.

6. Notify Unselected Candidates

Good personnel practice is that the Personnel Office informs candidates who are not selected, about your decision and thanks them for their interest. When possible, each candidate should be sent a personal letter. When large numbers are involved, a formal letter may be sent.

After all candidates have been notified, the interview process is concluded.

J.7. Qualities of a Good Interviewer

Right skill to conduct an effective job interview is an important aspect to hire the right person in a company.

i. Communication Skill

Interviewees will be more likely to open up to someone who shares their job vocabulary and can discuss job content intelligently.

ii. Knowledge of Jobs in the Industry

The interviewer must be acquainted with industry jobs in order to compare & contrast the available job position in the firm & in the industry as a whole.

iii. Judgment & Analytical Skill

The interviewer must not only be able to comprehend what the employee is saying, but also be able to probe for additional facts.

iv. Objectivity

There is no room in job analysis interviewing for preconceived ideas, personal biases, or extreme opinions.

v. Understanding of Human Behaviour

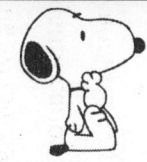

Thinking Time !!

Take a mock interview of your friend on any chosen topic, be it for a college entrance or selection in any sports team or for an Army s SSB and find out how good are you at taking interviews?

The success of the interview depends heavily on the interviewer's ability to motivate the potential employee to respond & encourage co-operation while minimising suspicion, hostility & embarrassment.

vi. Personality

Favourable personality traits for an interviewer include sincerity, integrity & the ability to get along with all types of people.

TEST YOUR GREY MATTER

Q 1) Describe the nature of Employment Interview. What purpose does it serve and what are its limitations?

Q 2) Discuss the utility of an employment interview. Enumerate various kinds of interviews.

Q 3) Differentiate between structured and unstructured interview.

Q 4) Design an interview procedure for filling a design engineer post in a manufacturing enterprise?

Q 4) What are the various steps involved in an interview process?

Q 6) What are the various skills and personality traits required to be a good interviewer?

Answers to questions given in the insight

1. All of them. Every month has at least 28 days.

2. 1 hour. If you take a pill at 1 o'clock, then another at 1.30 and the last at 2'clock, they will be taken in 1 hour.

3. 1 hour. It is a wind up alarm clock which cannot discriminate between a.m. and p.m.

4. 70. Dividing by half is the same as multiplying by 2.
5. 9 live sheep.
6. The match.
7. White.
8. 2 apples.
9. None. It was Noah, not Moses.
10. You are the driver.

17 Performance Appraisal

A. THE INSIGHT

The reason for you being here and reading this chapter is directly or indirectly a result of performance appraisal. Throughout our life we are appraised by someone or the other.......Be it our parents at home, teachers at college or boss in office. Our performance in our lower standards was appraised by the teachers which got us some marks and it was decided that we will be studying science and so we appeared for various entrance examinations. Somebody again evaluated our performance there......in some, we got good marks and in some we didn't......And the result is that we got into the college and are now studying Performance Appraisal.

B. HISTORY

- Roots of performance appraisal lie in the early 20th century and can be traced to Taylor's pioneering time and motion studies.

- But as a distinct and formal management studies used in the evaluation of work performance, appraisal really dates back to the time of the 2nd World War.

- Performance appraisal has been increasingly implemented by most modern organisation as a tool for employee assessment.

C. DEFINITION AND CONCEPT

1. **Performance** is an employee's accomplishment of assigned work measured against standards of the employee's position.

2. **Performance Appraisal** is the process of obtaining, analysing and recording information about the relative worth of an employee.

- Performance appraisal may be understood as the assessment of an individual's performance in a systematic way, the performance being measured against such factors as job knowledge, quality & quantity output, initiative, leadership abilities, supervision, co-operation, judgment etc.

- The focus of the performance appraisal is measuring and improving the actual performance of the employee and also the future potential of the employee. Its aim is to measure what an employee does.

- **According to Flippo**

  "Performance Appraisal is the systematic, periodic and an impartial rating of an employee's excellence in matters pertaining to his present job and his potential for a better job".

- It is a powerful tool to calibrate, refine and reward the performance of the Employee. It helps to analyze his achievements and evaluate his contribution towards the achievements of the overall organisation goals.

3. **Performance Management** refers to the integrated process by which organisation involves it employees in improving organisational effectiveness in the accomplishment of organisation mission & strategic goals. Performance Management consists of:

- Performance Planning.
- Monitoring Employee Performance.
- Employee Development.
- Evaluating Performance.
- Recognition.

D. PERFORMANCE APPRAISAL

Difference between Job Evaluation & Performance Appraisal

	Job Evaluation		Performance appraisal
(i)	Job Rated keeping in mind responsibility, qualification, experience, working conditions etc	(i)	Employee rated on the basis of performance.
(ii)	A job rated before employee is appointed.	(ii)	Employee rated after the employee has been hired and placed.
(iii)	Purpose is to establish wage differentials.	(iii)	Purpose is to decide promotion, rewards, punishment etc.
(iv)	It is not compulsory.	(iv)	Compulsory. It is done regularly for all employees.
(v)	Job Evaluation committee is consulted for the purpose of Evaluation.	(v)	Appraisal is done by the Employers themselves.

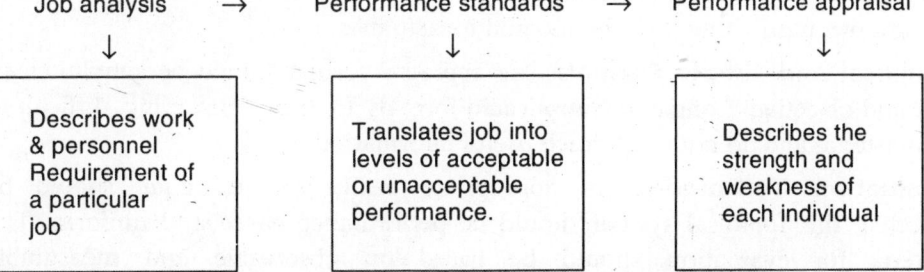

Job analysis → Performance standards → Performance appraisal

↓ ↓ ↓

Describes work & personnel Requirement of a particular job

Translates job into levels of acceptable or unacceptable performance.

Describes the strength and weakness of each individual

D.1. Characteristics of Performance Appraisal

- It is a step by step process.
- It is a Scientific & Objective study.
- It examines the employee's strengths & weaknesses.

- It is an ongoing & continuous process.
- It is a secure process for making correct decision on employees.

D.2. Objectives/Importance of Performance Appraisal

i. To review the performance of the employees over a given period of time.

ii. To judge the gap between the actual & desired performance.

iii. To help the management in exercising organisational control.

iv. Helps to strengthen the relationship & communication between superior-subordinates & management-employee.

v. To diagnose the strength & weakness of the individuals so as to identify the training & development needs of the future.

vi. To provide feedback to the employees regarding their past performance.

vii. Provide information to assist in the other personnel decisions in the organisation.

viii. Provide clarity on the expectations & responsibilities of the functions to be performed by the employees.

ix. To judge the effectiveness of other human resource functions of the organisation such as recruitment, selection, training & development.

x. To reduce the grievances of the employees.

D.3. Pre-Requisites for Effective & Successful Performance Appraisal

The essentials of an effective performance system are as follows:

i. **Documentation:** Means continuous noting and documenting the performance. It also helps the evaluators to give a proof and the basis of their ratings.

ii. **Standards/Goals:** The standards set should be clear, easy to understand, achievable, motivating, time bound and measurable.

iii. **Practical and Simple Format:** The appraisal format should be simple, clear, fair and objective. Long and complicated formats are time consuming, difficult to understand, and do not elicit much useful information.

iv. **Evaluation Technique:** An appropriate evaluation technique should be selected; the appraisal system should be performance based and uniform. The criteria for evaluation should be based on observable and measurable characteristics of the behaviour of the employee.

v. **Communication:** Communication is an indispensable part of the performance appraisal process. The desired behaviour or the expected results should be communicated to the employees as well as the evaluators. Communication also plays an important role in the review or feedback meeting. Open communication system motivates the employees to actively participate in the appraisal process.

vi. Feedback: The purpose of the feedback should be developmental rather than judgmental. To maintain its utility, timely feedback should be provided to the employees and the manner of giving feedback should be such that it should have a motivating effect on the employees' future performance.

vii. Personal bias: Interpersonal relationships can influence the evaluation and the decisions in the performance appraisal process. Therefore, the evaluators should be trained to carry out the processes of appraisals without personal bias.

D.4. Challenges of Performance Appraisal

The main **challenges** involved in the performance appraisal process are:

i. Determining the Evaluation Criteria

- Identification of the appraisal criteria is one of the biggest problems faced by the top management. The performance data to be considered for evaluation should be carefully selected.

- For the purpose of evaluation, the criteria selected should be **quantifiable or measurable.**

ii. Create a Rating Instrument

The purpose of the performance appraisal process is to judge the performance of the employees rather than the employee. The focus of the system should be on the development of the employees of the organisation and not on penalising them.

iii. Lack of Competence

Top management should choose the raters or the evaluators carefully. They should have the required expertise and the knowledge to decide the criteria accurately. They should have the experience and the necessary training to carry out the appraisal process objectively.

iv. Errors in Rating and Evaluation

- Many errors based on personal bias like stereotyping, **halo effect** (i.e. one trait of the employee which influences the evaluator's rating and he does not consider all other traits) etc. may creep into the appraisal process.

- Therefore the rater should exercise objectivity and fairness in evaluating and rating the **performance of the employees.**

v. Resistance

- The appraisal process may face resistance from the employees and the trade unions for the fear of negative ratings. Therefore, the employees should be communicated and clearly explained the purpose as well as the **process of appraisal**.

- The standards should be clearly communicated and every employee should be made aware that what exactly is expected from him/her.

D.5. Approaches to Performance Appraisal

a. Traditional Approach/Overall Approach

- Traditionally, performance appraisal has been used as just a method for determining and justifying the salaries of the employees. Then it was used as a tool for determining rewards (a rise in the pay) and punishments (a cut in the pay) for the past performance of the employees.

- This approach was a **Past Oriented** approach which focused only on the past performance of the employees i.e. during a past specified period of time.

- This approach did not consider the developmental aspects of the employee performance i.e. his **training and development** needs or career developmental possibilities.

- The primary concern of the traditional approach is to judge the performance of the organisation as a whole by the past performances of its employees. Therefore, this approach is also called as the **overall approach.**

b. Modern Approach

- In 1950s, the performance appraisal was recognised as a complete system in itself and the Modern Approach to performance appraisal was developed.

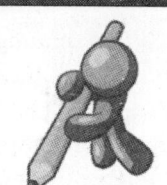

> **Wisdom Tooth**
>
> *Many opinions are better than one, especially when a company decides whom to promote and how to develop his management potential.*
>
> **William C. Bhyham**

- The modern approach to performance development has made the performance appraisal process more formal and structured.

- In this, performance appraisal is taken as a tool to identify better performing employees from others, employee's training needs, career development paths, rewards and bonuses and their promotions to the next levels.

- The modern approach to Performance appraisal is a future oriented approach and is developmental in nature. This recognizes employees as individuals and focuses on their development.

- Appraisals have become a continuous and periodic activity in the organisations. The results of performance appraisals are used to take various other HR decisions like promotions, demotions, transfers, training and development, reward outcomes.

- The modern approach to performance appraisals includes **a feedback process** that helps to strengthen the relationships between superiors and subordinates and improves communication throughout the organisation.

D.6. Process of Performance Appraisal

Following figure outlines the performance appraisal process. Each step in the process is crucial and is arranged logically.

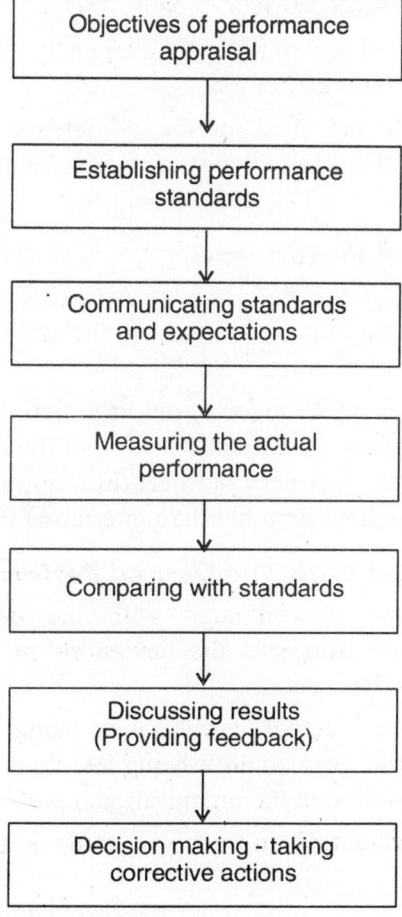

1. Objectives of Performance Appraisal

- The first basic step is to define the objectives of the appraisal.

- Objective of appraisal includes effecting promotions and transfers, assessing training needs, awarding pay hike, and the like.

2. Establishing Performance Standards

- The next step in the process of performance appraisal is the setting up of standards which will be used as the base to compare the actual performance of the employees.
- This step requires setting the criteria to judge the performance of the employees as successful or unsuccessful and the degrees of their contribution to the organisational goals and objectives.
- The standards set should be clear, easily understandable and in measurable terms.

3. Communicating the Standards

- Once set, it is the responsibility of the management to communicate the standards to all the employees of the organisation.
- The employees should be informed and the standards should be clearly explained to them. This will help them to understand their roles and to know what exactly is expected from them.

4. Measuring the Actual Performance

- The most difficult part of the Performance Appraisal process is measuring the actual performance of the employees, that is, the work done by the employees during the specified period of time.
- It is a continuous process which involves monitoring the performance throughout the year. This stage requires the careful selection of the appropriate techniques of measurement, taking care that personal bias does not affect the outcome of the process and providing assistance rather than interfering in an employees' work.

5. Comparing the Actual With The Desired Performance

- The actual performance is compared with the desired or the standard performance. The comparison tells the deviations in the performance of the employees from the standards set.
- The result can show the actual performance being more than the desired performance or, the actual performance being less than the desired performance depicting a negative deviation in the organisational performance.
- It includes recalling, evaluating and analysis of data related to the employees' performance.

6. Discussing Results

- The result of the appraisal is communicated and discussed with the employees on one-to-one basis.
- The focus of this discussion is on communication and listening. The results, the problems and the possible solutions are discussed with the aim of problem solving and reaching consensus.
- The feedback should be given with a positive attitude as this can have an effect on the employees' future performance.
- The purpose of the meeting should be to solve the problems faced and motivate the employees to perform better.

7. Decision Making

- The last step of the process is to take decisions which can be taken either to improve the performance of the employees, to take the required corrective actions, or to take the related HR decisions like rewards, promotions, demotions, transfers etc.

D.7. Attributes Considered In Evaluating Performance

PERSONAL QUALITIES	DEMONSTRATED PERFORMANCE
Adaptability	Professional knowledge
Appearance and bearing	Administrative ability
Decisiveness	Responsibility for staff development
Dependability	Foresight
Drive and determination	Delegation
Ingenuity	Motivation
Initiative	Morale
Integrity	Control
Loyalty	
Maturity	
Stamina	
Tenacity	
Verbal expression	
Written expression	

D.8. Common errors in Performance Evaluation

- When writing an evaluation for a person it is critically important for a manager to be aware of some common evaluation errors. These errors have a very negative effect on the quality of the evaluation.

- By being aware of the common errors, a person writing the evaluation can do a self check to make sure all evaluations are done fairly and equitably for all people.

Error	Definition	Example
Contrast Effect	Tendency of a rater to evaluate people in comparison with other individuals rather than against the standards for the job.	Think of the most attractive person you know and rate this person on a Scale of 1 to 10. Now think of your favourite glamorous movie star. Rerate your acquaintance. If you rated your friend lower the second time, contrast effect is at work.
First impression error	Tendency of a rater to make an initial positive or negative judgment of an employee and allow that first impression to colour or distort later information.	A new supervisor noticed an employee, who was going through a divorce, performing poorly. Within a month the employee's performance returned to its previous high level, but the supervisor's opinion of the individual's performance was affected by the initial negative impression.
Halo/horns effect	Inappropriate generalizations from one aspect of an individual's performance to all areas of that person's performance.	Sreedeep's outstanding writing ability caused his supervisor to rate him highly in unrelated areas where his performance was actually mediocre.
Central tendency	The inclination to rate people in the middle scale even when their performance clearly warrants a substantially higher or lower rating.	Because Jignesh had a concern that he would not be able to deal with confrontation during an appraisal session, he rated all of his employees as "Meets Expectations."
Negative and positive skew	The opposite of central tendency: the rating of all individuals as higher or lower than their performance warrants.	Abhishek rates all of his employees higher than he feels they actually deserve, in the hope that this will cause them to live up to the high rating. While Adwait sets impossibly high standards and is proud of never having met an employee who deserved a superior rating.

Attribution bias	The tendency to attribute performance failings to factors under the control of the individual and performance successes to external causes.	Ravi Mohan attributes the successes of his work group to the quality of his leadership and the failings to their bad attitudes and inherent laziness.
Recency effect	The tendency of minor events that have happened recently to have more influence on the rating than major events of many months ago.	Atul Prajapati kept no records of critical incidents. When he began writing the appraisals for his employees he discovered that he could only recall examples of either positive or negative performance for the last two months.
Stereotyping.	The tendency to generalize across groups and ignore individual differences	Saurabh Gomber was far better at work than his colleagues who were transferred to a new department but his boss rated him same as others and gave him a lower grade than he deserved.
Leniency	Rater tends to rate every employee at the upper end of the scale regardless of the actual performance of the employee.	Ravi Prakash does not give much weightage to actual performance of employee and rates everybody highly to avoid confrontations and decision making.

Thinking Time !!

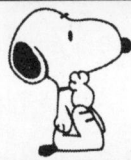

Make a table of above mentioned errors and write in the second column which one of them exists while your teacher evaluates you and your classmates. E.g. Is your teacher suffering from Halo Effect i.e. if any student is good in studies does he presupposes that he will be good in sports also?

TEST YOUR GREY MATTER

Q1) Define:
   i) Performance
   ii) Performance Appraisal
   iii) Performance Management
Q2) Differentiate between Performance Appraisal and Job Evaluation.
Q3) What are the major objectives of Performance Appraisal and how are they important for the organisation?
Q4) Enlist the difficulties or problems which are faced during Performance Appraisal.

Q5) Briefly describe the approaches of Performance Appraisal.

Q6) Describe the steps which are to be followed for effective Performance Appraisal.

Q7) "Accurate appraisal of performance is very difficult". Do you agree? Explain. Give a list of errors which may creep into the Performance Appraisal process.

D.9. Techniques of Performance Appraisal

The various methods and techniques used for Performance appraisal can be categorised as the following traditional and modern methods:

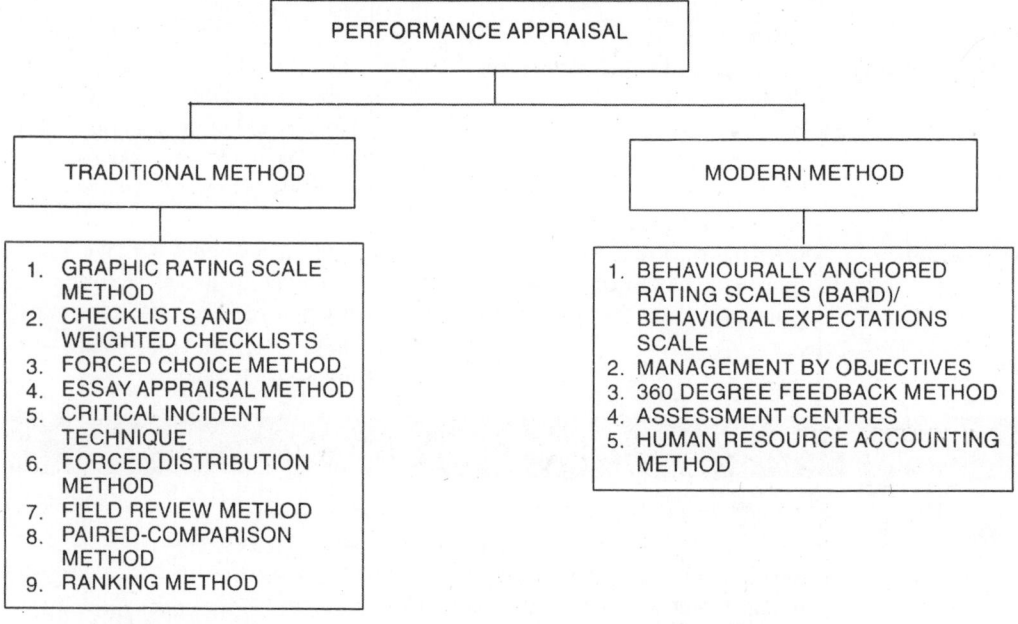

1. Traditional Methods of Performance Appraisal

a. Graphic Rating Scale Method

- This is the simplest and most popular technique for appraising employee performance.

- The typical **rating-scale** method consists of several numerical scales on each criterion such as dependability, initiative, output, attendance, attitude, co-operation etc.

- Each scale ranges from excellent to poor.

- The rater checks the appropriate performance level on each criterion, then computes the employee's total numerical score .The number of points scored may be linked to salary increase, whereby some points may amount to equal in rise of some percentage in salary.

Typical Graphic Rating Scale Method

Employee Name.................. Job title................

Department...................... Rate..............

Data..............................

	Poor	Fair	Satisfactory	Good	Excellent
Quality of work: Neatness, thoroughness and accuracy of work, knowledge of job					
Understanding: A clear understanding of the factors connected with the job.					
Attitude: Exhibits enthusiasm and cooperativeness on the job					
Dependability: Conscientious, thorough, reliable, accurate, with respect to attendance, reliefs, lunch breaks, etc.					
Quantity of work: Volume of work under normal working conditions					
Cooperation: Willingness and ability to work with others to produce desired goals.					

b. Checklists and Weighted Checklists

- A checklist represents, in its simplest form, a set of objectives or descriptive statements about the employee and his behaviour.

- If the rater believes strongly that the employee possesses a particular listed trait, he checks the item, otherwise, he leaves the item blank.

- A more recent variation of the checklist method is the **Weighted Checklist.** Under this, the value of each question may be weighted equally or certain questions may be weighted more heavily than others.

- **Advantages**
  i. Economy.
  ii. Ease of administration.

iii. Limited training of rater.

iv. Standardisation.

- **Disadvantages**
    i. Susceptibility to rater's biases (especially in halo effect).
    ii. Misinterpretation of checklist items.
    iii. Use of improper weights by HR department.

The following are some of the sample questions in the checklist.

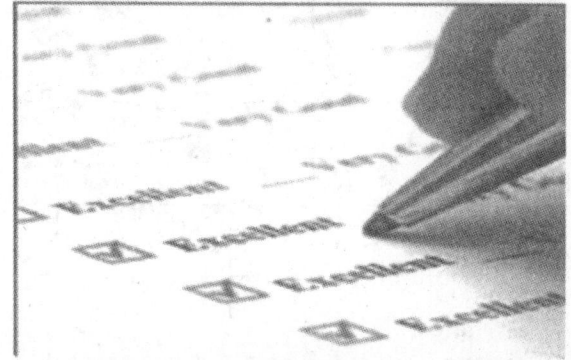

Checklist		
	Yes	No
Is the employee really interested in the task assigned?		
Is he respected by his colleagues (co-workers)?		
Does he give respect to his superiors?		
Does he follow instructions properly?		
Does he make mistakes frequently?		

c. Forced Choice Method

- This method was developed to eliminate bias and the prevalence of high ratings that might occur in some organisations.
- The primary purpose of the **forced choice method** is to correct the tendency of a rater to give consistently high or low ratings to all the employees.
- This method makes use of several sets of pair phrases, two of which may be positive and two negative and the rater is asked to indicate which of the four phrases is the most and least descriptive of a particular worker.
- Actually, the statement items are grounded in such ways that the rater cannot easily judge which statements apply to the most effective employee.

- The following box is a classic illustration of the forced choice items in organisations.

Table: Forced Choice Items

1. Least		Most
A	Does not anticipate difficulties	A
B	Grasps explanations easily and quickly	B
C	Does not waste time	C
D	Very easy to talk to	D
2. Least		Most
A	Can be a leader	A
B	Wastes time on unproductive things	B
C	At all times, cool and calm	C
D	Smart worker	D

d. Essay Appraisal Method

- Under this method, the rater is asked to express the strong as well as weak points of the employee's behaviour.

- This technique is normally used with a combination of the rating scale because the rater can elaborately present the scale by substantiating an explanation for his rating.

- While preparing the essay on the employee, the rater considers the following factors:

  i.   Job knowledge and potential of the employee.

  ii. Employee's understanding of the company's programmes, policies, objectives, etc.

  iii. The employee's relations with co-workers and superiors.

  iv. The employee's general planning, organising and controlling ability.

  v.   The attitudes and perceptions of the employee, in general.

- Essay evaluation is a non-quantitative technique.

- **Advantages**

  The essay provides a good deal of information about the employee and also reveals more about the evaluator. The strength of essay method depends on writing skills and analytical ability of the rater.

- **Disadvantages**

  i.   It is highly subjective; the supervisor may write a biased essay. The employees who are sycophants will be evaluated more favourably than other employees.

    ii. Some evaluators may be poor in writing essays on employee performance. They may become confused about what to say, how much they should state and the depth of the narrative. Others may be superficial in explanation and use flowery language which may not reflect the actual performance of the employee.

    iii. The appraiser is required to find time to prepare the essay. A busy appraiser may write the essay hurriedly without properly assessing the actual performance of the worker.

    iv. Writing essay is a time taking process. This becomes uneconomical from the view point of the firm, because the time of the evaluator (supervisor) is costly.

e. Critical Incident Technique

- Under this method, the manager prepares lists of statements of very effective and ineffective behaviour of an employee. These critical incidents or events represent the outstanding or poor behaviour of employees on the job.

- The manager maintains logs on each employee, whereby he periodically records critical incidents of the workers behaviour.

- At the end of the rating period, these recorded critical incidents are used in the evaluation of the workers' performance.

- An example of a good critical incident of a sales assistant is the following:

  - July 20 – The sales clerk patiently attended to the customer's complaint. He is polite, prompt, and enthusiastic in solving the customers' problem.

  - On the other hand the bad critical incident may appear as under:

  - July 20 – The sales assistant stayed 45 minutes over on his break during the busiest part of the day. He failed to answer the store manager's call thrice. He is lazy, negligent, stubborn and uninterested in work.

- **Advantages**
  - i. Evaluation is based on actual job behaviour.
  - ii. It reduces the recency bias, if rater records incidents throughout the rating period.
  - iii. This approach can increase the chance that the subordinates will improve because they learn more precisely what is expected of them.

- **Disadvantages**
  - i. Negative incidents may be more noticeable than positive incidents.
  - ii. The supervisors have a tendency to unload a series of complaints about incidents during an annual performance review session.

iii. It results in very close supervision which may not be liked by the employee.

iv. The recording of incidents may be a chore for the manager concerned, who may be too busy or forget to do it.

f. Forced distribution method

- One of the errors in rating is leniency – clustering a large number of employees around a high point on a rating scale. The force distribution method seeks to overcome the problem by compelling the rater to distribute the ratees on all points on the rating scale.

- The method operates under an assumption that the employee performance level conforms to a normal statistical distribution curve. Generally, it is assumed that employee performance levels conform to a **Bell –Shaped Curve. (**Bell curve is used for performance management. This theory was conceived by Hernstein & Murray in 1994.) With this method, a pre-determined percentage of employees are placed in each of the five categories as shown in the curve (Figure c).

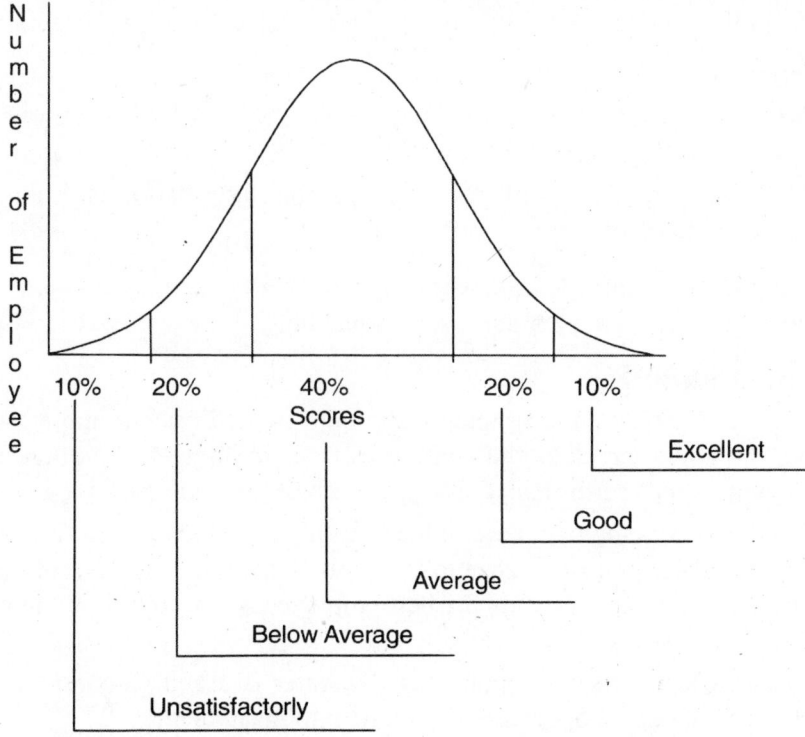

Figure c: force distribution on a bell-shaped curve

- **Disadvantages**
  i. This method always assumes that employee performance level always conforms to a normal (or some other) distribution.
  ii. Superior may resist placing any individual in the lowest (or the highest) group.
  iii. Difficulties can arise when rater has to explain to the employee why he or she was placed in one grouping and others in higher grouping.
  iv. In a small group, there may be no reasons to assume that bell- shaped distribution of performance really exists.

- **Advantage**

  One advantage of this method is that it seeks to eliminate the error of leniency.

g. Field Review Method

In this method, a senior member of the HR department or a training officer discusses and interviews the supervisors to evaluate and rate their respective subordinates.

- **Advantages**
  i. The method is primarily used for making promotional decisions at the managerial level.
  ii. Field reviews are also useful when comparable information is required from employees' in different units or locations.

- **Drawback** of this method is that it is a very time consuming method. But this method helps to reduce the superiors' personal bias.

h. Ranking method

- This is one of the oldest and simplest techniques of performance appraisal. In this method, the appraiser ranks the employees from the best to the poorest on the basis of their overall performance. It is quite useful for a comparative evaluation.
- In this method, all employees are judged on the same factors and they are rated on the overall basis with reference to their job performance instead of individual assessment of traits. In this way, the best employee is placed first in the rank and the poorest occupies the lowest rank.
- This system encounters a difficulty that the rater is asked to consider a whole man. Subjectivity of the appraiser may come into his judgement.

i. Paired-Comparison Method

- Although the Ranking Method implicitly requires that a man be compared to others on the list during the ranking process, this is not systematically built into the method. A procedure which does systematically force the rater to compare each man with every other man is known as the method of **Paired Comparison**.

- For example, consider the situation where 4 employees are being evaluated by a supervisor.

If we form all possible pairs of men, we shall have

N (N-1)/2 pairs formed; in our case, 4(4-1)/2 = 6pairs.

After the completion of comparison , the results can be tabulated , and the rank is created from the number of times each person is considered to be superior.

2. Modern Methods of Performance Appraisal

a. Behaviourally Anchored Rating Scales (Bars)/ Behavioural Expectations Scale

- This method represents the latest innovation in performance appraisal. It is a combination of the rating scale and critical incident techniques of employee performance evaluation.
- The critical incidents serve as anchor statements on a scale and the rating form usually contains six to eight specifically defined performance dimensions.
- The following chart represents an example of a sales trainee's competence and a behaviourally anchored rating scale.

Table: An Example of Behaviourally Anchored Rating Scale (BARS)

PERFORMANCE	POINTS	BEHAVIOUR
Extremely good	7	Can expect trainee to make valuable suggestions for increased sales and to have positive relationships with customers all over the country.
Good	6	Can expect to initiate creative ideas for improved sales.
Above average	5	Can expect to keep in touch with the customers throughout the year.
Average	4	Can manage, with difficulty, to deliver the goods in time.
Below average	3	Can expect to unload the trucks when asked by the supervisor.
Poor	2	Can expect to inform only a part of the customers.
Extremely poor	1	Can expect to take extended coffee breaks and roam around purposelessly.

How to construct BARS?

Developing BARS follows a general format which combines techniques employed in the critical incident method and weighted checklist ratings scales. Emphasis is pinpointed on pooling the thinking of people who will use the scales as both evaluators and evaluates. Following steps are followed:

Step 1: Collect critical incidents

❏ People with knowledge of the job to be probed, such as job holders and supervisors, describe specific examples of effective and ineffective behaviour related to job performance.

Step 2: Identify performance dimensions

❏ The people assigned the task of developing the instrument cluster the incidents into a small set of key performance dimensions. Generally between five and ten dimensions account for most of the performance.

❏ Examples of performance dimensions include technical competence, relationships with customers, handling of paper work and meeting day-to-day deadlines.

❏ While developing varying levels of performance for each dimension (anchors), specific examples of behaviour should be used, which could later be scaled in terms of good, average or below average performance.

Step 3: Reclassification of incidents

❏ Another group of participants who are knowledgeable about the job is instructed to retranslate or reclassify the critical incidents generated (in Step II) previously.

❏ They are given the definition of job dimension and told to assign each critical incident to the dimension that it best describes.

❏ At this stage, incidents for which there is not 75 per cent agreement are discarded as being too subjective.

Step 4: Assigning scale values to the incidents

❏ Each incident is then rated on a 'one-to-seven' or 'one-to-nine' scale with respect to how well it represents performance on the appropriate dimension.

❏ A rating of 'one' represents ineffective performance; the top scale value indicates very effective performance.

❏ The second group of participants usually assigns the scale values. Means and standard deviations are then calculated for the scale values assigned to each incident. Typically incidents that have standard deviations of 1.50 or less (on a 7-point scale) are retained.

Step 5: Producing the final instrument

- About six or seven incidents for each performance dimension – all having met both the retranslating and standard deviation criteria – will be used as behavioural anchors.
- The final BARS instrument consists of a series of vertical scales (one for each dimension) anchored (or measured) by the final incidents. Each incident is positioned on the scale according to its mean value.

Advantages

i. Because the above process typically requires considerable employee participation, its acceptance by both supervisors and their subordinates may be greater.

ii. **Proponents of BARS** also claim that such a system differentiates among behaviour, performance and results and consequently is able to provide a basis for setting developmental goals for the employee.

iii. As it is job-specific and identifies observable and measurable behaviour, it is a more reliable and valid method for performance appraisal.

b. Management By Objectives

- **Definition:** Management by Objectives (MBO) is a process of defining objectives for each employee and then comparing and directing their performance against the objectives which have been set.
- Management by Objectives was first outlined by **Peter Drucker** in 1954 in his book **'The Practice Of Management'**. According to Drucker, managers should avoid 'the activity trap' i.e. getting so involved in their day to day activities that they forget their main purpose or objective.

Concepts of MBO

i. **One of the MBO concepts** was that instead of just a few top-managers, all managers of a firm should participate in the strategic planning process, in order to improve the implementation ability of the plan.

ii. **Another concept of MBO** was that managers should implement a range of performance systems, designed to help the organisation stay on the right track.

Goals of MBO

- It aims to increase organisational performance by aligning goals and subordinate objectives throughout the organisation.
- Here, employees get strong input to identify their objectives, time lines for completion, etc. MBO includes ongoing tracking and feedback in the process to reach objectives.

Managerial Focus

MBO managers focus on the result, not the activity. They delegate tasks by **"negotiating a contract of goals"** with their subordinates without dictating a detailed roadmap for implementation. Management by Objectives (MBO) is about setting objectives and then breaking these down into more specific goals or key results.

Principles of MBO

a. Cascading of organisational goals and objectives.

b. Specific objectives for each member.

c. Participative decision making.

d. Explicit time period.

e. Performance evaluation and feedback.

MBO Process

The typical MBO process consists of:

1. Establishing a clear and precisely defined statement of objectives for the employee
2. Developing an action plan indicating how these objectives are to be achieved
3. Allowing the employee to implement this action plan
4. Appraising performance based on objective achievement
5. Taking corrective action when necessary
6. Establishing new objectives for the future

Important features/Advantages of MBO are

1. **Motivation** – Involving employees in the whole process of goal setting and increasing employee empowerment increases employee job satisfaction and commitment.

2. **Better communication and coordination** – Frequent reviews and interactions between superiors and subordinates helps to maintain harmonious relationships within the enterprise and also solve many problems faced during the period.

3. **Clarity of goals:** With MBO came the concept of **SMART goals** i.e. goals that are:

Specific
Measurable
Achievable
Realistic, and
Time bound.

The goals thus set are clear, motivating and there is a link between **organisational goals and performance targets** of the employees.

4. **Future Oriented:** The focus is on the future rather than on the past. Goals and standards are set for the performance of the future with periodic reviews and feedback.

Disadvantages/Limitations of MBO process

There are several limitations to the assumptive base underlying the impact of managing by objectives, including:

1. It over-emphasises the setting of goals over the working of a plan as a driver of outcomes.

2. It can lead to unrealistic expectations about what can and cannot be reasonably accomplished.

3. It underemphasises the importance of the environment or context in which the goals are set. That context may include the availability of resource, quality of resources etc.

4. It did not address the importance of successfully responding to obstacles and constraints as essential to reaching a goal. The model didn't adequately cope with the obstacles of:

   • Defects in resources, planning and methodology.

   • The impact of a rapidly changing environment, which could alter the landscape enough to make yesterday's goals and action plans irrelevant to the present.

c. 360 Degree Feedback Method

• 360 degree feedback, also known as **'multi-rater feedback'**, is the most comprehensive appraisal where the feedback about the employees' performance comes from all the sources that come in contact with the employee on his job.

• 360 degree respondents for an employee can be his/her peers, managers (i.e. superior), subordinates, team members, customers, suppliers/ vendors - anyone who comes into contact with the employee and can provide valuable insights and information or feedback regarding the **"on-the-job"** performance of the employee.

• Self assessment is an indispensable part of 360 degree appraisals and therefore 360 degree performance appraisal has high employee involvement and also have the strongest impact on behaviour and performance. It provides a "360-degree review" of the employees' performance and is considered to be one of the most credible performance appraisal methods.

Four integral components of 360 degree method:

i.   **Self appraisal**: It gives a chance to the employee to look at his/her strengths and weaknesses, his achievements, and judge his own performance.

ii. **Superior's appraisal**: It forms the traditional part of the 360 degree performance appraisal where the employee's responsibilities and actual performance is rated by the superior.

iii. **Subordinates appraisal**: It gives a chance to judge the employee on parameters like communication and motivating abilities, superior's ability to delegate the work, leadership qualities etc.

iv. **Peer Appraisal:** Also known as **Internal Customers**, the correct feedback given by peers can help to find employee' ability to work in a team, co-operation and sensitivity towards others.

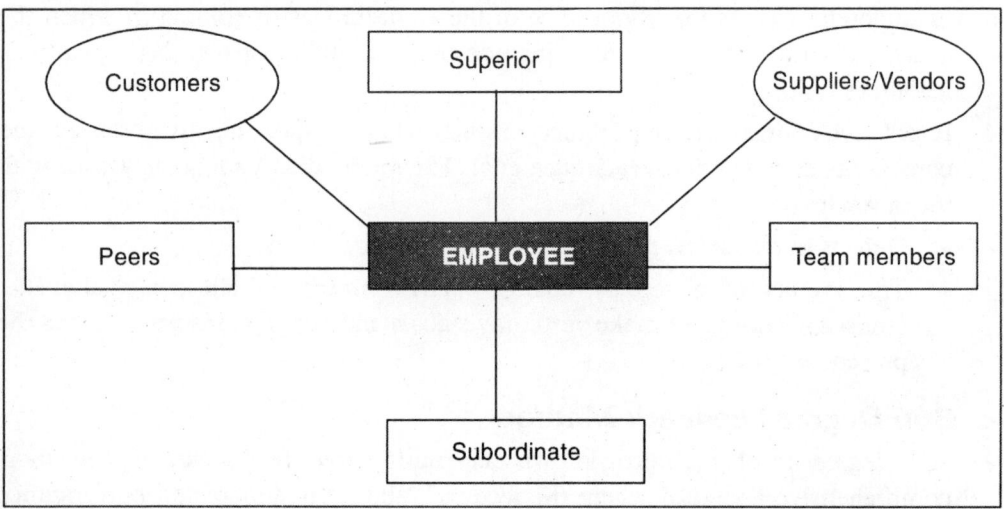

Disadvantages

i.   It is costly and requires time and energy commitment from the HR department.

ii. Outsourced vendors are required to customise and administer the survey form, which may not be always possible to do.

Advantages

i.   A good tool for matrix organisations as it is in line with the concept of a flat structure i.e. feedback comes from multiple sources of contact.

ii. It is helpful in assessing soft skills possessed by employees.

iii. It is effective in identifying and measuring interpersonal skills, customer satisfaction, and team–building skills.

d. Assessment Centres

- Assessment centre refers to a method to objectively observe and assess the people in action by experts or HR professionals with the help of various assessment tools and instruments.

- Assessment centres simulate the employees' on the job environment and facilitate the assessment of their on the job performance.

- An assessment centre typically involves the use of methods like social/informal events, tests and exercises, assignments being given to a group of employees to assess their competencies and on the **job behaviour** and potential to take higher responsibilities in the future.

- Generally, employees are given an assignment similar to the job they would be expected to perform if promoted. The trained evaluators observe and evaluate employees as they perform the assigned jobs and are evaluated on job related characteristics.

Components of Assessment Centre for Performance Appraisal

i. **Social/Informal Events:** An assessment centre has a group of participants and also a few assessors, which gives a chance to the employees to socialise with a variety of people and also to share information and know more about the organisation.

ii. **Information Sessions:** Information sessions are part of the assessment centres. They provide information to the employees about the organisation, their roles and responsibilities, the activities and the procedures etc.

iii. **Assignments:** Assignments in Assessment Centres include various tests and exercises which are specially designed to assess the competencies and the potential of the employees. These include various interviews, psychometric tests, management games etc. All these assignments are focused on the target job.

Common Features of all Assessment Centres

i. The final results are based on the pass/fail criteria.

ii. All the activities are carried out to fill the targeted job.

iii. Each session lasts from 1 to 5 days.

iv. The results are based on the assessment of the assessors with less emphasis on **self-assessment.**

v. Immediate review or feedback is not provided to the employees.

Disadvantages

i. It is very costly.

ii. Strong and unhealthy sense of competition among the assesses.

iii. Difficulty of conducting the test frequently.

iv. The possibility of overemphasising the test performance.

v. Assessment Centres require highly skilled observers as the observers may bring in their own perceptions and biases while evaluating.

Advantages

i. Assessment Centres not only help the organisation in placing the right candidate in the right job/assignment but also help in developing the participants.

ii. It appeals to the lay person's logic and therefore is regarded as a fair means of assessment by the participants.

iii. Assessment Centres can be customised for different kinds of jobs, competencies and organisational requirements.

iv. By involving the line managers in the procedure, assessment centres naturally gain support from them in the management decisions.

v. Their validity coefficient is higher than most other techniques used for predicting performance. This is so because it simulates real job challenges and evaluates the candidate on the same.

Essential Elements of Assessment Centres

i. **Job Analysis** – To understand job challenges and the competencies required for successful execution of the job.

ii. **Predefine competencies** - Modelling the competencies, which will be tested during the process.

iii. **Behavioural classification** - Behaviours displayed by participants must be classified into meaningful and relevant categories such as dimensions, attributes, characteristics, aptitudes, qualities, skills, abilities, competencies, and knowledge.

iv. **Assessment techniques** – These include a number of exercises to test the assesses of their potentials. Each competency is tested through at least 2 exercises for gathering adequate evidence for the presence of particular competence.

v. **Simulations** – The exercises should simulate the job responsibilities as closely as possible to eliminate potential errors in selection.

vi. **Observations** – Accurate and unbiased observation is the most critical aspect of an Assessment Centres.

vii. **Observers** – Multiple observers are used to eliminate subjectivity and biases from the process. They are given thorough training in the process prior to participating in the Assessment Centres.

viii.**Recording Behaviour** – A systematic procedure of recording must be used by the assessors for future reference. The recording could be in the form of hand written note, behavioural checklist, audio-video recording etc.

ix. **Reports** – Each observer must make a detailed report of his observation before going for the discussion of integration of scores.

x. **Data Integration** – The pooling of information from different assessors is done through statistical techniques.

Exercises in Assessment Centres

Following are the most widely used exercises in Assessment Centres. Every exercise unveils presence/absence of certain competency in the participant. The competencies that are normally evaluated through these different exercises are mentioned in column three.

TOOL	EXPLANATION	COMPETENCY
Case study interview	Requires candidates to read a large set of information and then answer questions relating to the subject matter	Analytical skills, assimilation of information, prioritization of information, time-management, working under pressure
Competency-based interview	Includes personal history questions and problem-solving tasks and scenarios	Analytical skills, business acumen, communication, interpersonal skills, personal attributes, teamwork
Fact-finding exercise	Includes research and retrieval of information on a given subject or interaction with the interviewer to obtain further information from them	Personal assertiveness, teamwork, Interpersonal effectiveness, drive for result
Group exercise	Includes problem solving within a committee or team	Time-management, analytical skills, business acumen
In-tray test	Includes prioritising documents, drafting replies to letters, and delegating important tasks	Analytical skills, creativity, lateral thinking, resourcefulness
Problem-solving task	includes building a structure with limited materials	Assimilation of information, presentation delivery, working under pressure
Presentation	Involves a 10 to 15 minute presentation on a pre-determined topic.	Assimilation of information, presentation delivery, working under pressure

Psychometric/ Personality/ Aptitude Tests	Includes a personality questionnaire and/or numerical, verbal, and diagrammatic reasoning tests.	Agreeableness, behavioural interaction, conscientiousness, extroversion /introversion, personal assertiveness, teamwork
Role-play exercise	Involves acting-out a business-related situation	Approach to business situations
Written exercise	Involves producing a concise written summary from a collection of documents.	Analytical skills, summarisation, written communication

Validity of Assessment Centres

Studying validity is studying the problem of whether or not a test measures what it intends to measure. Assessment Centres have **high predictive, face and content validity** because of the following reasons –

a. Designing of Assessment Centres is based on job analysis.

b. Observers are extensively trained.

c. Candidates are graded by using ratings of competencies

e. Human Resource Accounting Method

- **Definition:** American Accounting Association has defined Human Resource Accounting (HRA) as "a process of identifying and measuring data about human resources and communicating to the interested parties."

- Human resources are valuable assets for every organisation. Human resource accounting method tries to find the relative worth of these assets in the terms of money.

- In this method, the performance appraisal of the employees is judged in terms of cost and contribution of the employees. The cost of employees include all the expenses incurred on them like their compensation, recruitment and selection costs, induction and training costs etc. whereas their contribution includes the total value added (in monetary terms). The difference between the cost and the contribution will be the performance of the employees. Ideally, the contribution of the employees should be greater than the cost incurred on them.

Advantages of Accounting Method

1. It helps in giving valuable information to the management for effective planning and managing human resources.

2. It helps in measurement of standard cost of recruiting, selection, hiring and training people and organisation can select a person with highest expected realisable value.

3. It also provides necessary data to devise suitable promotion policy, congenial work environment and job satisfaction to the people.

Problems in Human Resource Accounting

1. There is no well set standard accounting practice for measuring the value of human resources.

2. The valuation of human resources is based on the assumption that the employee may remain with the organisation for a certain specified period.

3. There is a possibility that human resource accounting may lead to the dehumanisation in the organisation if the valuation is not done correctly.

4. There is also a possibility that trade union may oppose the use of HRA.

TEST YOUR GREY MATTER

Q1) List down the various types of Performance Appraisal methods in both Traditional Approach and Modern Approach and briefly describe at least one method of both the approaches?

Q2) Discuss the traditional methods of performance appraisal. How far are these methods relevant in present-day organisations?

Q3) Discuss the process of appraisal by Assessment Centres.

Q4) What do you mean by 360-degree appraisal? What are the relative merits and demerits of 360-degree appraisal?

Q5) What is 'Management By Objectives' method of performance appraisal and what are its advantages?

Q6) Describe the following methods of performance appraisal by giving their merits and demerits:

    (i)   Checklist Method.

    (ii)   Essay Appraisal Method.

    (iii) Critical Incident Technique.

    (iv) Forced Distribution Method.

    (v)   Field Review Method.

    (vi) Behaviourally Anchored Rating Scales (BARS)

CHAPTER

18

Training and Development

By the end of this chapter, you would be able to :

- Understand about training and development and their importance to the organisation.
- Know about different methods and processes of conducting training.
- Learn about learning and principles of learning.
- Study and understand about executive development and different ways of providing it.

The chapter contains :

- Nature of Training and Development
- Training, Development and Education
- Training
  - Objectives of Training
  - Features of Training
  - Importance of Training
  - The Benefits of Training
  - Disadvantages of Training
  - Training Process
  - Methods of Training
- Learning
  - Definition and Meaning
  - Learning Curve
  - Process of Learning
  - Principles of Learning
- Executive or Management Development
  - Objectives of Executive Development
  - Need and Importance of Executive Development
  - Techniques of Management Development

A. THE INSIGHT

"I want to talk about learning. But not the lifeless, sterile, futile, quickly forgotten stuff that is crammed into the mind of the poor helpless individual tied into his seat by ironclad bonds of conformity! I am talking about LEARNING - the insatiable curiosity that drives the adolescent boy to absorb everything he can see or hear or read about gasoline engines in order to improve the efficiency and speed of his 'cruiser'. I am talking about the student who says, "I am discovering, drawing in from the outside, and making that which is drawn in a real part of me." I am talking about any learning in which the experience of the learner progresses along this line: "No, no, that's not what I

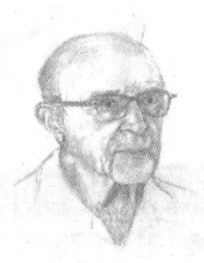

Carl Rogers 1983: 18-19

want"; "Wait! This is closer to what I am interested in, what I need"; "Ah, here it is! Now I'm grasping and comprehending what I need and what I want to know!"

B. NATURE OF TRAINING AND DEVELOPMENT

- Training And Development is an attempt to improve current or future employee's performance by increasing the employee's ability to perform through learning, usually by changing the employee's attitude or increasing his/her skills and knowledge.

- In simple terms, Training and Development refers to the imparting of specific skills, abilities and knowledge to an employee.

- The need for training and development is determined by the employee's performance deficiency, computed as follows:

  Training And Development Need = Standard Performance – Actual Performance

C. TRAINING, DEVELOPMENT AND EDUCATION

- Human Resource Development programmes are divided into three main categories: **Training, Development and Education.** Although some organisations categorise all learning under "Training" or "Training and Development," dividing it into three distinct categories makes the desired goals and objects more meaningful and precise.

- **Training** is the acquisition of technology, skill or knowledge which permits employees to perform their present job to standards. It improves human performance on the job the employee is presently doing or is being hired to do. It is also given when new technology in introduced into the workplace.

- **McFarland** defines several concepts used in the development of human resources. Although training and education are closely connected, these concepts differ in crucial ways. While the term **"training"** relates to imparting specific skills for specific objectives, the term **"education"** involves the development of the whole individual socially, intellectually and physically. Accordingly, training forms only a part of the entire educational process. And the term **"development"** can be defined as the nature and direction of change taking place among managerial personnel through educational and training process.

The following table draws a distinction between training and education more clearly:

Training	Education
Application	Theoretical orientation
Job Experience	Classroom learning
Specific Tasks	General concepts
Narrow perspective	Broad perspective

- Though training and education differ in nature and orientation, they are complementary. An employee, for example, who undergoes training, is presumed to have had some formal education. Furthermore, no training program is complete without an element of education. In fact, the distinction between training and education is getting increasingly blurred nowadays. As more and more employees are called upon to exercise judgment and to choose alternative solutions to the job problem, training programmes seek to broaden and develop the individual through education.

- **Development** refers to those learning opportunities which are designed to help employees grow. Development is not primarily skills-oriented. Instead, it provides general knowledge and attitudes, which will be helpful to employees in higher positions. Efforts towards development often depend on personal drive and ambition. Development activities, such as those supplied by management developmental programmes are generally voluntary.

- Let us try to understand the distinction between Training and Development through the following table:

LEARNING DIMENSION	TRAINING	DEVELOPMENT
Who	Non-managerial personnel	Managerial personnel
What	Technical / Mechanical Operation	Theoretical / conceptual ideas
Why	Specific job related information	General knowledge
When	Short- term focus	Long-term focus

D. TRAINING

Definition: It is a learning process that involves the acquisition of knowledge, sharpening of skills, concepts, rules, or changing of attitudes and behaviours to enhance the performance of employees.

- The major outcome of training is learning. Trainees learn new habits, refines skills and useful knowledge during their training programme, which helps them to improve their performance.

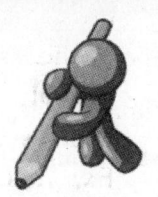

Wisdom Tooth

"There is nothing training cannot do; Nothing is above its reach: It can turn bad morals to good, it can destroy bad principles and create good ones, it can lift men to angelship."

- Mark Twain

D.1. Objectives of Training

- The overall training objective is to develop required knowledge, skills and attitudes of employees so that they can perform more productively and achieve the business goals.

- It is recognised that employees learn primarily from on-the-job experience. Therefore, in achieving this objective, the primary contribution is from on-the-job training and supporting contribution from the formal training effort.

Basic Objectives of Training are

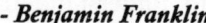

Wisdom Tooth

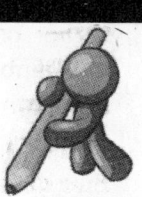

"Tell me and I forget, teach me and I remember, involve me and I learn"

- Benjamin Franklin

1. To impart basic knowledge and skill to new entrants and enable them to perform the job well.

2. To equip employee to meet the changing requirement of the job and organisation.

3. To teach the employees new techniques and ways of performing the job or operations.

4. To prepare employees for higher level task and build up a second line of competent managers.

5. To increase productivity and quality.

6. To increase efficiency.

D.2. Features of Training

1. Increases knowledge and skill for doing a job.

2. Bridge the gap between job needs and employee skills.

3. Job oriented process, vocational in nature.

4. Short-term activity designed especially for employees.

D.3. Importance of Training

i. Training is the corner-stone of sound management, it makes employees more effective and productive. It is an integral part of the whole management programme, with all its many activities functionally interrelated.

ii. New and changed techniques developed could be introduced and their advantage may be taken.

iii. It enables employees to develop and rise within the organisation, and increase their "market value", earning power and job security.

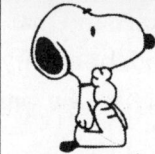

Thinking Time !!

Have you ever undergone any kind of training? Was it helpful to you? Share your experience with your friends.

iv. It enables the management to resolve sources of friction with employees. It moulds the employees' attitudes and helps them to achieve a better co-operation with the company and a greater loyalty to it.

v. Training heightens the morale of the employees and helps in reducing dissatisfaction, complaints, grievances and absenteeism and the rate of attrition.

vi. Trained employees make better and economical use of materials and equipment; therefore, wastage and spoilage are lessened, and the need for constant supervision is reduced.

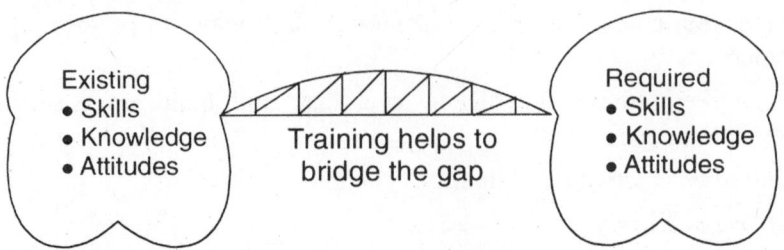

Existing
- Skills
- Knowledge
- Attitudes

Training helps to bridge the gap

Required
- Skills
- Knowledge
- Attitudes

D.4. Benefits of Training

1. Benefits to the Organisation

i. Leads to improved profitability and more positive attitudes towards profit orientation.

ii. Improves the job knowledge and skills at all levels of the organisation.

iii. Improves the morale of the work force.

iv. Helps people identify with organisational goals.

v. Helps create a better corporate image.

vi. Aids in organisational development.

vii. Aids in understanding and carrying out organisational policies.

viii. Organisation gets more effective decision making and problem solving.

ix. Aids in developing leadership skills, motivation, loyalty, better attitudes, and other aspects that successful workers and managers usually display.

x. Aids in increasing productivity and/or quality of work.

xi. Develops a sense of responsibility to the organisation for being competent and knowledgeable.

xii. Improves labour-management relations and creates an appropriate climate for growth, communication.

xiii. Reduces outside consulting costs by utilising competent internal consulting.

2. Benefits to the Individual

i. Helps the individual in making better decisions and effective problem solving.

ii. Through training and development, motivational variables of recognition, achievement, growth, responsibility and achievement, are internalised and operationalised.

iii. Aids in encouraging and achieving self-development and self-confidence.

iv. Helps a person handle stress, tension, frustration and conflict.

v. Provides information for improving leadership knowledge, communication skills, and attitudes.

vi. Increases job satisfaction and recognition.

vii. Moves a person towards personal goals while improving interaction skills.

viii. Develops a sense of growth in learning.

ix. Helps a person develop speaking and listening skills; also writing skills when exercises are required.

x. Helps eliminate fear in attempting new tasks.

D.5. Disadvantages Of Training

i. Can be a financial drain on resources as training could be expensive.

ii. Equips staff to leave for a better job.

iii. Often takes people away from their job for varying periods of time.

D.6. Training Process

There are six steps in the training process. All those involved in training need to be aware of the key stages in the training process, often referred to as the training cycle:

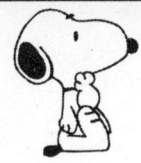

Thinking Time !!

Make a list of areas in which you require training and you think it will be helpful to you.

It could be Cricket or Public Speaking or anything you could possibly think of.

Training cycle based on a human resource development plan

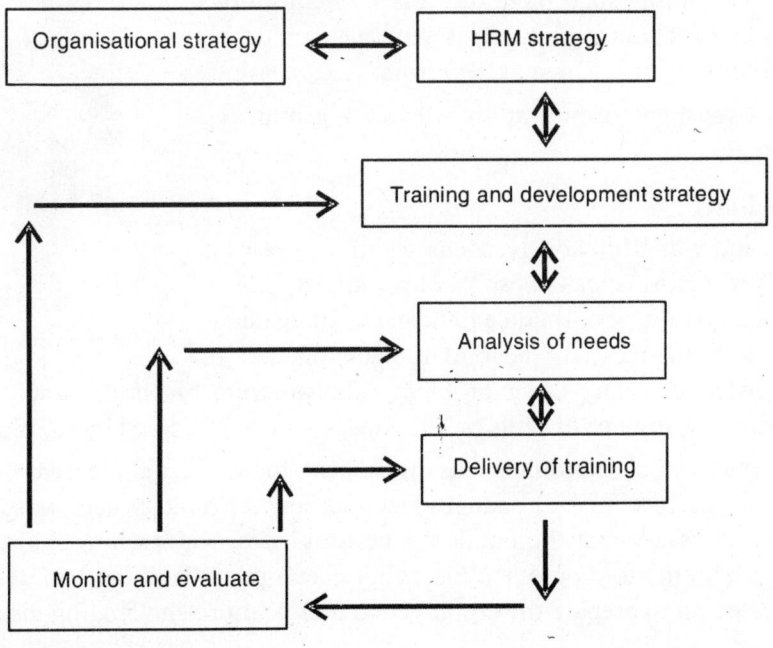

Steps In The Training Process

1. Organisational objectives
2. Assessment of Training needs
3. Establishment of Training goals
4. Devising training programme
5. Implementation of training programme
6. Evaluation of results

D.6.1. Organisational Objectives and Strategies

- The first step in the training process in an organisation is the assessment of its objectives and strategies.

- What business are we in? At what level of quality do we wish to provide this product or service? Where do we want to be in the future? It is only after answering these related questions that the organisation must assess the strengths and weaknesses of its human resources.

D.6.2. Needs Assessment

- Needs assessment presents problems and future challenges to be met through training and development.

- Organisations spend vast sums of money (usually as a percentage of turnover) on training and development. Before committing such huge resources, organisations that implement training programs without conducting needs assessment may be making errors.

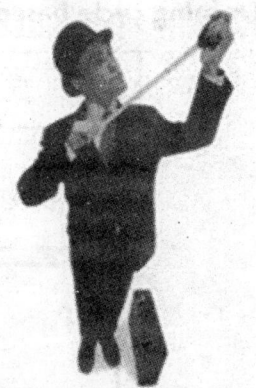

- Needs assessment occurs at two levels - **group and individual.**

Individual

- An individual obviously needs training when his or her performance falls short of standards, that is, when there is performance deficiency. Inadequacy in performance may be due to lack of skill or knowledge or any other problem. The problem of performance deficiency caused by absence of skills or knowledge can be remedied by training.

- Assessment of training needs must also focus on anticipated skills of an employee. Technology changes fast and new technology demands new skills. It is necessary that the employee be trained to acquire new skills. This will help him/her to progress in his or her career path. Training and development is essential to prepare the employee to handle more challenging tasks.

❑ Individuals may also require new skills because of possible job transfers. Although job transfers are common, as organisational personnel demands vary, they do not necessarily require elaborate training efforts. Employees commonly require only an orientation to new facilities and jobs.

Group

Assessment of training needs occurs at the group level too. Any change in the organisation's strategy necessitates training of groups of employees.

Needs Assessment Methods

- Several methods are available for the purpose of needs assessment. As shown below some are useful for organisational-level needs assessment and others for individual needs assessment.

- **Methods used in training needs assessment**

Group or organisational analysis	Individual Analysis
• Organisational goals and objectives.	• Performance appraisal
• Personnel /skills inventories	• Work sampling
• Organisational climate indices	• Interviews
• Efficiency indices	• Questionnaires
• Exit interview	• Attitude survey
• MBO or work planning systems	• Training progress
• Quality circles	• Rating scales.
• Customer survey/satisfaction data	
• Consideration of current and projected changes	

Benefits of Needs Assessment

As pointed above, needs assessment helps diagnose the causes of performance deficiency in employees. Causes require remedial actions. This being a generalised statement there are certain specific benefits of needs assessment. They are:

i. Trainers may be informed about the broader needs of the training group and their sponsoring organisations.

ii. The sponsoring organisations are able to reduce the perception gap between the participant and his or her boss about their needs and expectations from the training programmes.

iii. Trainers are able to design their course inputs closer to the specific needs of the participants.

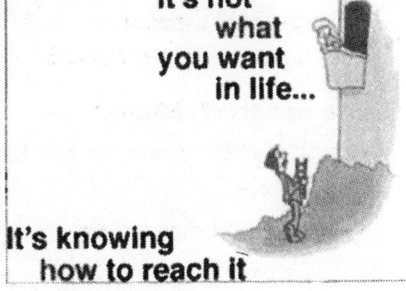

It's not
what
you want
in life...

It's knowing
how to reach it

D.6.3. Training and Development Objectives

- Once training needs are assessed, training and development goals must be established.
- Without clearly set goals, it is not possible to design a training and development programme and, after it has been implemented there will be no way of measuring its effectiveness.
- Goals must be tangible, verifiable, and measurable.
- This is easy where skills training is involved. For example, a successful trainee will be expected to type 55 words per minute with two or three errors per page.
- Nevertheless, clear behavioural standards of expected results are necessary so that the programme can be effectively designed and results can be evaluated.

D.6.4. Designing Training and Development Programme

Every training and development programme must address certain vital issues:
i.   Who are the trainees?
ii. Who are the trainers?
iii. What methods and techniques are to be used for training?
iv. What should be the level of learning?
v.   What learning principles are needed?
vi. Where is the program conducted?

i. Who are the trainees?

- Trainees should be selected on the basis of self nomination, recommendations of supervisors or by the HR department itself.
- It is preferred to have two or more target audiences, as bringing several target audiences together can also facilitate group processes such as problem solving and decision-making.
- For example, employees and their supervisors may effectively learn together about a new work process and their respective roles.

ii. Who are the trainers?

- Several people including the following may conduct training and development programmes:
  1) Immediate supervisors
  2) Co-workers, as in buddy systems,
  3) Members of the personnel staff,
  4) Specialists in other parts of the company,

5) Outside consultants,

6) Industry associations, and faculty members at universities.

iii. What methods and techniques are to be used for training?

● Many methods of training are used to train employees. The most commonly used methods are categorized into two groups- (i) On–The-Job (ii) Off-The-Job Methods.

It is dealt with in detail, later in the chapter.

iv. What should be the level of learning?

● The inputs passed on to trainees in training and development program are education, skills, ethics etc. There are three basic levels at which these inputs can be taught.

● At the **lowest level**, the employees must acquire fundamental knowledge. This means developing a basic understanding of a field and becoming acquainted with the language, concepts and relationships involved in it.

● The **goal of the next level** is skill development, or acquiring the ability to perform in a particular skill area.

● The **highest level** aims at increased operational proficiency. This involves obtaining additional experience and improving skills that have already been developed.

v. What learning principles are needed?

● Learning and learning principles are mentioned later in this chapter.

vi. Where is the program conducted?

● A final consideration is where the training should be conducted. And the decision comes down to the following choices:

❑ At the job itself.

❑ On site but not the job –for example, in training class room in the company.

❑ Off the site, such as in a university or college class room, resorts etc.

D.6.4.1 Methods and Techniques of Training

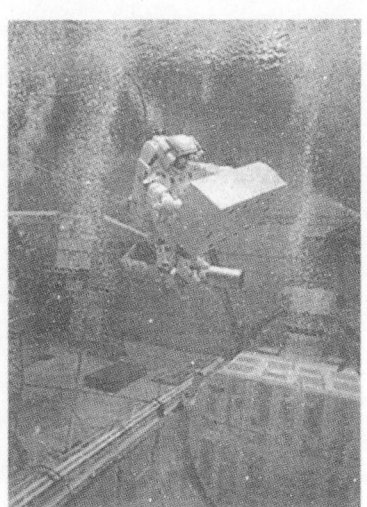

An astronaut in training for an extra-vehicular activity mission using an underwater simulation environment.

● A multitude of methods of training are used to train employees. Training methods are categorised into two groups

a. On the job training.

b. Off-the job methods.

- On the job training refers to methods that are applied in the workplace, while the employee is actually working. Off-the-job methods are used away from workplaces.

a. On-The-Job Training

Definition: Cannell (1997:28) defines on-the-job training as:

"Training that is planned and structured, that takes place mainly at the normal workstation of the trainee-although some instruction may be provided in a special training area on site - and where a manager, supervisor, trainer or peer colleague spends significant time with a trainee to teach a set of skills that have been specified in advance."

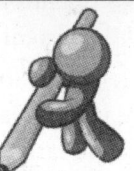

Wisdom Tooth

"I hated every minute of training, but I said, Don t quit. Suffer now and live the rest of your life as a champion."

Muhammad Ali

Advantages

i. Tailor-made course content using REAL company situations/examples.

ii. It is usually less expensive than off -the-job training.

iii. Learning will take place using the equipment which will be actually used.

iv. Trainees become accustomed more rapidly.

Disadvantages

i. Possibility of poor instruction and insufficient time.

ii. Trainee may be exposed to bad work practices.

iii. A large amount of spoiled work and scrap material may be produced.

iv. Valuable equipment may be damaged.

v. Training takes place under production conditions that are stressful, i.e. noisy, busy, confusing and exposing the trainee to comments by other workers.

Types of On the Job Training

i. Orientation training

ii. Job-instruction training

iii. Apprentice training

iv. Internships training

v. Job rotation

vi. Coaching

i. Orientation Training

- Induction or orientation training program is designed for new employees (including transferred, re-hired and seasonal/temporary employees) of the organisation.

- This program familiarises the new employee with the culture, accepted practices and performance standards of the organisation.

- Induction training is very essential for any company because it helps an individual/new recruit to grow within a company and motivates him/her. It inculcates in the employee, more confidence to progress.

- It is during induction that a new recruit gets to know about the organisation's employment philosophy, physical work environment, employee's rights, employee's responsibilities, organisation, culture and values along with key business processes.

Objectives of an Orientation Programme

a. To build up confidence among the new employees regarding organisation performance, reliability etc and himself so that they may become an efficient employee.

b. To infuse a feeling of loyalty and belongingness to the organisation among the new joiners.

c. To describe the information of facilities like cafeteria, library etc.

d. To explain the terms and conditions of the organisation.

ii. Job-Instruction Training

- Job Instruction Technique (JIT) uses a strategy with focus on knowledge (factual and procedural), skills and attitudes development.

- **Procedure of Job Instruction Technique (JIT)**

  JIT consists of four steps:

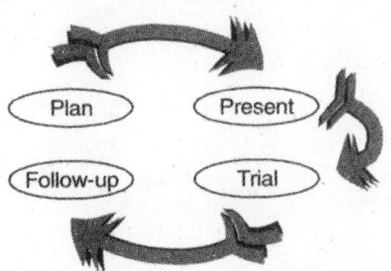

1. **Plan:** This step includes a written breakdown of the work to be done because the trainer and the trainee must understand that documentation is a must and important for the familiarity of work.

2. **Present:** In this step, trainer provides the synopsis of the job while presenting the participants the different aspects of the work. When the trainer is finished, the trainee demonstrates how to do the job and why it is that done in that specific manner. Trainee actually demonstrates the procedure while emphasising the key points and safety instructions.

3. **Trial:** This step is actually a kind of rehearsal step, in which trainee tries to perform the work and the trainer is able to provide instant feedback. In this step, the focus is on improving the method of instruction because a trainer considers that any error that occurs may be a function of training, not the trainee. This step allows the trainee to see the after effects of using an incorrect method. The trainer then helps the trainee by questioning and guiding to identify the correct procedure.

4. **Follow-up:** In this step, the trainer checks the trainee's job frequently after the training program is over to prevent bad work habits from developing.

iii. Apprentice Training

- Combines classroom instruction with on-the-job training
- Trainee is placed under the supervision of an experienced person who teaches him the necessary skills and observes his performance.
- Traditionally used in craft jobs.
- Apprentice earns less than the master craftsperson who is the instructor.

iv. Internships Training

- Interns and assistants work on real preservation projects according to their abilities and interests, and the needs of the clients.
- Internship training has become very popular nowadays throughout the world because of cooperation between employers and vocational and professional institutions.
- Under this training programme, professional and vocational institutions enter into arrangement with organisations for providing practical knowledge to their students through actual work experience.
- All engineering, management and other professional students undergo this training programme for at least 4-6 weeks. During this training, employer pays stipend to the students and also may provide other facilities such as accommodation etc.

v. Job Rotation

In Job Rotation, trainee is required to move from one job to another to broaden experience before assuming a permanent position.

Advantages
a. Helps new employees understand variety of jobs and broaden their horizon.
b. Helps in understanding problems faced by other managers, departments etc.
c. Trainee also learns about different aspects and viewpoints of work and applies them in his domain of work.
d. It equips trainee to work in any aspect and domain of the organisation. Thus, provides a good career opportunity.

Disadvantages
a. The supervision or feedback the trainee receives is often inconsistent.
b. Some of the experience is not useful for the permanent position.
c. It is a long term and expensive procedure.

vi. Coaching

- In this type of program, the trainee may have one person who acts as a tutor to him.
- The coach attempts to help the trainee by providing feedback, setting goals, and discussing any problem that may occur.
- Coaching not only provides the subordinate with necessary skills for doing the assignment but also gives him diversified knowledge to grow.

Advantages
a. Can be used for different levels within the organisation.
b. It provides the opportunity for practical learning.

Disadvantages
a. It depends on the skill and knowledge of the coach.
b. Employee cannot learn beyond the limits of his coach.
c. Coach may not be able to provide sufficient time.

b. Off -The -Job Training

Definition: Off-the-job training is the one, which takes place away from normal work situations and is generally theoretical in nature. It is associated more with knowledge than skills.

Advantages

i.   A specialist instructor enables delivery of high quality training.

ii.   Wider range of facilities and equipment are available.

iii. The trainee can learn the job in planned stages.

iv.   It is free from the pressures and distractions of company life.

v.   It is easier to calculate the cost of off-the-job training because it is more self-contained.

vi.   Cross-fertilisation of ideas between different companies.

Disadvantages

i.   Can result in transfer of learning difficulties when a trainee changes from training equipment to production equipment.

ii.   No training can be entirely off-the-job as some aspects of the task can only be learned by doing them in the normal production setting, with its own customs and network of personal relationships.

iii. Can be more expensive.

Types Of Off-The –Job Training

i.   Vestibule

ii.   Demonstration and Example

iii. Lecture

iv.   Audio-Visuals including television, films etc.

v.   Programmed instruction

vi.   Computer Based Training

vii. Games and Simulation- includes Business Games, Case Studies, In-Basket Technique, Role Plays, Behaviour-Modelling

viii. Conference.

i. Vestibule Training

- This training method attempts to duplicate on-the-job-situation in a company classroom.

- It is a classroom training that is often imparted with the help of equipment and machines, which are identical to those in use in the place of work. Here, training is generally given in the form of lectures, conferences, case studies, role-play etc.
- This technique enables the trainees to concentrate on learning new skills rather than on performing actual job.
- This type of training is efficient to train semi-skilled personnel, particularly when many employees have to be trained for the same kind of work at the same time.
- It is often used to train bank tellers, inspectors, machine operators, typists etc.

Advantages of Vestibule Training

a. As training is given in a separate room, distractions are minimised.

b. A trained instructor, who knows how to teach, can be more effectively utilised.

c. The correct method can be taught without interrupting production.

d. It permits the trainee to practice without the fear of the supervisor's/ co-worker's observation and their possible ridicule.

ii. Demonstrations and Example

- In this type of training method, the trainer describes and displays how to do something by actually performing the activity himself & explaining why & what he is doing.
- This method is very effective in teaching because it is much easier to show a person how to do a job than tell him or give him instruction about a particular job.
- This training is done in combination with lectures, pictures, text materials etc.

iii. Lectures

- Lecture is a verbal presentation of information by an instructor to a large audience.

Advantages

a) This method can be used for very large groups,

b) The cost per trainee is low as it can reach large number of people at once.

c) It is mainly used in colleges and universities.

Limitations

a) The method violates the principle of learning by practice.

b) It constitutes a one-way communication.

c) There is no feedback from the audience.

d) Inability to identify and correct misunderstandings

e) Its application is restricted in training factory employees.

- Continued lecturing method can be made effective it if is combined with other methods of training.

iv. Audio-Visuals

- Audio-visuals include television slides, overheads, video-types and films.
- These can be used to provide a wide range of realistic examples of job conditions and situations in a condensed period of time.
- The quality of the presentation can be controlled and will remain equal for all training groups.
- Audio-visuals constitute a one-way system of communication with no scope for the audience to raise doubts for clarification.
- There is no flexibility of presentation from audience to audience.

v. Programmed Instruction (PI)

- This is a method where training is offered without the intervention of a trainer. Information is provided to the trainee in blocks, either in a book form or through a teaching machine.
- PI involves:
  a. Presenting questions, facts, or problems to the learner.
  b. Allowing the person to respond.
  c. Providing feedback on the accuracy of his or her answers.
  d. If the answers are correct, the learner proceeds to the next block. If not, he or she repeats the same.

Features of Programmed Instruction

Some of the features of programmed instructions are:
a. It provides immediate feedback to trainee's response.
b. It frequently reviews the content.
c. It programs small learning steps that result in fewer response errors.
d. It allows trainees to move through the content at their own speed or capability.
e. It requires frequent active responses by the trainees.

vi. Computer Based Training (CBT)

- With the worldwide expansion of companies and changing technologies, the demands for knowledge and skilled employees have increased more than ever, which in turn, is putting pressure on HR department to provide training at lower costs. Many organisations are now implementing CBT as an alternative to classroom based training to accomplish those goals.

- Some of the benefits of Computer Based Training are:

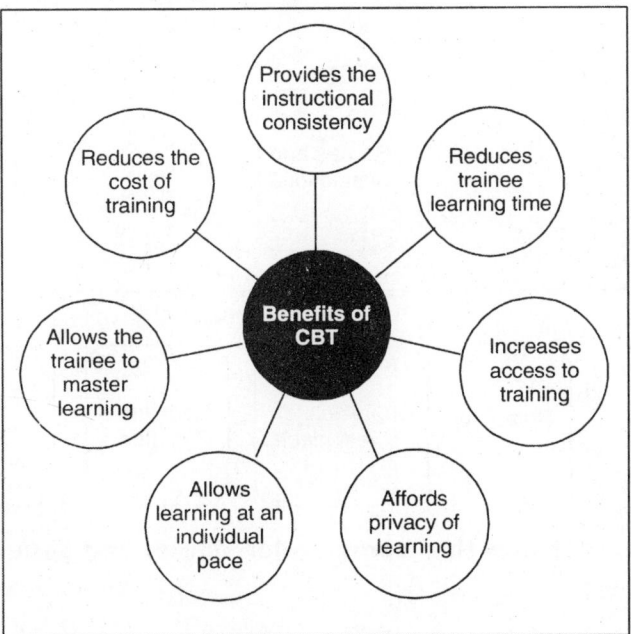

- According to a recent survey, about 75% of the organisations are providing training to employees through Intranet or Internet.
- Internet is not a method of training, but has become the technique of delivering training. The growth of electronic technology has created alternative training delivery systems.

vii.   Games and Simulations

- **Games and Simulations** are usually played for enjoyment but sometimes are also used as an educational tool for training purposes.
- Training games and simulations are different from work as they are designed to reproduce or simulate events, circumstances, processes that take place in a trainees' job.
- **Training Game:** A Training Game is defined as a spirited activity or exercise in which trainees compete with each other according to the defined set of rules.
- **Simulation:** Simulation is creating computer versions of real-life. Simulation is about imitating or making judgment or presenting how events might occur in a real situation.

- Training games and simulations are now seen as an effective tool for training because of their key components, which are:
  a. Challenge
  b. Rules
  c. Interactivity

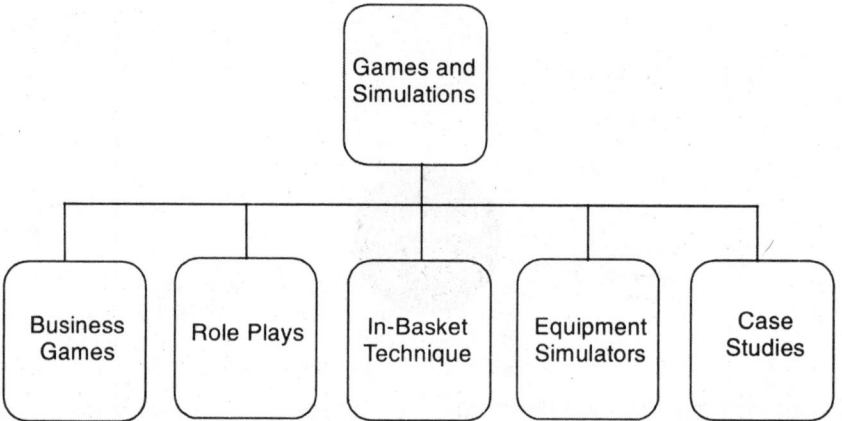

- **The various methods that come under Games and Simulations are**

1. Business Games
2. Case Studies
3. In-Basket Technique
4. Role Plays
5. Behaviour-Modelling

vii-1. Business Games

- Business games are simulators that try to present the way an industry, company, organisation, consultancy, or subunit of a company functions.

- Basically, they are based on a set of rules, procedures, plans, relationships, principles derived from research.

- In business games, trainees are given some information that describe a particular situation and are then asked to make decisions that will best suit the company and then the system provides the feedback about the impact of their decisions. Again, on the basis of the feedback they are asked to make the decisions. This process continues until some meaningful results come out or some predefined state of the organisation exists or a specified number of trials are completed.

- As an example, if the focus is on an organisation's financial state, the game may end when the organisation reaches a desirable or defined profitability level.

- Some of the benefits of business games are:
  a. It develops leadership skills
  b. It improves application of total quality principles
  c. It develops skills in using quality tools
  d. It strengthens management skills
  e. It demonstrates principles and concepts
  f. It explores and solves complex problems

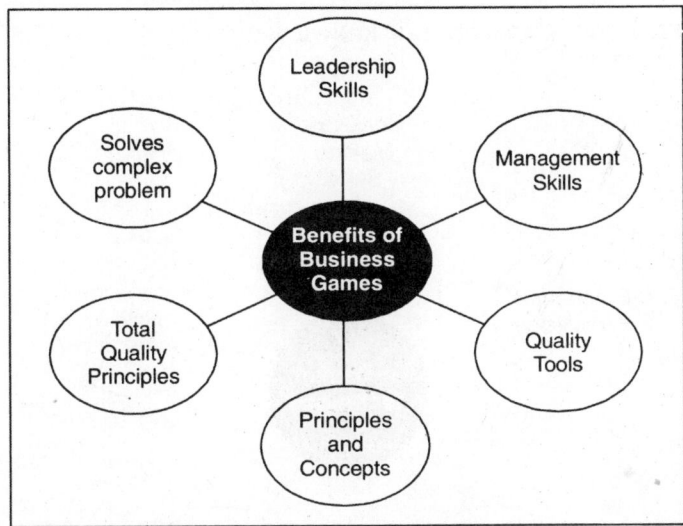

- Business games simulate a whole organisation and provide much better perspective than any other training method. They allow trainees to see how their decisions and actions impact the related areas.

vii.2. Case Study

- This method was developed in 1800's At the Harvard Law School.
- The case study is based upon the belief that managerial competence can best be attained through the study, contemplation and discussion of concrete cases.
- When the trainees are given cases to analyse, they are asked to identify the problem and recommend a tentative solution for it.
- The case study is primarily useful as a training technique for supervisors and is especially valuable as a technique of developing discussion-making skills, and for broadening the perspective of the trainee.
- In case study method the trainee is expected to master the facts, should be acquainted with the content of the case, define the objective sought in dealing with the issues in the case, identify the problem, develop alternative courses of

action, define the controls needed to make the action effective and role play the action to test its effectiveness and find conditions that may limit it.

Case Study method focuses on

a. Building decision making skills

b. Assessing and developing Knowledge, Skills and Attitudes (KSAs)

c. Developing communication and interpersonal skills

d. Developing management skills

e. Developing procedural and strategic knowledge

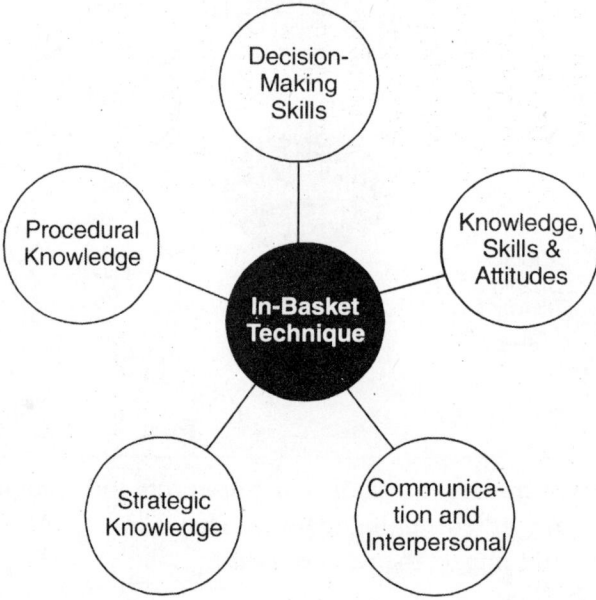

vii.3. In-Basket Technique

It provides trainees with a log of written text or information and requests, such as memos, messages, and reports, which would be handled by manager, engineer, reporting officer, or administrator.

Procedure of the In-Basket Technique

• In this technique, trainee is given some information about the role to be played such as description, responsibilities, general context about the role.

• The trainee is then given the log of materials that make up the in-basket and asked to respond to materials within a particular time period.

• After all the trainees complete in-basket, a discussion with the trainer takes place.

- In this discussion the trainee describes the justification for the decisions.
- The trainer then provides feedback, reinforcing decisions made suitably or encouraging the trainee to increase alternatives for those made unsuitably.

A variation on the technique is to run multiple, simultaneous in-baskets in which each trainee receives a different but organised set of information. It is important that trainees must communicate with each other to accumulate the entire information required to make a suitable decision.

This technique focuses on:
a. Building decision making skills.
b. Assessing and developing Knowledge, Skills and Attitudes (KSAs).
c. Developing communication and interpersonal skills.
d. Developing procedural knowledge.
e. Developing strategic knowledge.

vii.4. Role Play

Role play is a simulation in which each participant is given a role to play. Trainees are given some information related to the description of the role, concerns, objectives, responsibilities, emotions, etc. Then, a general description of the situation, and the problem that each one of them faces is given. For instance, the situation could be, strike in a factory, managing conflict, two parties in a conflict, scheduling vacation days, etc. Once the participants read their role descriptions, they act out their roles by interacting with one another.

Role Plays help in
a. Developing interpersonal skills.
b. Developing communication skills.
c. Conflict resolution.
d. Group decision making.
e. Developing insight into one's own behaviour and its impact on others.

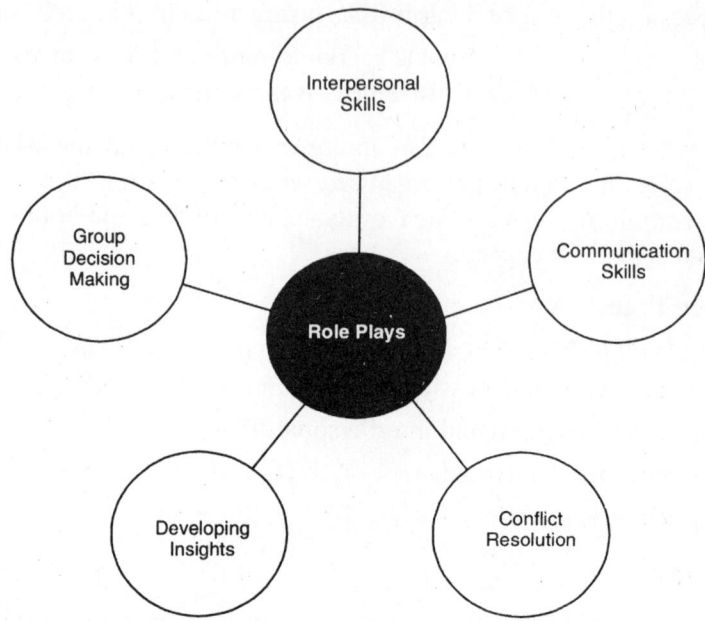

Various types of Role Plays are

a. Multiple Role Play

In this type of role play, all trainees are in groups, with each group acting out the role play simultaneously. After the role play, each group analyses the interactions and identifies the learning points.

b. Single Role Play

One group of participants plays the role for the rest, providing demonstrations of the situation. Other participants observe the role play, analyse their interactions with one another and learn from the play.

c. Role Rotation

It starts as a single role play. After the interaction of participants, the trainer will stop the role play and discuss what happened so far. Then the participants are asked to exchange characters. This method allows a variety of ways to approach the roles.

d. Spontaneous Role Play

In this kind of role play, one of the trainees plays himself while the other trainees play people with whom the first participant interacted before.

vii.5. Behaviour Modelling

- **Definition**: A training technique in which trainees are first shown good management techniques in a film, are asked to play roles in a simulated situation, and are then given feedback and praise by their supervisors.

- Behaviour Modelling involves

  1. Showing trainees the right (or "model") way of doing something,

  2. Letting each person practice the right way to do it, and then

  3. Providing feedback regarding each trainee's performance.

- The basic behaviour modelling procedure can be outlined as follows:

  ❑ **Modelling:** First, trainees watch films or videotapes that show a model person behaving effectively in a problem situation. In other words, trainees are shown the right way to behave in a simulated but realistic situation. The film might thus show a supervisor effectively disciplining a subordinate, if teaching 'how to discipline' is the aim of the training.

  ❑ **Role playing:** Next, the trainees are given roles to play in a simulated situation; here they practice and rehearse the effective behaviours demonstrated by the models.

  ❑ **Social reinforcement:** The trainer provides reinforcement in the form of praise and constructive feedback based on how the trainee performs in the role playing situation.

  ❑ **Transfer of training:** Finally, trainees are encouraged to apply their new skills when they are back on their jobs.

- Measures of learning and skill development were highest for behaviour modelling, followed by the computer-assisted training, and then by conventional instruction.

viii. Conference

- In this method, the participating individuals confer to discuss points of common interest to each other.

- This lays emphasis on small group discussion, on organised subject matter and on the active participation of the members involved.

- There are three types of conferences,

  1. **Direct Discussion:** Here trainer guides the discussion in such a way that the facts, principles or concepts are explained.

  2. **Training Conference:** The instructor gets the group to pool its knowledge and past experience and brings different points of view to bear on the problem.

3. Seminar Conference: In this method instructor defines the problem, encourages and ensures the full participation in the discussion.

D.6.5. Implementation of Training Program

- Once the training programme has been designed, it needs to be implemented.
- **Problems of Implementation:**
    1. Most Managers are too busy to engage in training efforts.
    2. Availability of trainers is a problem.
- **Programme implementation involves action on the following lines**
    1. Deciding the location and organising training and other facilities.
    2. Scheduling the training programme.
    3. Conducting the programme.
    4. Monitoring the progress of trainees.

D.6.6. Evaluation of Training

- The process of examining a training program is called training evaluation.
- Training evaluation checks, whether training has had the desired effect.
- Training evaluation ensures whether candidates are able to implement their learning in their respective workplaces, or in the regular work routines.
- Purposes of Training Evaluation:

The five main purposes of training evaluation are:

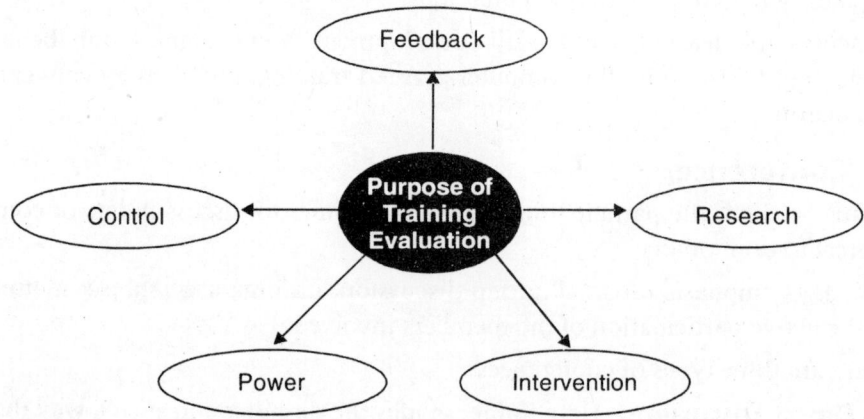

i. Feedback

It helps in giving feedback to the candidates by defining the objectives and linking it to learning outcomes.

ii. Research

It helps in ascertaining the relationship between acquired knowledge, transfer of knowledge at the work place, and training.

iii. Control

It helps in controlling the **training program** because if the training is not effective, then it can be dealt with accordingly.

iv. Power games

At times, the top management (higher authoritative employee) uses the evaluative data to manipulate it for its own benefits.

v. Intervention

It helps in determining whether the actual outcomes are aligned with the expected outcomes.

Process of Training Evaluation

1. Before Training

- The learner's skills and knowledge are assessed before the training program.
- At the start of training, candidates generally perceive it as a waste of resources because most of the times, candidates are unaware of the objectives and learning outcomes of the program. Once aware, they are asked to give their opinions on the methods used and whether those methods confirm to the candidates preferences and learning style.

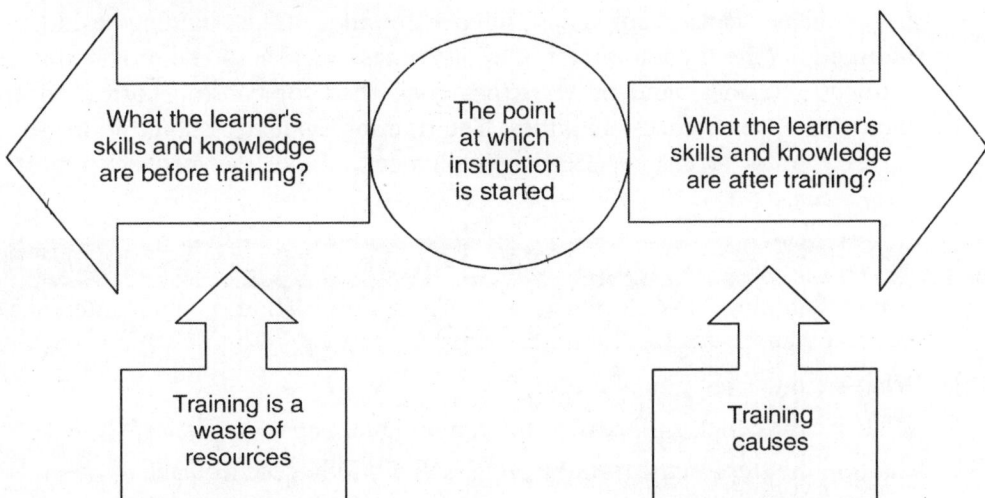

2. During Training

It is the phase in which instruction is started. This phase usually consists of short tests at regular intervals

3. After Training

It is the phase when learner's **skills and knowledge** are assessed again to measure the effectiveness of the training. This phase is designed to determine whether the training has had the desired effect at individual, department and organisational levels. There are various evaluation techniques for this phase.

Techniques of Evaluation

i. **Questionnaires:** Comprehensive questionnaires could be used to obtain opinions, reactions, views of trainees.

ii. **Tests:** Standard tests could be used to find out whether trainees have learnt anything during and after the training.

iii. **Interviews:** Interviews could be conducted to find out the usefulness of training offered to operatives.

iv. **Studies:** Comprehensive studies could be carried out eliciting the opinions and judgments of trainers, superiors and peer groups about the training.

v. **Human resource factors:** Training can also be evaluated on the basis of employee satisfaction, which in turn can be examined on the basis of decrease in employee attrition, absenteeism, accidents, grievances, discharges, dismissals, etc.

vi. **Feedback:** After the evaluation, the situation should be examined to identify the probable causes for gaps in performance. The training evaluation information (about costs, time spent, outcomes, etc.) should be provided to the instructors, trainees and other parties concerned for control, correction and improvement of trainees' activities. The training evaluator should follow it up sincerely so as to ensure effective implementation of the feedback report at every stage.

TEST YOUR GREY MATTER

Q1) Define Training, Development and Education. What is the difference between them?

Q2) What are the objectives of training?

Q3) What are the benefits of training to an individual and organisation?

Q4) Mention the steps in the training process and briefly describe each of them.

Q5) How are the training needs assessed?

Q6) What are the factors which should be considered while designing a training program?

Q7) Enumerate the methods of training.

Q8) What is On-the-Job training? Give its advantages and disadvantages?

Q9) Describe Apprentice and Internship training. What are their advantages?

Q10) What is Off-the-Job training? Give its advantages and disadvantages?

Q11) Describe Vestibule and Games and Simulation form of training?

Q12) Why is training evaluation necessary? How is it done?

E. LEARNING

E.1. Meaning and Definition of Learning

Definition: **Learning** is defined as "a relatively permanent change in behaviour that occurs as a result of prior experience."

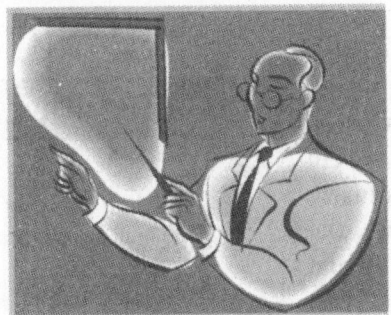

Learning

- The ability to learn is one of the most outstanding human characteristics. Learning occurs continuously throughout a person's lifetime.

- An individual's way of perceiving, thinking, feeling, and doing may change as a result of a learning experience. Thus, **learning can be defined** as a change in behaviour as a result of experience. This can be physical and overt, or it may involve complex intellectual or attitudinal changes which affect behaviour in more subtle ways.

E.2. Process of Learning

Learning theory may be described by psychologists and educators to explain how people acquire skills, knowledge and attitudes.

There are four theories which explain how learning occurs

1. Classical conditioning
2. Operant conditioning
3. Social learning theory
4. Cognitive theory

1. Classical Conditioning

- Classical conditioning is based on the premise that a physical event – termed a stimulus – that initially does not elicit a particular response gradually acquires the capacity to elicit that response as a result of repeated pairing with a stimulus that elicits a reaction.

- Learning of this type is quite common and seems to play an important role in such reactions as strong fears, taste aversions, some aspects of sexual behaviour and even racial or ethnic prejudice.

- **Pavlov Experiment**: In 1904 Ivan Pavlov a Nobel Prize winning psychologist from Russia, identified it as an important behavioural process. He conducted an experiment on a dog and tried to relate the dog's salivation and the ringing of a bell. He began to feed his dogs in association with the ringing of a bell. After a certain time the dogs were shown to salivate profusely in association with the ringing bell where the actual sight or smell of food was not present. Pavlov regarded

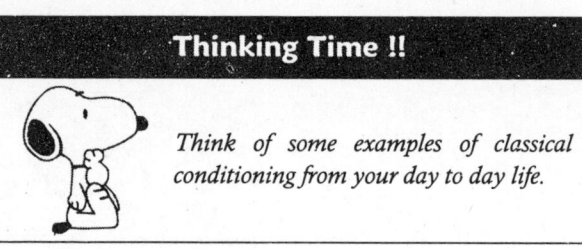

Thinking Time !!

Think of some examples of classical conditioning from your day to day life.

this salivation as being a conditioned reflex and designated the process by which the dogs had picked up this reflex classical conditioning.

2. Operant conditioning

- Operant conditioning also called instrumental conditioning refers to the process that our behaviour produces certain consequences. If our actions have pleasant effects, then we will be more likely to repeat them in the future. If, however, our actions have unpleasant effects, we are less likely to repeat them in the future. Thus, according to this theory, behaviour is the function of its consequences.

- American psychologist B.F. Skinner defined operant conditioning as:

It is the process of shaping behaviour by means of reinforcement and punishment.

- **Example:** A lion in a circus learns to stand up on a chair and jump through a hoop to receive a food treat. This example is operant conditioning because standing on a chair and jumping through a hoop is voluntary behaviour. The food serves as a positive reinforcement because it is given and it increases the behaviour.

3. Social Learning Theory/Observational Learning

- Social learning theory, also called as Observational Learning, occurs by observing others - parents, teachers, film stars and other popular figures in public life.

- The learner picks up whatever the role model does or does not do.

Thinking Time !!

Who is your Role model and why? What are the characteristics of your nature which you deliberately learned from others? (It includes Rajnikant s way of lighting his cigarettes and wearing his goggles)

- The Social Learning Theory is based on the belief that human behaviour is determined by a constant reciprocal relationship between cognitive factors (i.e. knowledge, beliefs, and expectations), environmental factors (i.e. social norms), and behavioural factors (i.e. self-efficacy, skills).

- With Social Learning Theory, a person is encouraged to observe and model positive behaviour, increase one's confidence and attitude to use new skills, and receive support from others or the environment to implement those skills.

- **Examples of Social learning theory** :Advertisements are prime examples of Social Learning Theory. We watch them, then copy them.

4. Cognitive Theory

- Contemporary perspective about learning is that it is a cognitive process. Cognitive process assumes that people are conscious, active participants in how they learn.

- Cognitive theory of learning assumes that the organism learns the meaning of various objects and events and learned responses depending on the meaning assigned to stimuli.

- Cognitive processes include executive functions of recognizing expectancies, planning and monitoring performance, encoding and chunking information, and producing internal and external responses.

E.3. Learning Curve

- A highly useful learning concept which is valid for a wide range of situation is the learning curve, a diagrammatic presentation of the amount learned in relation to time.

- A typical learning curve will show on the Y-axis the amount learnt and the passage of time on the X-axis.

Amount learned

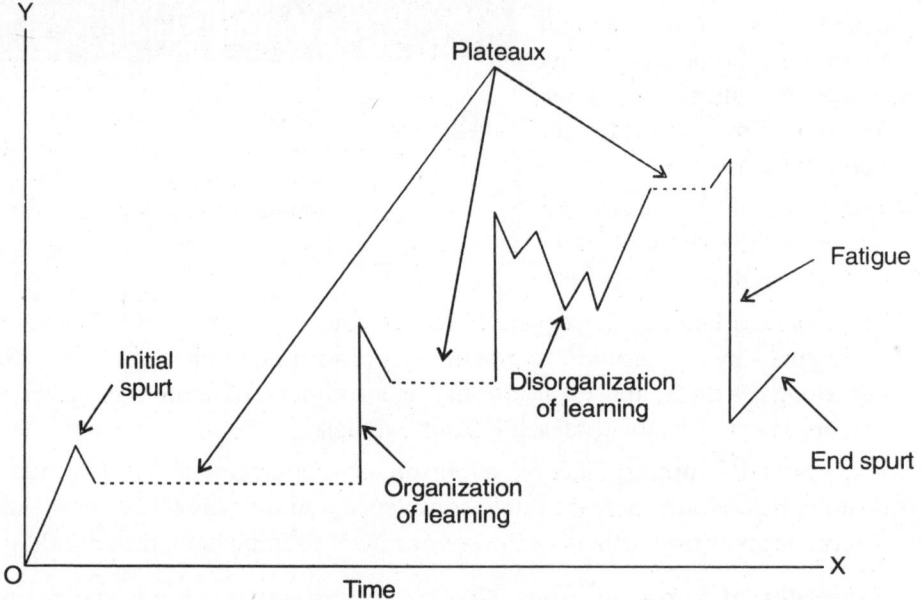

Figure: Learning Curve

Characteristics of learning curves

i. Initial Spurt

- At the beginning, it is natural that the rate of learning exhibits spurt. Usually, the graph levels off at some stage, indicating that maximum performance has been achieved.

- It is because at the beginning of the learning process, the subject is highly motivated and seems to exhibit a significant surge of effort.

- Many experienced trainers exploit this initial spurt by selecting the most important items to be communicated and presenting them as a package to the students at the beginning of the training unit.

- In many ways, it is possible to exemplify the initial spurt with the saying **"The First Step Is the Best Step"**.

ii. Learning Plateau

- At some point in the learning process there is a flattening off in terms of the improvement, a plateau.

- Frequently, the process of learning is marked by discontinuities and involves escalating from one plateau to another.

- Most learners are only too aware of the experience of finding themselves on a plateau, which manifests itself in the feeling that they are never going to get anywhere.

iii. Organisation of Learning

- Jumping from one plateau to another is called organisation of learning.

- Organisation of learning is achieved when the learner discovers a new and more effective method of performing particular tasks.

- For example, when he learns to apply calculus to solve problems of business.

iv. Disorganisation of Learning

It is an actual fall in performance. This arises when the subject has to choose between alternative methods of tackling a task.

v. End spurt

- When the training season draws to an end and the subject realises this, there occurs resurgence of interest and effort to learn more. This revival is called the end spurt.

- The end spurt is preceded by fatigue which is likely to set in with the passage of time.

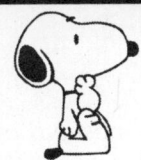

Thinking Time !!

At which stage of learning curve are you at present, while reading this chapter? Take the help of the curve to improve your learning.

E.4. Principles of Learning

- Principles of learning are highly useful for the trainer in order to impart maximum knowledge and skills to the trainees.

- Blind adherence to these principles can cause more harm than good and so each principle should, therefore, be interpreted and applied carefully in full consideration of the particular task being learned.

- The most important among them are:

  a. Motivation

  b. Reinforcement, punishment and extinction.

  c. Whole versus part learning

  d. Learning curves

  e. Meaningfulness of material

  f. Learning styles

a. Motivation

- The concept of motivation is basic, because without motivation learning does not take place or, at least, is not apparent.
- Motivation may be seen at different levels of complexity of a situation. A thirsty rat will learn the path through a maze to a dish of water; it is not likely to do so well, or even more purposefully at all, if it is satisfied.
- On a broader level, a college student must have the need and drive to accomplish a task and reach a specific goal.
- Refer Chapter 5 on Motivation for details.

b. Reinforcement, Punishment and Extinction

- Reinforcement, punishment and extinction play a key role in learning process.
- Reinforcement is used to enhance desirable behaviour; punishment and extinction are employed to minimise undesirable behaviour.

Reinforcement

There are two types of reinforcement: positive and negative.

i. Positive Reinforcement

- It is the process of getting something nice after showing a desired behaviour. This is done to repeat the same behaviour.

- **Example of Positive Reinforcement:** When a manager praises an employee for successfully completing a task on schedule, this is positive reinforcement. This encourages the employee and increases the possibility of completing his work on time.

ii. Negative Reinforcement

- In negative reinforcement, an unpleasant event that precedes a behaviour is removed when the desired behaviour occurs. This procedure increases the likelihood that the desired behaviour will occur.

- Negative reinforcement strengthens and increases behaviour by the threat of and the use of an undesirable consequence or the termination or withdrawal of an undesirable consequence.

Punishment

- Punishment is the attempt to eliminate or weaken undesirable behaviour.
- It is used in two ways.
  i. One way to punish a person is to apply a negative consequence called **Punishers** – following an undesirable behaviour. For example, a professional athlete who is excessively offensive to an official (undesirable behaviour) may be ejected from a game (punished).
  ii. The other way to punish a person is to withhold a positive consequence following an undesirable behaviour. For example, a sales representative who makes a few visits to companies (undesirable behaviour) is likely to receive less commission (positive reinforcement) at the end of the month.

Extinction

- An alternate to punishing undesirable behaviour is extinction.
- Extinction is the weakening of a behaviour by ignoring it or making sure it is not reinforced.
- The rationale for using extinction is that a behaviour not followed by any reinforcer is weakened.
- In other words, if rewards are withdrawn for behaviour that was previously reinforced, the behaviours probably will become less frequent and die out. But extinction needs time and patience to be effective.

c. Whole Versus Part Learning

- A great deal of work has been done in psychology of learning to decide whether learning a whole job is superior to breaking the job into parts and learning the parts.
- In part learning, the individual is not only required to learn each individual part but must be able to combine the separate parts so that the whole performance can be accomplished.
- No overall conclusion, however, has been reached in this field.

d. Learning Curve

- Discussed earlier in this chapter

e. Meaningfulness of Material

- A definite relationship has been established between learning and meaningfulness of the subject learnt.
- The more meaningful the material, the better does learning proceed.
- Learning of nonsense syllables proceeds more slowly than that of prose or poetry.
- Thus trainers apply certain techniques that increase meaning for the trainees.
- Organising meaningfulness units, creating association with already familiar terms, and providing a conceptual basis of logical reason for the material are some of the practical possibilities.

f. Learning Styles

- The final principle of learning is the learning style.
- Learning style refers to the ability of an individual to learn.
- A manager's long-term success depends more on the ability to learn than on the mastery of the specific skills or technical knowledge.
- There are four styles people use when learning:

Accommodation, Divergence, Assimilation And Convergence

- The four styles are based on dimensions: feeling versus thinking and doing versus observing.

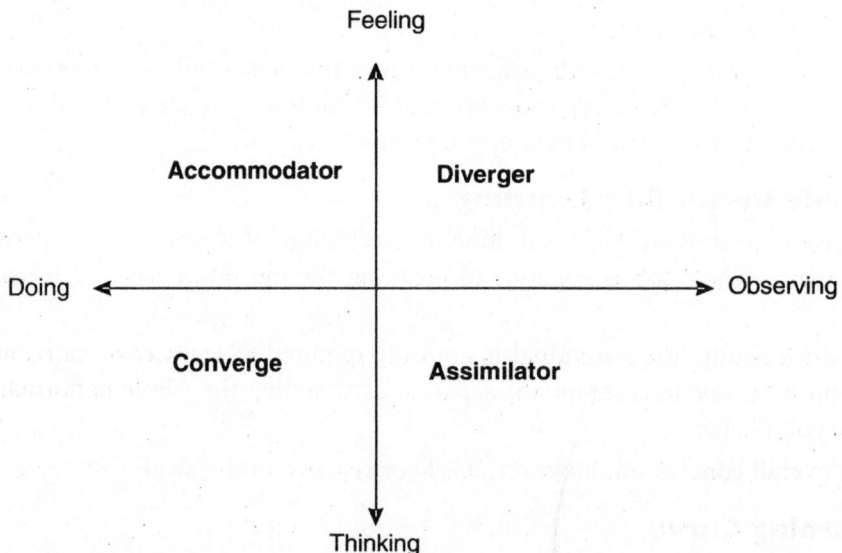

a. Accommodator

- An accommodator learns by doing and feeling.

- He tends to learn primarily from hands-on experience.
- He tends to act on gut feeling rather than on logical analysis.
- An accommodator tends to rely more heavily on people for information while making decisions.
- He seeks action-oriented careers such as marketing, politics, public relations and management.

b. Diverger

- A diverger learns by observing and feeling.
- The diverger has the ability to view concrete situations from different angles.
- When solving problems, diverger enjoys brainstorming.
- He takes time and analyses many alternatives.
- Diverger is imaginative and sensitive to the needs of the other people.
- He seeks careers in entertainment, arts and services sector.

c. Converger

- A converger learns by doing and thinking.
- The converger seeks practical use for information.
- When presented with problems and making decisions, the converger tends to focus on solutions.
- Converger tends to prefer dealing with technical tasks and problems rather than social and interpersonal issues.
- Converger seeks technical careers in various scientific fields and work at engineering, production supervision, IT and managerial jobs.

d. Assimilator

- An assimilator learns by observing and thinking.
- The assimilator is effective at understanding a wide range of information and putting it into concise and logical form.
- It is more important for the assimilator that an idea or theory is logical than practical.
- Assimilator tends to be more concerned with abstract idea and concept than with people. He tends to seek careers in education, information and science.

F. EXECUTIVE OR MANAGEMENT DEVELOPMENT

- Management development is any attempt to improve managerial performance by imparting knowledge, changing attitudes, or increasing skills. So, it is the result of not only participating in formal courses of instruction but also of actual job experience

- The ultimate aim of such a development program is to enhance the future performance of the organisation itself.

- For this reason, the general management development process consists of

1. Assessing the company's need (for instance, to fill future executive openings, or to boost competitiveness)

2. Appraising the manager's performance, and

3. Developing the managers (and future managers) themselves.

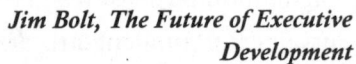

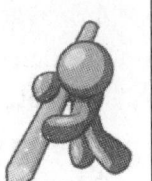

> **Wisdom Tooth**
>
> *"It has become obvious that an organisation s executive and leadership talent is its greatest and most sustainable source of competitive advantage...*
>
> *Cultivating the next generation of business leaders is imperative."*
>
> **Jim Bolt, The Future of Executive Development**

- Thus, the management development program may be aimed at filling a specific position, such as CEO, perhaps with one of two potential candidates.

- When an executive position is to be filled, the process is usually called succession planning.

- Succession planning refers to the process through which senior-level openings are planned and eventually filled.

F.1. Objectives of Executive Development

i. To increase the efficiency of performance of existing executives by developing their managerial skills.

ii. To ensure adequate reserve of managerial talents at all levels for the long term survival and growth of organisation.

iii. To encourage the executives to adopt the latest technology and process and thus to prevent obsolescence of executives.

iv. To provide opportunities to managers for their career advancements - as a motivational tool.

v. In order to introduce change in organisation by introducing change agents and thus to influence behaviour of workers through the developed workers.

vi. To establish harmony and coordination in the changed circumstance

vii. To increase proficiency in management techniques such as work study, inventory control, operations research and quality control.

viii.   To inculcate knowledge of human motivation and human relationship.

ix. To establish friendly human relationship and effective communication system in the organisation

x. To develop unity of management team.

F.2. Needs and Importance of Executive Development

The need of executive development in the modern times arises because of the following factors:-

i.   To keep the executives abreast of the changes and development in their respective fields.

ii. To improve thought process and analytical ability.

iii. To broaden the outlook of the executive regarding his role position and responsibilities.

iv. To understand the conceptual issues relating to economic, social, and technical areas.

v. To understand the problems of human relations and improve human relating skills.

vi. To simulate creative thinking.

vii. To specialize in overall view of the functions of the organisation and equip them to co-ordinate each other's efforts efficiently.

F.3. Techniques of Management Development

There are two type of methods by which managers can acquire the knowledge, skills, and attitude and make themselves competent managers.

The methods are mention below:-

On-The-Job Methods, viz.

i.   Coaching

ii. Understudy

iii. Job rotation

iv. Multiple management

Off-The-Job Methods, viz.

i.   Outside Seminars

ii. In-house development centres

iii. Conference training

iv. Sensitivity Training

v. Simulation Exercise

vi. Transactional Analysis

On The Job Development Techniques

i. **Coaching:** Discussed earlier in types of on job training.

ii. **Job rotation:** Discussed earlier in types of on job training.

iii. **Under study:**

- This method supplies the organisation a person with as much competence as the superior to fill his post which may be vacant because of promotion, retirement, or transfer.

- Superior will teach him what his entire job involves and gives him a feel of what his job is.

- Decision making skills, leadership skills can also be taught by involving them in discussions of daily operating problems and assigning him the task of supervising two or three people.

iv. Multiple Management

- Multiple management is a system in which permanent advisory committees of managers study the problems of the company and make recommendations to higher management. It is also called junior-board of executive management.

- These committees discuss the actual problems and different alternative solutions after which the decision is taken.

- This method has the advantages of being relatively inexpensive, developing teamwork and group decision-making among managers, enabling the managers to see the problems from organisational rather than departmental point of view.

Off The Job Development Techniques

i. Outside Seminars

There are special seminars and conferences offered, aimed at developing executives. For example, the American management association provides thousands of courses in areas ranging from accounting and controls to assertiveness training, basic financial skills, information systems, project management, and total quality management.

ii. In-House Development Centres

Some employers have in-house development centres. These centres usually combine classroom learning (lectures and seminars, for example) with other techniques like assessment centres, in–basket exercise, and role-playing to help develop employee and other managers.

iii. Conference

Discussed earlier in types of off job training.

iv. Sensitivity

- Sensitivity training is about making people understand about themselves and others reasonably, which is done by developing in them social sensitivity and behavioural flexibility.
- Social sensitivity in one word is empathy. It is the ability of an individual to sense what others feel and think from their own point of view.
- Behavioural flexibility is ability to behave suitably in light of understanding.
- Procedure of Sensitivity Training:

Sensitivity Training Program requires three steps:

a. Unfreezing the old values

It requires that the trainees become aware of the inadequacy of the old values. This can be done when the trainee faces dilemma in which his old values is not able to provide proper guidance. The first step consists of a small procedure:

- An unstructured group of 10-15 people is formed.
- Unstructured group without any objective looks to the trainer for its guidance
- But the trainer refuses to provide guidance and assume leadership
- Soon, the trainees are motivated to resolve the uncertainty
- Then, they try to form some hierarchy. Some assume leadership role which may not be liked by other trainees
- Then, they start realising what they wish to do and realise alternative ways of dealing with the situation

b. Development of new values

- With the trainer's support, trainees begin to examine their interpersonal behaviour and give each other feedback.
- The reasoning of the feedback is discussed which motivates trainees to experiment with a range of new behaviours and values. This process constitutes the second step in the change process of the development of these values.

c. Refreezing the new ones

- This step depends upon how much opportunity the trainees get to practice their new behaviours and values at their work place.

v. Simulation exercise

The various methods that come under Simulations Exercise are:

1. **Business Games**: Discussed earlier in types of Off the Job Training.

2. **Case Studies:** Discussed earlier in types of Off the Job Training.
3. **In-Basket Technique:** Discussed earlier in types of Off the Job Training.
4. **Role Plays:** Discussed earlier in types of Off the Job Training.

vi. Transactional Analysis

- Eric Berne (1910-1970) is the founder of Transactional Analysis.
- Transactional analysis, commonly known as TA, is an integrative approach to the theory of psychology and psychotherapy. Integrative because it has elements of psychoanalytic, humanist and cognitive approaches.
- According to the International Transactional Analysis Association:

"TA is a theory of personality and a systematic psychotherapy for personal growth and personal change."

Philosophy of TA

i. People are OK; thus each person has validity, importance, equality of respect.

ii. Everyone (with only few exceptions, such as the severely brain-damaged) has the capacity to think.

iii. People decide their story and destiny, and these decisions can be changed

Some core models and concepts are part of TA as follows:–

The Ego-State (or Parent-Adult-Child, PAC) model

At any given time, a person experiences and manifests his personality through a mixture of behaviours, thoughts and feelings. Typically, according to TA, there are three ego-states that people consistently use:

- **Parent ("Exteropsyche"):** A state in which people behave, feel, and think in response to an unconscious mimicking of how their parents (or other parental figures) acted, or how they interpreted their parent's actions. For example, a person may shout at someone out of frustration because they learned from an influential figure in childhood, the lesson that this seemed to be a way of relating that worked.

- **Adult ("Neopsyche"):** A state of the ego which is most like a computer processing information and making predictions devoid of major emotions that cloud its operation. Learning to strengthen the adult is a goal of TA. While a person is in the adult ego state, he/she is directed towards an objective appraisal of reality.

- **Child ("Archaeopsyche"):** A state in which people behave, feel and think similarly to how they did in childhood. For example, a person who receives a poor evaluation at work may respond by looking at the floor, and crying, as they used to do when scolded as a child. Conversely, a person who receives a good evaluation may respond with a broad smile and a joyful gesture of thanks. The child is the source of emotions, creation, recreation, spontaneity and intimacy.

Transactions and Strokes

Transactions

- They are basic units of social interaction.
- They are flows of communication, and more specifically the unspoken psychological flow of communication that runs in parallel between two people.
- Transactions occur simultaneously at both explicit and psychological levels.
- In Transactional Analysis the learner identifies the ego states that both the initiator and respondent exhibit in the transaction.

Strokes

- They are the unit of recognition, attention or responsiveness that one person gives another.
- Strokes can be positive (nicknamed "Warm Fuzzies") or negative ("Cold Pricklies").
- A key idea is that people hunger for recognition, and that lacking positive strokes, will seek whatever kind they can, even if it is recognition of a negative kind.

TEST YOUR GREY MATTER?

Q1) What is learning? What are theories of learning?

Q2) Describe Cognitive and Operant Conditioning methods of learning?

Q3) Describe Learning Curve? What are its various characteristics?

Q4) What are the basic principles of learning? Explain.

Q5) What do you mean by learning styles? Give details of each one of them.

Q6) Define Executive Development. Why is it important for the organisation?

Q7) Mention various objectives of employee development.

Q8) Describe various On-the-Job and Off-the-Job techniques of Employee Development program.

Q9) Write short note on:

    i) Transactional Analysis.

    ii) Sensitivity training.